ANNALS *of* THE NEW YORK ACADEMY OF SCIENCES

T0344712

EDITOR-IN-CHIEF
Douglas Braaten

ASSOCIATE EDITOR
Rebecca E. Cooney

PROJECT MANAGER
Steven E. Bohall

EDITORIAL ADMINISTRATOR
Daniel J. Becker

Artwork and design by Ash Ayman Shairzay

The New York Academy of Sciences
7 World Trade Center
250 Greenwich Street, 40th Floor
New York, NY 10007-2157

annals@nyas.org
www.nyas.org/annals

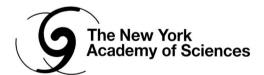

**The New York
Academy of Sciences**

Published by Blackwell Publishing
On behalf of the New York Academy of Sciences

Boston, Massachusetts
2011

ANNALS *of* THE NEW YORK ACADEMY OF SCIENCES

VOLUME
1243

ISSUE

The Year in Diabetes and Obesity

ISSUE EDITORS

Rexford S. Ahima[a] and Alvin C. Powers[b]

University of Pennsylvania[a] and Vanderbilt University[b]

TABLE OF CONTENTS

Ann. N.Y. Acad. Sci. ISSN 0077-8923

ANNALS OF THE NEW YORK ACADEMY OF SCIENCES
Issue: *The Year in Diabetes and Obesity*

Central nervous control of energy and glucose balance: focus on the central melanocortin system

Yong Xu,[1] Joel K. Elmquist,[2] and Makoto Fukuda[2]

[1]Children's Nutrition Research Center, Department of Pediatrics, Baylor College of Medicine, Houston, Texas. [2]Division of Hypothalamic Research, Department of Internal Medicine, University of Texas Southwestern Medical Center, Dallas, Texas

Addresses for correspondence: Yong Xu, Ph.D., M.D., Children's Nutrition Research Center, Department of Pediatrics, Baylor College of Medicine, One Baylor Plaza, Houston, TX 77030. yongx@bcm.edu. Makoto Fukuda, Ph.D., Division of Hypothalamic Research, Department of Internal Medicine, University of Texas Southwestern Medical Center at Dallas, 5323 Harry Hines Boulevard, Dallas, TX 75390-9077. Makato.Fukuda@UTSouthwestern.edu

Studies have suggested that manipulations of the central melanocortin circuitry by pharmacological agents produce robust effects on the regulation of body weight and glucose homeostasis. In this review, we discuss recent findings from genetic mouse models that have further established the physiological relevance of this circuitry in the context of glucose and energy balance. In addition, we will discuss distinct neuronal populations that respond to central melanocortins to regulate food intake, energy expenditure, insulin sensitivity, and insulin secretion, respectively. Finally, multiple hormonal and neural cues (e.g., leptin, estrogen, and serotonin) that use the melanocortin systems to regulate energy and glucose homeostasis will be reviewed. These findings suggest that targeting the specific branches of melanocortin circuits may be potential avenues to combat the current obesity and diabetes epidemics.

Keywords: melanocortins; leptin; estrogen; serotonin; body weight

Introduction

The use of genetic mouse models has catalyzed substantial advances in the understanding about how the central nervous system (CNS) provides a coordinated control of energy and glucose homeostasis. While numerous molecules in the brain and neural structures play key roles in regulating energy and glucose balance and deserve attention, the current review will focus on the central melanocortin system. As illustrated below, the physiological significance of the central melanocortin system has gone beyond the regulation of feeding and body weight. Current evidence indicates that central melanocortins also regulate insulin sensitivity and glucose homeostasis through distinct CNS populations expressing melanocortin receptors. We will also review evidence supporting the role of the melanocortin system as the key mediator for multiple metabolic cues, such as leptin, estrogens, and serotonin.

The central melanocortin system

The central melanocortin system comprises neurons that produce endogenous melanocortins and the downstream neurons that express melanocortin receptors.[1-3] The melanocortin neurons include those expressing pro-opiomelanocortin (POMC) and those expressing neuropeptide Y (NPY) and agouti-related peptide (AgRP), which are both located in the arcuate nucleus (ARC). While POMC neurons synthesize and secrete an anorexigenic peptide, α-melanocyte–stimulating hormone (α-MSH), to activate melanocortin receptors, NPY/AgRP neurons release orexigenic peptides, NPY, and AgRP.[1-3] Notably, AgRP is the endogenous antagonist of the melanocortin receptors.[1-3] POMC and NPY/AgRP populations have been long believed to be the primary central regulators of energy homeostasis.[4,5]

The anorexigenic property of POMC neurons has been well established, as the deletion of POMC gene causes hyperphagia and obesity.[6] However, neither single deletion of AgRP or NPY nor double deletion of AgRP and NPY in mice leads to abnormality in food intake and body weight.[7] These results are not in agreement with pharmacological studies showing that treatment of AgRP or NPY leads to an increase in food intake.[8,9] It has been argued that the lack of phenotypes in animals with gene mutations at the embryonic stage could result from possible

doi: 10.1111/j.1749-6632.2011.06248.x
Ann. N.Y. Acad. Sci. 1243 (2011) 1–14 © 2011 New York Academy of Sciences.

genetic compensations during early development. To circumvent this issue and establish the role of NPY/AgRP neurons in the control of body weight, several groups have used distinct genetic mouse models to achieve selective ablation of NPY/AgRP neurons during adulthood. For example, Palmiter and colleagues used a mouse model with the Cre-inducible diphtheria toxin receptor (DTR). Crossing these mice with AgRP-Cre transgenic mice generated mice with DTR expressed only in AgRP-expressing cells. Injections of diphtheria toxin into these mice results in selective ablation of NPY/AgRP neurons. They found that ablation of NPY/AgRP neurons during adulthood leads to rapid decreases in food intake and body weight.[10] Similarly, Barsh and colleagues crossed AgRP-Cre transgenic mice to a loxP-flanked mitochondrial transcription factor A (Tfam) allele to selectively delete Tfam from AgRP cells, which causes progressive loss of this population as animals grow.[11] These mice with NPY/AgRP ablation display modest lean phenotypes.[11] Finally, targeted expression of a neurotoxic ataxin-3 to AgRP-expressing neurons resulted in loss of the NPY/AgRP neurons and decreases in food intake and body weight.[12] Results from these three different models with genetic ablation of NPY/AgRP neurons all support a physiological role of these neurons in promoting feeding and body weight gain. This notion has been further supported by recent studies using genetic tools to selectively manipulate electrophysiological properties of NPY/AgRP neurons. For example, Aponte and colleagues generated mice expressing the light-activated cation channel, channelrhodopsin-2 (ChR2), only in NPY/AgRP neurons.[13] Light stimulation in these mice induces rapid activation of NPY/AgRP neurons, which results in increased feeding.[13] Similarly, Krashes and colleagues used Designer-Receptors-Exclusively-Activated-by-Designer-Drugs (DREADD)[14,15] to rapidly depolarize or hyperpolarize NPY/AgRP neurons in mice.[16] While depolarization of NPY/AgRP neurons promotes eating, hyperpolarization of these neurons inhibits eating.[16] Collectively, these genetic mouse models with NPY/AgRP ablation or stimulation/inhibition during adulthood demonstrate a physiological role of NPY/AgRP neurons in the control of energy homeostasis. The discrepancy between these recent studies[10–13,16] and those with early embryonic gene deletion[7] may indicate

that other neuronal populations (e.g., POMC neurons) undergo adaptive changes to compensate for the loss of NPY/AgRP during early development.

It is important to note that NPY/AgRP ablation or stimulation/inhibition models cannot rule out the possibility that other neuropeptides or neurotransmitters released by these neurons may contribute to the regulation of energy homeostasis. Indeed, Aponte and colleagues demonstrated that increased feeding induced by activation of NPY/AgRP neurons does not require the melanocortin receptors,[13] suggesting that these neurons may release neurotransmitters other than AgRP to regulate feeding. NPY released from these NPY/AgRP neurons could certainly be one of these neurotransmitters. Alternatively, NPY/AgRP neurons also release GABA, a classic neurotransmitter that has been implicated in the control of body weight.[10,17] To evaluate the physiological relevance of GABA release from NPY/AgRP neurons, Tong and colleagues generated a mouse model carrying loxP-flanked alleles encoding the vesicular GABA transporter (VGAT), which is required for presynaptic release of GABA.[18] Crossing these loxed VGAT mice with knockin AgRP-IRES-Cre mice produced mice with selective deletion of VGAT in NPY/AgRP neurons. Mice lacking VGAT in NPY/AgRP neurons have reduced GABA release, and these mice display reduced body weight primarily due to increased energy expenditure.[19] These findings provide genetic evidence that GABA release from NPY/AgRP neurons is required to maintain normal energy homeostasis. It has been suggested that NPY/AgRP neurons provide a direct GABAergic input to POMC neurons, which forms a neural network to mediate actions of various metabolic signals.[10,17,20,21] This notion is further supported by the observations that the inhibitory postsynaptic currents (both at the basal condition and after ghrelin treatment) recorded from identified POMC neurons are significantly attenuated in mice lacking VGAT in NPY/AgRP neurons. In addition, the orexigenic effects of ghrelin are significantly blunted in these mutant mice.[19] In addition to this GABAergic AgRP-POMC network, recent evidence from the Palmiter group demonstrated that GABA released from NPY/AgRP neurons also acts on neurons in the parabrachial nucleus to maintain normal feeding behavior.[22]

Neurons expressing melanocortin receptors receive inputs from POMC neurons and NPY/AgRP neurons to regulate energy and glucose home-ostasis. In particular, melanocortin receptor 3 and 4 (MC3Rs and MC4Rs) have been demonstrated to be the most relevant melanocortin receptors in the context of energy and glucose homeosta-sis.[5,23,24] For example, MC3Rs are required to me-diate melanocortin actions on energy expenditure, as MC3R knockout mice show decreased energy ex-penditure and increased sensitivity to diet-induced obesity.[23,25] Effects of MC3Rs on food intake are not yet fully understood. Initial characterization of MC3R knockout mice showed that mutants eat less when fed with chow, and no difference in food in-take was observed when fed with a high-fat diet (HFD).[23,25] However, Butler and colleagues recently reported that MC3R knockout mice eat more dur-ing the light cycle, but not in the dark cycle.[26] This suggests that MC3Rs may be involved in the circa-dian control of feeding behavior. Similarly, Butler and colleagues recently demonstrated that MC3R knockout mice, when subjected to a light-cycle feed-ing paradigm, exhibit hyperinsulinemia and glucose intolerance compared to wild-type controls.[27] These findings support the notion that MC3Rs in the brain are important for the circadian control of glucose and energy homeostasis.

MC4Rs are also involved in the regulation of en-ergy and glucose homeostasis. For example, muta-tions in MC4R gene in mice[5] or humans[28,29] lead to obesity. Data obtained from MC4R knockout mice indicate that central MC4R signals contribute to the control of body weight balance by regulating both food intake and energy expenditure.[5,30,31] Re-cent evidence also demonstrated that the central melanocortin system directly controls peripheral lipid and glucose metabolism, effects that are in-dependent of its role in food intake and energy ex-penditure.[32] An interesting question is which MC4R populations in the CNS are responsible for each of these distinct functions, given that MC4Rs are expressed in multiple relevant CNS sites.[33–35] The Lowell and Elmquist laboratories developed a loxTB MC4R null mouse model whose MC4R expression is globally disrupted by a loxP-flanked transcrip-tional blocking cassette (loxTB) inserted into the MC4R gene.[36] These loxTB MC4R null mice dis-play hyperphagia, lower energy expenditure, obe-sity, hyperinsulinemia, and hyperglycemia,[36] phe-notypes identical to those seen in the conventional MC4R knockout mice.[5] Uniquely, the loxTB cas-sette can be removed by the Cre-recombinase, which results in reactivation of MC4R expression. The loxTB MC4R null mice were crossed with SIM1-Cre transgenic mice to restore MC4R expression only in SIM1 neurons in the paraventricular nu-cleus of the hypothalamus (PVH) and the amyg-dala.[36] This manipulation markedly improves the obesity seen in loxTB MC4R null mice. Notably, the hyperphagia is completely rescued, while reduced energy expenditure, hyperglycemia, and hyperin-sulinemia are unaffected.[36] These findings demon-strate that MC4Rs expressed by SIM1 neurons in the PVH and the amygdala control food intake, but not energy expenditure and glucose/insulin balance.

We have recently crossed the loxTB MC4R null mice with the ChAT-IRES-Cre and Phox2b-Cre mice, respectively.[37] The ChAT-IRES-Cre restored MC4R expression in all cholinergic neurons, which include both the sympathetic preganglionic neurons in the intermediolateral column (IML) and the parasympathetic preganglionic neurons in the dorsal motor nucleus of the vagus (DMV); the Phox2b-Cre led to selective reexpression of MC4Rs in autonomic control neurons, including the parasympathetic preganglionic neurons in the DMV.[37] We found that while MC4Rs in cholinergic neurons (both sympathetic and parasympathetic neurons) are sufficient to increase energy expendi-ture and partially rescue the obesity seen in loxTB MC4R mice, reexpression of MC4Rs in Phox2b neurons (parasympathetic neurons) does not signif-icantly affect energy expenditure and body weight.[37] Therefore, these findings suggest that MC4Rs ex-pressed in the sympathetic preganglionic neurons in the IML are important for the control of energy expenditure. Further, we found that reexpression of MC4Rs in cholinergic neurons attenuates both hyperglycemia and hyperinsulinemia.[37] In addition, euglycemic–hyperinsulinemic clamp studies revealed that hepatic insulin action and insulin-mediated suppression of hepatic glucose production are improved in mice with MC4Rs reexpressed in cholinergic neurons.[37] In contrast, restoration of MC4Rs in Phox2b neurons only attenuates hyperinsulinemia, but has fewer effects on glucose levels.[37] Based on these findings, we suggest that MC4Rs expressed in the sympathetic preganglionic neurons in the IML are involved in the regulation of insulin sensitivity in liver and hepatic glucose production, whereas MC4Rs expressed by parasympathetic neurons in the DMV may control insulin secretion from the pancreas.

Leptin

Leptin is a circulating adipokine that plays critical roles in the regulation of body mass and body composition.[38] Leptin contributes to the regulation of body weight by influencing both food intake[39,40] and energy expenditure.[41–43] Biological actions of leptin are thought to be primarily mediated by the long-form leptin receptor (also known as LEPR-B).[44] Accumulating evidence indicates that leptin produces antiobesity effects by acting via LEPR-B in the brain.[45] For example, CNS-specific deletion of LEPR-B results in marked obesity.[46,47] In contrast, transgenic, brain-specific reconstitution of LEPR-B in LEPR-deficient (db/db) mice ameliorates obesity.[48–50]

LEPR-B is abundantly expressed in several sites within the hypothalamus, including the ARC, the dorsomedial nucleus of the hypothalamus, the lateral hypothalamic area, and the ventromedial hypothalamic nucleus (VMH).[51–56] Taking advantage of the Cre-loxP genetic animal models that allow manipulations of LEPR-B in a cell- or site-specific manner, the relative importance of leptin action at these different sites is beginning to be understood.

The melanocortin pathway is downstream of leptin actions. Particularly, leptin directly depolarizes POMC neurons.[21,57] Furthermore, fasted rodents (a condition of reduced leptin levels) and leptin-deficient (ob/ob) mice both have decreased hypothalamic POMC mRNA content, which can be normalized by exogenous leptin administration.[58–60] These findings support the possibility that leptin acts on LEPR-B expressed by POMC neurons to regulate body weight balance. To directly test this possibility, we have previously crossed the loxP-flanked LEPR-B allele with the POMC-Cre transgene, which resulted in selective deletion of endogenous LEPR-B from POMC neurons.[20] We demonstrated that this deletion causes modest obesity primarily because of decreased energy expenditure.[20,61] Bjørbæk and colleagues have recently crossed actin-driven loxTB LEPR-B alleles with the POMC-Cre transgene, which results in reexpression of LEPR-B in all POMC neurons (including those that do not endogenously express LEPR-B) on the db/db background.[62] The reexpression leads to a modest reduction in body weight.[62] Collectively, the deletion and

reexpression models provide consistent evidence to support that POMC neurons are one physiologically relevant site that mediates leptin actions on body weight control. Of note, while selective deletion of LEPR-R from POMC neurons does not significantly affect food intake,[20,61] reexpression of LEPR-R in all POMC neurons partially rescue hyperphagia seen in db/db mice.[62] This discrepancy can be interpreted to suggest that LEPR-B is only expressed in POMC neurons that regulate energy expenditure but are not major regulators of food intake. Alternatively, the lack of feeding phenotype in deletion models is due to compensatory effects of other brain regions expressing LEPR-B.

Indeed, leptin has been shown to act on a subset of neurons in the VMH, namely steroidogenic factor 1 (SF1) neurons. SF1 is a transcription factor that is expressed exclusively in the VMH within the brain.[63] Deletion of SF1 in mice disrupts VMH structure[64] and leads to obesity.[65] We found that leptin directly depolarizes SF1 neurons via LEPR-B-mediated mechanisms.[66] In addition, selective deletion of LEPR-B in SF1 neurons produces modest obesity,[66,67] indicating that LEPR-B expressed by SF1 neurons is also required to maintain normal body weight. Interestingly, mice lacking LEPR-B only in SF1 neurons show impaired thermogenic responses to acute HFD challenge,[66] suggesting that leptin actions via SF1 neurons are required to mediate the appropriate thermogenic responses to overnutrition.

Actions of leptin in the CNS have been implicated in glycemic control (as reviewed in Refs. 68 and 69). Many of these leptin regulations on glucose homeostasis appear to be mediated by LEPR-B expressed in the hypothalamus. For example, it has been shown that while partial restoration of LEPR-B in the ARC on the LEPR-B null background only modestly decreases body weight, such manipulation remarkably improves hyperinsulinemia and completely normalizes hyperglycemia seen in LEPR-B null mice.[70] Similarly, LEPR-B reexpression in all POMC neurons on the db/db background produces robust improvements in the glucose/insulin profile, while body weight is only modestly reduced.[62] Moreover, SF1-specific deletion of LEPR-B causes insulin resistance before onset of obesity.[67] Consistent with findings that acute infusion of leptin in the third cerebral ventricle markedly inhibits liver glycogenolysis and suppresses glucose production in rodents,[71] phenotypes observed in these genetic mouse models support that leptin actions in the ARC (e.g., POMC neurons) and in SF1 neurons are required to regulate insulin sensitivity and glucose homeostasis and that these effects are likely independent of leptin effects on body weight and adiposity.

In addition to the aforementioned hypothalamic neurons, emerging evidence suggests that leptin may also act on extra-hypothalamic sites to regulate feeding behavior and body weight balance. For example, Hayes and colleagues have recently shown that knock-down of LEPR-B in the nucleus of solitary tract (NTS) and area postrema (AP) via stereotaxic injections of AAV-shRNA leads to increased susceptibility to diet-induced obesity.[72] Development of obesity in these animals is not due to alterations in energy expenditure, but rather to impaired satiation and increased food intake.[72] Consistently, Scott and colleagues. demonstrated that selective deletion of LEPR-B in the NTS produces hyperphagia in mice.[73] Thus, these results suggest that LEPR-B expressed in the NTS/AP is required to mediate the anorexigenic effects of leptin.

Leptin modulates multiple intracellular signaling cascades that in turn lead to alteration of gene expression profiles and changes of neuronal electrophysiological activity. As LEPR-B is a member of the class I cytokine receptor superfamily that commonly activates Janus kinase/signal transducer and activator of transcription (JAK/STAT) pathway,[44] the JAK/STAT3 pathway is thought to be a central mediator of leptin actions. Indeed, leptin rapidly induces tyrosine phosphorylation on both JAK2 and STAT3 in the hypothalamus. Knock-in mice in which the STAT3 binding site on LEPR-B (Tyr 1138) is mutated display hyperphagic and obese phenotypes as db/db mice that completely lack LEPR-B.[74] In addition, deletion of STAT3 from the entire population of the leptin-responsive cells results in hyperphagia and obesity.[75] Interestingly, no deficits in reproduction and glucose homeostasis were observed in these mouse lines, suggesting that other signaling pathways rather than STAT3 may be involved.

Leptin also modulates other signaling pathways, including the PI3K/Akt pathway,[76–79] the mTOR/S6K pathway,[80,81] and the AMPK pathway.[82] Leptin increases the levels of PIP3, [83,84] a catalyzed product of PI3K. Pharmacological and genetic studies have shown that the PI3K pathway is required to mediate leptin actions to acutely suppress food intake[85] and to depolarize POMC neurons.[76–78] The hypothalamic mTOR/S6K pathway is another indispensable signaling mechanism mediating leptin anorexigenic actions.[86] Leptin inhibits $5'$-AMP-activated protein kinase (AMPK) in the hypothalamus. Expression of the constitutively active form of AMPK attenuates leptin's anorexigenic effects.[82] However, the molecular links between LEPR-B and PI3K, mTOR/S6K, or AMPK are not fully understood.

Leptin signaling is negatively regulated by suppressor of cytokine signaling-3 (SOCS-3)[87] and protein tyrosine phosphatase 1B (PTP1B).[88,89] SOCS-3 and PTP1B are increased within the hypothalamus in a state of excess nutrition/obesity.[89–92] Over-expression of SOCS-3 or PTP1B *in vitro* attenuates leptin-induced STAT3 activation.[88,89] Mice with brain-specific SOCS-3 deletion are protected from diet-induced obesity and leptin resistance.[93,94] PTP1B knockout mice are likewise resistant to diet-induced obesity.[88,89,95] Deletion of SOCS3 from POMC neurons results in increased leptin sensitivity and improves glucose homeostasis despite normal body weight gain.[96] In addition, mice lacking PTP1B only in POMC neurons show reduced body weight, enhanced leptin sensitivity, and increased energy expenditure.[97] Interestingly, a direct comparison among brain-specific knockout mice of SOCS-3, PTP1B, or both suggests that brain functions of SOCS-3 and PTP1B do not completely overlap in terms of control of energy homeostasis.[98] Collectively, SOCS-3 and PTP1B contribute to cellular leptin resistance.

Estrogens

Ovarian estrogens exert important antiobesity effects in women and female mammals. For example, lower levels of estrogens in postmenopausal women are associated with an increased risk for developing obesity.[99–101] Ovariectomized (OVX) animals with reduced estrogen signaling develop obesity and hyperadiposity.[102–104] Although OVX induces a transient increase in food intake, the hyperphagia does not seem to account for the development of obesity.[104] Further, OVX rats gain weight to a similar extent when they are pair-fed compared to estradiol-treated rats,[105,106] suggesting that endogenous estrogens regulate body weight homeostasis primarily by modulating energy expenditure. However, estradiol replacement was shown to decrease food intake and increase energy expenditure in rodents,[107] indicating that exogenous estrogens may promote a negative energy balance by influencing both energy intake and energy expenditure. Importantly, estrogens are also thought to play a role in regulating fat distribution. For example, female humans and rodents distribute relatively more fat in subcutaneous depot, while males have more fat stored in visceral depot, which is more likely to cause metabolic syndromes such as insulin resistance.[108–110] Estrogens appear to account for this sexual dimorphism because the differences in the fat distribution between premenopausal females and age-matched men are abolished between postmenopausal females and age-matched men.[111]

Estrogen receptor-α (ERα), one of the estrogen receptors, is believed to mediate most estrogenic effects on energy homeostasis. For example, female mice with a targeted deletion in the ERα gene (ERαKO) develop obesity and hyperadiposity, primarily due to decreased energy expenditure.[112] Although no hyperphagia is observed in ERαKO mice,[112–114] ERα is clearly required to mediate normal satiation process because estradiol-induced hypophagia and CCK-induced satiation in wild-type mice are blocked in ERαKO mice.[114]

ERα is expressed in brain regions implicated in the regulation of energy balance. These include the PVH, medial preoptic area (MPOA), ARC, VMH, and NTS, etc.[115,116] In earlier attempts to determine the effects of estrogen on food intake and body weight in these CNS regions, intranuclear microinjections and lesions were often used. However, due to the inherent difficulty in precisely placing cannulae or producing lesions in small but complex brain regions, findings obtained from these studies are difficult to reproduce and interpret.[117–122]

Recently, the role of estrogens and ERα in the VMH in the regulation of energy balance has been reexamined using the ERα silencing approach.[123] In this study, ERα in the VMH is knocked down with an AAV-shRNA.[123] Animals with impaired ERα signaling in the VMH are less sensitive to estradiol-induced weight loss and develop obesity characteristic of increased visceral fat.[123] The obesity syndrome is likely caused by decreased physical activity and impaired diet-induced thermogenesis, whereas food intake of these animals is not directly affected.[123] We recently generated mice with ERα

deleted in VMH SF1 neurons.[124] We found that deletion of ERα in VMH SF1 neurons in female mice, while not affecting food intake, significantly reduces basal metabolic rate and diet-induced thermogenesis, which consequently results in increased body weight and hyperadiposity.[124] Interestingly, a significant increase in visceral fat deposition (versus subcutaneous fat deposition) was observed in these mutant females.[124] Finally, we showed that the decreased energy expenditure and increased visceral fat distribution in mice lacking ERα in SF1 neurons presumably results from decreased sympathetic tone (as demonstrated by decreased plasma norepinephrine levels).[124] Our findings are largely consistent with those obtained from the VMH-specific ERα knock-down model. Collectively, these results support the hypothesis that ERα signaling in VMH neurons (e.g., SF1 neurons) plays an important role in regulating energy expenditure and fat distribution.

A recent study demonstrated that NPY/AgRP neurons are required to mediate the anorexigenic effects of estrogens. In this study, Xu and colleagues showed that hypothalamic expression of NPY and AgRP in wild-type mice is tightly regulated across the estrus cycle, with the lowest levels during the estrus, which coincides with the plasma estrogen peak and feeding nadir.[125] They further showed that central estradiol administration suppresses fasting-induced c-Fos activation in NPY/AgRP neurons and blunts the refeeding response.[125] Importantly, the cyclic changes in food intake and estradiol-induced anorexia are blunted in mice with degenerated NPY/AgRP neurons.[125] This study indicates that NPY/AgRP neurons are functionally required for the cyclic changes in feeding across estrous cycles. Surprisingly, these authors also found that ERα is not expressed in NPY/AgRP neurons,[125] suggesting that estrogen may regulate these neurons indirectly via presynaptic neurons that express ERα (e.g., POMC neurons).

Indeed, POMC neurons coexpress ERα.[124,126,127] In addition, estrogens regulate excitability of POMC neurons. Using electron microcopy, Horvath and colleagues have reported that the number of excitatory synaptic inputs to ARC POMC neurons rises as mice enter proestrus when estrogen levels are high.[107] Further, central estradiol administration rapidly increases the excitatory synapses on POMC neurons, an effect that is also reflected by increased miniature excitatory postsynaptic current recorded from POMC neurons.[107] These synaptological rearrangements in POMC neurons are tightly paralleled with the effects of estradiol on food intake and body weight.[107] Similarly, Ronnekleiv and colleagues reported that estradiol administration in hypothalamic slices activates POMC neurons by rapidly uncoupling GABA$_B$ receptors from the G protein–gated inwardly rectifying K$^+$ channels.[128] Importantly, we recently demonstrated that female mice lacking ERα in POMC neurons only develop hyperphagia.[124] These observations, together with the findings from the Horvath and Ronnekleiv groups, indicate that estrogen/ERα signals in POMC neurons are physiologically relevant in the regulation of food intake.[124]

Serotonin

Central serotonin (5-HT) systems play critical roles in the suppression of feeding. Brain 5-HT is primarily synthesized by neurons in the dorsal raphe nucleus (DRN) in the midbrain, which have projections to the hypothalamus.[129] 5-HT release from the DRN is rapidly enhanced after each meal,[130] suggesting that increased 5-HT bioavailability may participate in the regulation of feeding behavior. Indeed, fenfluramine, a pharmacological agent that increases serotonin content by stimulating synaptic release of serotonin and blocking its reuptake into presynaptic terminals,[131] shows a potent anorexigenic activity in rodents and humans.[132–134] Conversely, treatments that suppress central serotoninergic signaling produce hyperphagia and weight gain in humans and rodents.[135–138] At least 14 serotonin receptors have been cloned, and many of these receptors have been implicated in the regulation of food intake and body weight.[139] In particular, the 5-HT$_{2C}$ receptor (5-HT$_{2C}$R), which is exclusively expressed in the CNS,[139] has been shown to mediate a significant portion of the anorexigenic effects of central serotonin systems. For example, relatively selective 5-HT$_{2C}$R agonists, including mCPP, promote satiety and produce hypophagia. These effects are blocked by 5-HT$_{2C}$R antagonists or in 5-HT$_{2C}$R knockout animals.[140–144] Notably, deletion of 5-HT$_{2C}$Rs causes hyperphagia and obesity in mice,[144,145] indicating that the endogenous 5-HT$_{2C}$R signal is a physiological regulator of feeding. In addition, mutations in the 5-HT$_{2C}$R gene have been recently linked to several obesity con-

ditions seen in humans. For instance, commonly used atypical antipsychotic drugs (e.g., clozapine and olanzapine) have been reported to cause serious weight gain, which may be associated with their 5-HT$_{2C}$R antagonist properties and with polymorphisms in 5-HT$_{2C}$R gene.[146,147] Furthermore, a splicing variant of 5-HT$_{2C}$R with impaired function has been suggested to contribute to hyperphagia and obesity in patients with Prader–Willi syndrome.[148]

Recent studies have demonstrated that 5-HT$_{2C}$Rs are also involved in glycemic control, actions that are independent of their effects on food intake and body weight. For example, deletion of 5-HT$_{2C}$Rs in ob/ob mice leads to synergistic impairment of glucose balance, while such double deletion does not lead to more severe obese phenotypes compared to ob/ob mice.[149] In addition, mCPP administration at a subthreshold dose (1 mg/kg), which does not affect food intake and body weight, ameliorates insulin resistance and glucose intolerance in mice with diet-induced obesity.[150] Collectively, these findings indicate that both endogenous 5-HT$_{2C}$Rs and exogenous drugs that activate 5-HT$_{2C}$Rs exert antiobesity and antidiabetic effects.

5-HT$_{2C}$Rs are widely expressed in the brain,[151] and the physiological relevant sites of 5-HT$_{2C}$Rs that regulate body weight and glucose balance are difficult to identify due to the lack of commercially available 5-HT$_{2C}$R–selective drugs. Using neuroanatomy, electrophysiology, and genetic mouse models, several groups have demonstrated that POMC neurons are one of the physiologically important targets of 5-HT$_{2C}$R signals in the context of energy homeostasis. For example, POMC neurons coexpress 5-HT$_{2C}$Rs[152] and receive inputs from 5-HT–immunoreactive nerve terminals from the DRN.[153] These anatomical findings are further supported by electrophysiological studies showing that 5-HT compounds, including fenfluramine and mCPP, activate POMC neurons, effects that are blocked by 5-HT$_{2C}$R antagonists.[152,154] In addition, 5-HT$_{2C}$R agonists increase POMC expression in the ARC.[150,155] Collectively, these findings indicate that a 5-HT$_{2C}$R–melanocortin circuit may provide the anatomical basis to mediate the anorexigenic actions of 5-HT compounds (e.g., fenfluramine).

The physiological relevance of this 5-HT$_{2C}$R–melanocortin circuitry is established using genetic mouse models. First of all, we showed that the anorexigenic action of fenfluramine is blunted in Ay mice[101] or MC4R knockout mice,[156] suggesting that the intact central melanocortin system is required to mediate the pharmacological actions of 5-HT. Recently, we generated a loxTB 5-HT$_{2C}$R null mouse model in which expression of 5-HT$_{2C}$Rs is disrupted globally by inserting a loxP-flanked transcriptional blocker cassette.[157] Crossing these loxTB 5-HT$_{2C}$R null mice with transgenic POMC-Cre mice produced 2C/POMC mice in which 5-HT$_{2C}$R is expressed only in POMC neurons. We found that loxTB 5-HT$_{2C}$R null mice predictably develop hyperphagia and obesity and show attenuated anorexigenic responses to fenfluramine and mCPP.[158] All of these deficiencies are normalized in 2C/POMC mice.[158] Notably, energy expenditure is not affected in either loxTB 5-HT$_{2C}$R null mice or 2C/POMC mice.[158] These results highlight the physiological functions of the 5-HT$_{2C}$R–melanocortin circuitry in the control of food intake and body weight. We recently demonstrated that while the anorexigenic effects of fenfluramine are abolished in mice with global MC4R deficiency, these effects can be restored in mice with MC4Rs reexpressed only in SIM1 neurons in the PVH and the amygdala.[159] These observations further support the model that 5-HT compounds (e.g., fenfluramine) act on 5-HT$_{2C}$Rs expressed by POMC neurons to stimulate secretion of α-MSH, which in turn activates MC4Rs expressed by SIM1 neurons in the PVH and amygdala to suppress food intake.

The 5-HT$_{2C}$R–melanocortin circuitry is also physiologically relevant in the regulation of insulin sensitivity and glucose homeostasis. For example, it has been shown that mCPP improves glucose tolerance and insulin sensitivity in wild-type mice with diet-induced obesity, while such antidiabetic effects are blunted in mice lacking MC4Rs.[150] In addition, young loxTB 5-HT$_{2C}$R null mice develop insulin resistance in the liver, phenotypes that are independent of hyperphagia and obesity.[160] Notably, insulin resistance is normalized by reexpression of 5-HT$_{2C}$Rs only in POMC neurons (2C/POMC mice).[160] In addition, we demonstrated that while the global deletion of 5-HT$_{2C}$Rs abolishes antidiabetic effects of mCPP, such effects are restored in 2C/POMC mice.[160] Collectively, these findings demonstrate that 5-HT$_{2C}$Rs expressed by POMC neurons are physiological regulators of insulin sensitivity and glucose homeostasis.

In addition to 5-HT$_{2C}$Rs, 5-HT$_{1B}$ receptors (5-HT$_{1B}$Rs) are another important target of 5-HT action on feeding. Specifically, high-affinity 5-HT$_{1B}$R agonists and fenfluramine produce substantial reductions in food intake, effects that are attenuated by pharmacological blockade 5-HT$_{1B}$Rs.[161–163] In addition, 5-HT$_{1B}$R knockout mice show increased body weight and food intake[164] and are less sensitive to fenfluramine-induced anorexia.[165] 5-HT$_{1B}$Rs are widely expressed in the brain, with particularly high levels in the olfactory tubercle, caudate putamen, cortex, hypothalamus, hippocampal formation, thalamus, DRN, and cerebellum.[156,166,167] NPY/AgRP neurons in the ARC may be one of the physiologically relevant targets of 5-HT$_{1B}$Rs to regulate food intake. First, we demonstrated that 5-HT–positive terminals establish synaptic contacts on both cell body and axon terminals of NPY/AgRP neurons,[105] and 5-HT$_{1B}$Rs are expressed by a subset of NPY/AgRP neurons.[105] We further showed that 5-HT and selective 5-HT$_{1B}$R agonists hyperpolarize NPY neurons and decrease their firing rate, effects that are blocked by the 5-HT$_{1B}$R antagonist.[105] Given that NPY/AgRP neurons provide a strong inhibitory GABAergic projection to POMC neurons[19,21,168] and that 5-HT$_{1B}$Rs expressed on axon terminals have been demonstrated to suppress GABA release,[169,170] the direct inhibitory effects of 5-HT$_{1B}$Rs on NPY/AgRP neurons may lead to indirect activation (disinhibition) of POMC neurons. Indeed, we observed that fenfluramine and 5-HT$_{1B}$R agonists potently suppress the inhibitory postsynaptic currents in POMC neurons. Finally, we showed that the anorexigenic effects of fenfluramine and the 5-HT$_{1B}$R agonist are blunted in MC4R knockout mice or Ay mice.[105] Collectively, these findings support a model that 5-HT directly inhibits NPY/AgRP neurons via 5-HT$_{1B}$Rs. This action indirectly activates POMC neurons, and this 5-HT$_{1B}$R–NPY/AgRP–POMC circuitry may at least partly mediate the anorexigenic effects of 5-HT.

As discussed above, current evidence indicates that the central melanocortin pathway plays essential roles in multiple aspects of energy and glucose homeostasis. These include food intake, energy expenditure, insulin sensitivity, and insulin secretion. Remarkably, many of these functions are mediated by distinct CNS regions expressing melanocortin receptors (Fig. 1). Further, multiple hormones and/or

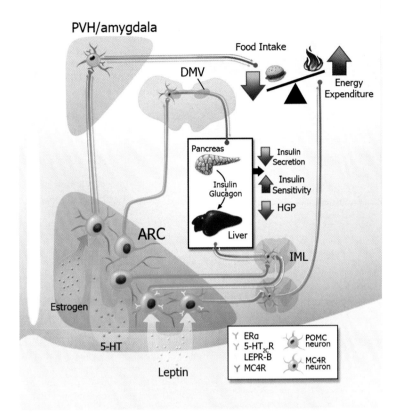

Figure 1. A schematic model for functional segregation of the central melanocortin system. Current evidence suggests that several subsets of POMC neurons exist in the ARC that project to and act on distinct downstream MC4R populations to suppress food intake, to increase energy expenditure, to decrease insulin secretion, or to increase insulin sensitivity, respectively. Multiple metabolic cues, including estrogens, 5-HT, and leptin, directly act on distinct or partially overlapping POMC subsets to regulate different aspects of energy and glucose homeostasis.

neurotransmitters, including leptin, serotonin, and estrogen, have been shown to directly act on POMC neurons to regulate energy and glucose balance (Fig. 1). Interestingly, the physiological functions of these signals, while all acting through POMC neurons, are not necessarily identical. For example, leptin directly acts on POMC neurons to regulate energy expenditure and glucose homeostasis.[20] On the other hand, estrogens, via actions on ERα in POMC neurons, suppress food intake, but do not directly regulate energy expenditure.[124] 5-HT acts on 5-HT$_{2C}$Rs in POMC neurons to regulate both feeding[158] and insulin sensitivity,[160] but does not affect energy expenditure. Collectively, these results suggest that several subsets of POMC neurons exist that project to and act on distinct downstream MC4R populations to exert different functions. Multiple

metabolic cues may be integrated by distinct or partially overlapping POMC subsets. Supporting this notion, we have recently found that acute electrophysiological responses to leptin, insulin, and 5-HT$_{2C}$R agonists are largely segregated in distinct subsets of POMC neurons.[57,171]

In conclusion, the past two decades have been an exciting time in the field of obesity and diabetes research. We have witnessed an explosion of knowledge regarding the control of energy balance and glucose homeostasis. This includes genetic, pharmacological, and neuroanatomic studies. While the increase in our knowledge is impressive, it is somewhat disappointing that the number of treatments for obesity and its complications have not kept up with the pace of discovery. Hopefully, the ever-increasing knowledge base will lead to rational strategies in the

years that follow to deal with the increasing inci-
dences of obesity and diabetes.

Acknowledgments

We thank Ms. Xiaorui Zhang for the illustration.
YX is supported by R00DK085330, R01DK093587,
P30 DK079638–03, the Naman Family Fund for Basic Research, and the Curtis Hankamer Basic Research Fund; JKE is supported by RL1 DK081185,
R37DK53301, and R01DK071320; MF is supported
by the American Heart Association.

Conflicts of interest

The authors declare no conflicts of interest.

References

1. Elmquist, J.K., C.F. Elias & C.B. Saper. 1999. From lesions to leptin: hypothalamic control of food intake and body weight. *Neuron* **22:** 221–232.
2. Cone, R.D. 2005. Anatomy and regulation of the central melanocortin system. *Nat. Neurosci.* **8:** 571–578.
3. Williams, D.L. & M.W. Schwartz. 2005. The melanocortin system as a central integrator of direct and indirect controls of food intake. *Am. J. Physiol. Regul. Integr. Comp. Physiol.* **289:** R2–R3.
4. Cone, R.D. 1999. The Central Melanocortin System and Energy Homeostasis. *Trends Endocrinol. Metab.* **10:** 211–216.
5. Huszar, D. *et al.* 1997. Targeted disruption of the melanocortin-4 receptor results in obesity in mice. *Cell* **88:** 131–141.
6. Yaswen, L. *et al.* 1999. Obesity in the mouse model of pro-opiomelanocortin deficiency responds to peripheral melanocortin. *Nat. Med.* **5:** 1066–1070.
7. Qian, S. *et al.* 2002. Neither agouti-related protein nor neuropeptide Y is critically required for the regulation of energy homeostasis in mice. *Mol Cell Biol.* **22:** 5027–5035.
8. Ollmann, M.M. *et al.* 1997. Antagonism of central melanocortin receptors in vitro and in vivo by agouti-related protein. *Science* **278:** 135–138.
9. Pierroz, D.D. *et al.* 1996. Chronic administration of neuropeptide Y into the lateral ventricle inhibits both the pituitary-testicular axis and growth hormone and insulin-like growth factor I secretion in intact adult male rats. *Endocrinology* **137:** 3–12.
10. Gropp, E. *et al.* 2005. Agouti-related peptide-expressing neurons are mandatory for feeding. *Nat. Neurosci.* **8:** 1289–1291.
11. Xu, A.W. *et al.* 2005. Effects of hypothalamic neurodegeneration on energy balance. *PLoS Biol.* **3:** e415.
12. Bewick, G.A. *et al.* 2005. Post-embryonic ablation of AgRP neurons in mice leads to a lean, hypophagic phenotype. *FASEB J.* **19:** 1680–1682.
13. Aponte, Y., D. Atasoy & S.M. Sternson. 2011. AGRP neurons are sufficient to orchestrate feeding behavior rapidly and without training. *Nat. Neurosci.* **14:** 351–355.
14. Alexander, G.M. *et al.* 2009. Remote control of neuronal activity in transgenic mice expressing evolved G protein-coupled receptors. *Neuron* **63:** 27–39.
15. Ferguson, S.M. *et al.* 2011. Transient neuronal inhibition reveals opposing roles of indirect and direct pathways in sensitization. *Nat. Neurosci.* **14:** 22–24.
16. Krashes, M.J. *et al.* 2011. Rapid, reversible activation of AgRP neurons drives feeding behavior in mice. *J. Clin. Invest.* **121:** 1424–1428.
17. Flier, J.S. 2006. AgRP in energy balance: will the real AgRP please stand up? *Cell Metab.* **3:** 83–85.
18. Wojcik, S.M. *et al.* 2006. A shared vesicular carrier allows synaptic corelease of GABA and glycine. *Neuron* **50:** 575–587.
19. Tong, Q. *et al.* 2008. Synaptic release of GABA by AgRP neurons is required for normal regulation of energy balance. *Nat. Neurosci.* **11:** 998–1000.
20. Balthasar, N. *et al.* 2004. Leptin receptor signaling in POMC neurons is required for normal body weight homeostasis. *Neuron* **42:** 983–991.
21. Cowley, M.A. *et al.* 2001. Leptin activates anorexigenic POMC neurons through a neural network in the arcuate nucleus. *Nature* **411:** 480–484.
22. Wu, Q., M.P. Boyle & R.D. Palmiter. 2009. Loss of GABAergic signaling by AgRP neurons to the parabrachial nucleus leads to starvation. *Cell* **137:** 1225–1234.
23. Chen, A.S. *et al.* 2000. Inactivation of the mouse melanocortin-3 receptor results in increased fat mass and reduced lean body mass. *Nat. Genet.* **26:** 97–102.
24. Fan, W. *et al.* 2000. The central melanocortin system can directly regulate serum insulin levels. *Endocrinology* **141:** 3072–3079.
25. Butler, A.A. *et al.* 2000. A unique metabolic syndrome causes obesity in the melanocortin-3 receptor-deficient mouse. *Endocrinology* **141:** 3518–3521.
26. Butler, A.A. 2006. The melanocortin system and energy balance. *Peptides* **27:** 281–290.
27. Sutton, G.M. *et al.* 2010. Central nervous system melanocortin-3 receptors are required for synchronizing metabolism during entrainment to restricted feeding during the light cycle. *FASEB J.* **24:** 862–872.
28. Vaisse, C. *et al.* 1998. A frameshift mutation in human MC4R is associated with a dominant form of obesity. *Nat. Genet.* **20:** 113–114.
29. Yeo, G.S. *et al.* 1998. A frameshift mutation in MC4R associated with dominantly inherited human obesity. *Nat. Genet.* **20:** 111–112.
30. Chen, A.S. *et al.* 2000. Role of the melanocortin-4 receptor in metabolic rate and food intake in mice. *Transgenic Res.* **9:** 145–154.
31. Ste Marie, L. *et al.* 2000. A metabolic defect promotes obesity in mice lacking melanocortin-4 receptors. *Proc. Natl. Acad. Sci. USA* **97:** 12,339–12,344.
32. Nogueiras, R. *et al.* 2007. The central melanocortin system directly controls peripheral lipid metabolism. *J. Clin. Invest.* **117:** 3475–3488.
33. Kishi, T. *et al.* 2003. Expression of melanocortin 4 receptor mRNA in the central nervous system of the rat. *J. Comp. Neurol.* **457:** 213–235.

34. Liu, H. *et al.* 2003. Transgenic mice expressing green flu-orescent protein under the control of the melanocortin-4 receptor promoter. *J. Neurosci.* **23:** 7143–7154.

35. Mountjoy, K.G. *et al.* 1994. Localization of the melanocortin-4 receptor (MC4-R) in neuroendocrine and autonomic control circuits in the brain. *Mol. Endocrinol.* **8:** 1298–1308.

36. Balthasar, N. *et al.* 2005. Divergence of melanocortin pathways in the control of food intake and energy expenditure. *Cell* **123:** 493–505.

37. Rossi, J. *et al.* 2011. Melanocortin-4 receptors expressed by cholinergic neurons regulate energy balance and glucose homeostasis. *Cell Metab.* **13:** 195–204.

38. Leibel, R.L., W.K. Chung & S.C. Chua, Jr. 1997. The molecular genetics of rodent single gene obesities. *J. Biol. Chem.* **272:** 31,937–31,940.

39. Alingh Prins, A. *et al.* 1986. Daily rhythms of feeding in the genetically obese and lean Zucker rats. *Physiol. Behav.* **38:** 423–426.

40. McLaughlin, C.L. & C.A. Baile. 1981. Ontogeny of feeding behavior in the Zucker obese rat. *Physiol. Behav.* **26:** 607–612.

41. Trayhurn, P., P.L. Thurlby & W.P. James. 1977. Thermogenic defect in pre-obese ob/ob mice. *Nature* **266:** 60–62.

42. Dauncey, M.J. 1986. Activity-induced thermogenesis in lean and genetically obese (ob/ob) mice. *Experientia* **42:** 547–549.

43. Dauncey, M.J. & D. Brown. 1987. Role of activity-induced thermogenesis in twenty-four hour energy expenditure of lean and genetically obese (ob/ob) mice. *Q. J. Exp. Physiol.* **72:** 549–559.

44. Tartaglia, L.A. 1997. The leptin receptor. *J. Biol. Chem.* **272:** 6093–6096.

45. Halaas, J.L. *et al.* 1997. Physiological response to long-term peripheral and central leptin infusion in lean and obese mice. *Proc. Natl. Acad. Sci. USA* **94:** 8878–8883.

46. Cohen, P. *et al.* 2001. Selective deletion of leptin receptor in neurons leads to obesity. *J. Clin. Invest.* **108:** 1113–1121.

47. McMinn, J.E. *et al.* 2005. Neuronal deletion of Lepr elicits diabesity in mice without affecting cold tolerance or fertility. *Am. J. Physiol. Endocrinol. Metab.* **289:** E403–E411.

48. Kowalski, T.J. *et al.* 2001. Transgenic complementation of leptin-receptor deficiency. I. Rescue of the obesity/diabetes phenotype of LEPR-null mice expressing a LEPR-B transgene. *Diabetes* **50:** 425–435.

49. Chua, S.C., Jr. *et al.* 2004. Transgenic complementation of leptin receptor deficiency. II. Increased leptin receptor transgene dose effects on obesity/diabetes and fertility/lactation in lepr-db/db mice. *Am. J. Physiol. Endocrinol. Metab.* **286:** E384–E392.

50. de Luca, C. *et al.* 2005. Complete rescue of obesity, diabetes, and infertility in db/db mice by neuron-specific LEPR-B transgenes. *J. Clin. Invest.* **115:** 3484–3493.

51. Elmquist, J.K. *et al.* 1997. Leptin activates neurons in ventrobasal hypothalamus and brainstem. *Endocrinology* **138:** 839–842.

52. Elmquist, J.K. *et al.* 1998. Leptin activates distinct projections from the dorsomedial and ventromedial hypothalamic nuclei. *Proc. Natl. Acad. Sci. USA* **95:** 741–746.

53. Fei, H. *et al.* 1997. Anatomic localization of alternatively spliced leptin receptors (Ob-R) in mouse brain and other tissues. *Proc. Natl. Acad. Sci. USA* **94:** 7001–7005.

54. Mercer, J.G. *et al.* 1996. Localization of leptin receptor mRNA and the long form splice variant (Ob-Rb) in mouse hypothalamus and adjacent brain regions by in situ hybridization. *FEBS Lett.* **387:** 113–116.

55. Schwartz, M.W. *et al.* 1996. Identification of targets of leptin action in rat hypothalamus. *J. Clin. Invest.* **98:** 1101–1106.

56. Scott, M.M. *et al.* 2009. Leptin targets in the mouse brain. *J. Comp. Neurol.* **514:** 518–532.

57. Williams, K.W. *et al.* 2010. Segregation of acute leptin and insulin effects in distinct populations of arcuate proopiomelanocortin neurons. *J. Neurosci.* **30:** 2472–2479.

58. Mizuno, T.M. *et al.* 1998. Hypothalamic pro-opiomelanocortin mRNA is reduced by fasting and [corrected] in ob/ob and db/db mice, but is stimulated by leptin. *Diabetes* **47:** 294–297.

59. Schwartz, M.W. *et al.* 1997. Leptin increases hypothalamic pro-opiomelanocortin mRNA expression in the rostral arcuate nucleus. *Diabetes* **46:** 2119–2123.

60. Thornton, J.E. *et al.* 1997. Regulation of hypothalamic proopiomelanocortin mRNA by leptin in ob/ob mice. *Endocrinology* **138:** 5063–5066.

61. Hill, J.W. *et al.* 2010. Direct insulin and leptin action on pro-opiomelanocortin neurons is required for normal glucose homeostasis and fertility. *Cell Metab.* **11:** 286–297.

62. Huo, L. *et al.* 2009. Leptin-dependent control of glucose balance and locomotor activity by POMC neurons. *Cell Metab.* **9:** 537–547.

63. Ikeda, Y. *et al.* 1995. The nuclear receptor steroidogenic factor 1 is essential for the formation of the ventromedial hypothalamic nucleus. *Mol. Endocrinol.* **9:** 478–486.

64. Dellovade, T.L. *et al.* 2000. Disruption of the gene encoding SF-1 alters the distribution of hypothalamic neuronal phenotypes. *J. Comp. Neurol.* **423:** 579–589.

65. Majdic, G. *et al.* 2002. Knockout mice lacking steroidogenic factor 1 are a novel genetic model of hypothalamic obesity. *Endocrinology* **143:** 607–614.

66. Dhillon, H. *et al.* 2006. Leptin directly activates SF1 neurons in the VMH, and this action by leptin is required for normal body weight homeostasis. *Neuron* **49:** 191–203.

67. Bingham, N.C. *et al.* 2008. Selective loss of leptin receptors in the ventromedial hypothalamic nucleus results in increased adiposity and a metabolic syndrome. *Endocrinology* **149:** 2138–2148.

68. Morton, G.J. & M.W. Schwartz. 2011. Leptin and the central nervous system control of glucose metabolism. *Physiol. Rev.* **91:** 389–411.

69. Kalra, S.P. 2011. Pivotal role of leptin-hypothalamus signaling in the etiology of diabetes uncovered by gene therapy: a new therapeutic intervention? *Gene Ther.* **18:** 319–325.

70. Coppari, R. *et al.* 2005. The hypothalamic arcuate nucleus: a key site for mediating leptin's effects on glucose homeostasis and locomotor activity. *Cell Metab.* **1:** 63–72.

71. Pocai, A. *et al.* 2005. Central leptin acutely reverses diet-induced hepatic insulin resistance. *Diabetes* **54:** 3182–3189.

72. Hayes, M.R. *et al.* 2010. Endogenous leptin signaling in the caudal nucleus tractus solitarius and area postrema is

required for energy balance regulation. *Cell Metab.* **11:** 77–83.

73. Scott, M.M. *et al.* 2011. Leptin receptor expression in hindbrain Glp-1 neurons regulates food intake and energy balance in mice. *J. Clin. Invest.* **121:** 2413–2421.

74. Bates, S.H. *et al.* 2003. STAT3 signalling is required for leptin regulation of energy balance but not reproduction. *Nature* **421:** 856–859.

75. Piper, M.L. *et al.* 2008. Specific physiological roles for signal transducer and activator of transcription 3 in leptin receptor-expressing neurons. *Mol. Endocrinol.* **22:** 751–759.

76. Plum, L. *et al.* 2006. Enhanced PIP3 signaling in POMC neurons causes KATP channel activation and leads to diet-sensitive obesity. *J. Clin. Invest.* **116:** 1886–1901.

77. Niswender, K.D. *et al.* 2003. Insulin activation of phosphatidylinositol 3-kinase in the hypothalamic arcuate nucleus: a key mediator of insulin-induced anorexia. *Diabetes* **52:** 227–231.

78. Hill, J.W. *et al.* 2008. Acute effects of leptin require PI3K signaling in hypothalamic proopiomelanocortin neurons in mice. *J. Clin. Invest.* **118:** 1796–1805.

79. Fukuda, M. *et al.* 2008. Monitoring FoxO1 localization in chemically identified neurons. *J. Neurosci.* **28:** 13,640–13,648.

80. Cota, D. *et al.* 2008. The role of hypothalamic mammalian target of rapamycin complex 1 signaling in diet-induced obesity. *J. Neurosci.* **28:** 7202–7208.

81. Blouet, C., H. Ono & G.J. Schwartz. 2008. Mediobasal hypothalamic p70 S6 kinase 1 modulates the control of energy homeostasis. *Cell Metab.* **8:** 459–467.

82. Minokoshi, Y. *et al.* 2004. AMP-kinase regulates food intake by responding to hormonal and nutrient signals in the hypothalamus. *Nature* **428:** 569–574.

83. Metlakunta, A.S., M. Sahu & A. Sahu. 2008. Hypothalamic phosphatidylinositol 3-kinase pathway of leptin signaling is impaired during the development of diet-induced obesity in FVB/N mice. *Endocrinology* **149:** 1121–1128.

84. Xu, A.W. *et al.* 2005. PI3K integrates the action of insulin and leptin on hypothalamic neurons. *J. Clin. Invest.* **115:** 951–958.

85. Xu, Y. *et al.* PI3K signaling in the ventromedial hypothalamic nucleus is required for normal energy homeostasis. *Cell Metab.* **12:** 88–95.

86. Cota, D. *et al.* 2006. Hypothalamic mTOR signaling regulates food intake. *Science* **312:** 927–930.

87. Bjorbaek, C. *et al.* 1998. Identification of SOCS-3 as a potential mediator of central leptin resistance. *Mol. Cell.* **1:** 619–625.

88. Cook, W.S. & R.H. Unger. 2002. Protein tyrosine phosphatase 1B: a potential leptin resistance factor of obesity. *Dev. Cell.* **2:** 385–387.

89. Zabolotny, J.M. *et al.* 2002. PTP1B regulates leptin signal transduction in vivo. *Dev. Cell.* **2:** 489–495.

90. Munzberg, H., J.S. Flier & C. Bjorbaek. 2004. Region-specific leptin resistance within the hypothalamus of diet-induced obese mice. *Endocrinology* **145:** 4880–4889.

91. Enriori, P.J. *et al.* 2007. Diet-induced obesity causes severe but reversible leptin resistance in arcuate melanocortin neurons. *Cell Metab.* **5:** 181–194.

92. White, C.L. *et al.* 2008. HF diets increase hypothalamic PTP1B and induce leptin resistance through both leptin-dependent and independent mechanisms. *Am. J. Physiol. Endocrinol. Metab.* **296:** E291–E299.

93. Mori, H. *et al.* 2004. Socs3 deficiency in the brain elevates leptin sensitivity and confers resistance to diet-induced obesity. *Nat. Med.* **10:** 739–743.

94. Howard, J.K. *et al.* 2004. Enhanced leptin sensitivity and attenuation of diet-induced obesity in mice with haploinsufficiency of Socs3. *Nat. Med.* **10:** 734–738.

95. Bence, K.K. *et al.* 2006. Neuronal PTP1B regulates body weight, adiposity and leptin action. *Nat. Med.* **12:** 917–924.

96. Kievit, P. *et al.* 2006. Enhanced leptin sensitivity and improved glucose homeostasis in mice lacking suppressor of cytokine signaling-3 in POMC-expressing cells. *Cell Metab.* **4:** 123–132.

97. Banno, R. *et al.* 2010. PTP1B and SHP2 in POMC neurons reciprocally regulate energy balance in mice. *J. Clin. Invest.* **120:** 720–734.

98. Briancon, N. *et al.* 2010. Combined neural inactivation of suppressor of cytokine signaling-3 and protein-tyrosine phosphatase-1B reveals additive, synergistic, and factor-specific roles in the regulation of body energy balance. *Diabetes* **59:** 3074–3084.

99. Carr, M.C. 2003. The emergence of the metabolic syndrome with menopause. *J. Clin. Endocrinol. Metab.* **88:** 2404–2411.

100. Flegal, K.M. *et al.* 2002. Prevalence and trends in obesity among US adults, 1999–2000. *JAMA* **288:** 1723–1727.

101. Freedman, D.S. *et al.* 2002. Trends and correlates of class 3 obesity in the United States from 1990 through 2000. *JAMA* **288:** 1758–1761.

102. Drewett, R.F. 1973. Sexual behaviour and sexual motivation in the female rat. *Nature* **242:** 476–477.

103. Blaustein, J.D. & G.N. Wade. 1976. Ovarian influences on the meal patterns of female rats. *Physiol. Behav.* **17:** 201–208.

104. Wallen, W.J., M.P. Belanger & C. Wittnich. 2001. Sex hormones and the selective estrogen receptor modulator tamoxifen modulate weekly body weights and food intakes in adolescent and adult rats. *J. Nutr.* **131:** 2351–2357.

105. Roy, E.J. & G.N. Wade. 1977. Role of food intake in estradiol-induced body weight changes in female rats. *Horm. Behav.* **8:** 265–274.

106. Mueller, K. & S. Hsiao. 1980. Estrus- and ovariectomy-induced body weight changes: evidence for two estrogenic mechanisms. *J. Comp. Physiol. Psychol.* **94:** 1126–1134.

107. Gao, Q. *et al.* 2007. Anorectic estrogen mimics leptin's effect on the rewiring of melanocortin cells and Stat3 signaling in obese animals. *Nat. Med.* **13:** 89–94.

108. Bjorntorp, P. 1997. Hormonal control of regional fat distribution. *Hum. Reprod.* **1**(12 Suppl): 21–25.

109. Bjorntorp, P. 1997. Obesity. *Lancet* **350:** 423–426.

110. Bjorntorp, P. 1997. Body fat distribution, insulin resistance, and metabolic diseases. *Nutrition* **13:** 795–803.

111. Kotani, K. *et al.* 1994. Sexual dimorphism of age-related changes in whole-body fat distribution in the obese. *Int. J. Obes. Relat. Metab. Disord.* **18:** 207–212.

112. Heine, P.A. *et al.* 2000. Increased adipose tissue in male and female estrogen receptor-alpha knockout mice. *Proc. Natl. Acad. Sci. USA* **97:** 12,729–12,734.

113. Ohlsson, C. *et al.* 2000. Obesity and disturbed lipoprotein profile in estrogen receptor-alpha-deficient male mice. *Biochem. Biophys. Res. Commun.* **278:** 640–645.

114. Geary, N. *et al.* 2001. Deficits in E2-dependent control of feeding, weight gain, and cholecystokinin satiation in ER-alpha null mice. *Endocrinology* **142:** 4751–4757.

115. Osterlund, M. *et al.* 1998. Differential distribution and regulation of estrogen receptor-alpha and -beta mRNA within the female rat brain. *Brain Res. Mol. Brain Res.* **54:** 175–180.

116. Merchenthaler, I. *et al.* 2004. Distribution of estrogen receptor alpha and beta in the mouse central nervous system: in vivo autoradiographic and immunocytochemical analyses. *J. Comp. Neurol.* **473:** 270–291.

117. Butera, P.C. & R.J. Beikirch. 1989. Central implants of diluted estradiol: independent effects on ingestive and reproductive behaviors of ovariectomized rats. *Brain Res.* **491:** 266–273.

118. Palmer, K. & J.M. Gray. 1986. Central vs. peripheral effects of estrogen on food intake and lipoprotein lipase activity in ovariectomized rats. *Physiol. Behav.* **37:** 187–189.

119. Butera, P.C., D.M. Willard & S.A. Raymond. 1992. Effects of PVN lesions on the responsiveness of female rats to estradiol. *Brain Res.* **576:** 304–310.

120. Hrupka, B.J., G.P. Smith & N. Geary. 2002. Hypothalamic implants of dilute estradiol fail to reduce feeding in ovariectomized rats. *Physiol. Behav.* **77:** 233–241.

121. Dagnault, A. & D. Richard. 1994. Lesions of hypothalamic paraventricular nuclei do not prevent the effect of estradiol on energy and fat balance. *Am. J. Physiol.* **267:** E32–E38.

122. Wade, G.N. & I. Zucker. 1970. Modulation of food intake and locomotor activity in female rats by diencephalic hormone implants. *J. Comp. Physiol. Psychol.* **72:** 328–336.

123. Musatov, S. *et al.* 2007. Silencing of estrogen receptor alpha in the ventromedial nucleus of hypothalamus leads to metabolic syndrome. *Proc. Natl. Acad. Sci. USA* **104:** 2501–2506.

124. Xu, Y. *et al.* 2011. Distinct hypothalamic neurons mediate estrogenic effects on energy homeostasis and reproduction. *Cell Metab.* **14:** 453–465.

125. Olofsson, L.E., A.A. Pierce & A.W. Xu. 2009. Functional requirement of AgRP and NPY neurons in ovarian cycle-dependent regulation of food intake. *Proc. Natl. Acad. Sci. USA* **106:** 15,932–15,937.

126. Miller, M.M. *et al.* 1995. Effects of age and long-term ovariectomy on the estrogen-receptor containing subpopulations of beta-endorphin-immunoreactive neurons in the arcuate nucleus of female C57BL/6J mice. *Neuroendocrinology* **61:** 542–551.

127. de Souza, F.S. *et al.* 2011. The estrogen receptor alpha colocalizes with proopiomelanocortin in hypothalamic neurons and binds to a conserved motif present in the neuron-specific enhancer nPE2. *Eur. J. Pharmacol.* **660:** 181–187.

128. Malyala, A. *et al.* 2008. PI3K signaling effects in hypothalamic neurons mediated by estrogen. *J. Comp. Neurol.* **506:** 895–911.

129. Lechin, F., B. van der Dijs & G. Hernandez-Adrian. 2006. Dorsal raphe vs. median raphe serotonergic antagonism. Anatomical, physiological, behavioral, neuroendocrinological, neuropharmacological and clinical evidences: relevance for neuropharmacological therapy. *Prog. Neuropsychopharmacol. Biol. Psychiatry* **30:** 565–585.

130. De Fanti, B.A., J.S. Hamilton & B.A. Horwitz. 2001. Meal-induced changes in extracellular 5-HT in medial hypothalamus of lean (Fa/Fa) and obese (fa/fa) Zucker rats. *Brain Res.* **902:** 164–170.

131. Rowland, N.E. & J. Carlton. 1986. Neurobiology of an anorectic drug: fenfluramine. *Prog. Neurobiol.* **27:** 13–62.

132. Foltin, R.W. & T.H. Moran. 1989. Food intake in baboons: effects of a long-acting cholecystokinin analog. *Appetite* **12:** 145–152.

133. McGuirk, J. *et al.* 1991. Differential effects of d-fenfluramine, l-fenfluramine and d-amphetamine on the microstructure of human eating behaviour. *Behav. Pharmacol.* **2:** 113–119.

134. Rogers, P.J. & J.E. Blundell. 1979. Effect of anorexic drugs on food intake and the micro-structure of eating in human subjects. *Psychopharmacology (Berl)* **66:** 159–165.

135. Blundell, J.E. & M.B. Leshem. 1974. Central action of anorexic agents: effects of amphetamine and fenfluramine in rats with lateral hypothalamic lesions. *Eur. J. Pharmacol.* **28:** 81–88.

136. Geyer, M.A. *et al.* 1976. Behavioral studies following lesions of the mesolimbic and mesostriatal serotonergic pathways. *Brain Res.* **106:** 257–269.

137. Ghosh, M.N. & S. Parvathy. 1973. The effect of cyproheptadine on water and food intake and on body weight in the fasted adult and weanling rats. *Br. J. Pharmacol.* **48:** 328P–329P.

138. Saller, C.F. & E.M. Stricker. 1976. Hyperphagia and increased growth in rats after intraventricular injection of 5,7-dihydroxytryptamine. *Science* **192:** 385–387.

139. Vickers, S.P. & C.T. Dourish. 2004. Serotonin receptor ligands and the treatment of obesity. *Curr. Opin. Investig. Drugs* **5:** 377–388.

140. Vickers, S.P. *et al.* 1999. Reduced satiating effect of d-fenfluramine in serotonin 5-HT(2C) receptor mutant mice. *Psychopharmacology (Berl)* **143:** 309–314.

141. Kennett, G.A. & G. Curzon. 1991. Potencies of antagonists indicate that 5-HT1C receptors mediate 1–3(chlorophenyl)piperazine-induced hypophagia. *Br. J. Pharmacol.* **103:** 2016–2020.

142. Kennett, G.A. *et al.* 1997. SB 242084, a selective and brain penetrant 5-HT2C receptor antagonist. *Neuropharmacology* **36:** 609–620.

143. Clifton, P.G., M.D. Lee & C.T. Dourish. 2000. Similarities in the action of Ro 60–0175, a 5-HT2C receptor agonist and d-fenfluramine on feeding patterns in the rat. *Psychopharmacology (Berl).* **152:** 256–267.

144. Tecott, L.H. *et al.* 1995. Eating disorder and epilepsy in mice lacking 5-HT2c serotonin receptors. *Nature* **374:** 542–546.

145. Nonogaki, K. *et al.* 1998. Leptin-independent hyperphagia and type 2 diabetes in mice with a mutated serotonin 5-HT2C receptor gene. *Nat. Med.* **4:** 1152–1156.

146. Templeman, L.A. *et al.* 2005. Polymorphisms of the 5-HT2C receptor and leptin genes are associated with antipsychotic drug-induced weight gain in Caucasian subjects with a first-episode psychosis. *Pharmacogenet. Genomics* **15:** 195–200.

147. Reynolds, G.P., Z.J. Zhang & X.B. Zhang. 2002. Association of antipsychotic drug-induced weight gain with a 5-HT2C receptor gene polymorphism. *Lancet* **359:** 2086–2087.

148. Kishore, S. & S. Stamm. 2006. The snoRNA HBII-52 regulates alternative splicing of the serotonin receptor 2C. *Science* **311:** 230–232.

149. Wade, J.M. *et al.* 2008. Synergistic impairment of glucose homeostasis in ob/ob mice lacking functional serotonin 2C receptors. *Endocrinology* **149:** 955–961.

150. Zhou, L. *et al.* 2007. Serotonin 2C receptor agonists improve type 2 diabetes via melanocortin-4 receptor signaling pathways. *Cell Metab.* **6:** 398–405.

151. Molineaux, S.M. *et al.* 1989. 5-HT1c receptor is a prominent serotonin receptor subtype in the central nervous system. *Proc. Natl. Acad. Sci. USA* **86:** 6793–6797.

152. Heisler, L.K. *et al.* 2002. Activation of central melanocortin pathways by fenfluramine. *Science* **297:** 609–611.

153. Kiss, J., C. Leranth & B. Halasz. 1984. Serotoninergic endings on VIP-neurons in the suprachiasmatic nucleus and on ACTH-neurons in the arcuate nucleus of the rat hypothalamus. A combination of high resolution autoradiography and electron microscopic immunocytochemistry. *Neurosci. Lett.* **44:** 119–124.

154. Qiu, J. *et al.* 2007. Serotonin 5-hydroxytryptamine2C receptor signaling in hypothalamic proopiomelanocortin neurons: role in energy homeostasis in females. *Mol. Pharmacol.* **72:** 885–896.

155. Lam, D.D. *et al.* 2008. Serotonin 5-HT2C receptor agonist promotes hypophagia via downstream activation of melanocortin 4 receptors. *Endocrinology* **149:** 1323–1328.

156. Heisler, L.K. *et al.* 2006. Serotonin reciprocally regulates melanocortin neurons to modulate food intake. *Neuron* **51:** 239–249.

157. Zigman, J.M. *et al.* 2005. Mice lacking ghrelin receptors resist the development of diet-induced obesity. *J. Clin. Invest.* **115:** 3564–3572.

158. Xu, Y. *et al.* 2008. 5-HT2CRs expressed by proopiomelanocortin neurons regulate energy homeostasis. *Neuron* **60:** 582–589.

159. Xu, Y. *et al.* 2010. A serotonin and melanocortin circuit mediates d-fenfluramine anorexia. *J. Neurosci.* **30:** 14,630–14,634.

160. Xu, Y. *et al.* 2010. 5-HT(2C)Rs expressed by proopiomelanocortin neurons regulate insulin sensitivity in liver. *Nat. Neurosci.* **13:** 1457–1459.

161. Halford, J.C. & J.E. Blundell. 1996. The 5-HT1B receptor agonist CP-94,253 reduces food intake and preserves the behavioural satiety sequence. *Physiol. Behav.* **60:** 933–939.

162. Lee, M.D. & K.J. Simansky. 1997. CP-94, 253: a selective serotonin1B (5-HT1B) agonist that promotes satiety. *Psychopharmacology (Berl)* **131:** 264–270.

163. Lee, M.D. *et al.* 1998. Infusion of the serotonin1B (5-HT1B) agonist CP-93,129 into the parabrachial nucleus potently and selectively reduces food intake in rats. *Psychopharmacology (Berl)* **136:** 304–307.

164. Bouwknecht, J.A. *et al.* 2001. Male and female 5-HT(1B) receptor knockout mice have higher body weights than wildtypes. *Physiol. Behav.* **74:** 507–516.

165. Lucas, J.J. *et al.* 1998. Absence of fenfluramine-induced anorexia and reduced c-Fos induction in the hypothalamus and central amygdaloid complex of serotonin 1B receptor knock-out mice. *J. Neurosci.* **18:** 5537–5544.

166. Bonaventure, P. *et al.* 1998. Detailed mapping of serotonin 5-HT1B and 5-HT1D receptor messenger RNA and ligand binding sites in guinea-pig brain and trigeminal ganglion: clues for function. *Neuroscience* **82:** 469–484.

167. Bruinvels, A.T. *et al.* 1994. Localization of 5-HT1B, 5-HT1D alpha, 5-HT1E and 5-HT1F receptor messenger RNA in rodent and primate brain. *Neuropharmacology* **33:** 367–386.

168. Roseberry, A.G. *et al.* 2004. Neuropeptide Y-mediated inhibition of proopiomelanocortin neurons in the arcuate nucleus shows enhanced desensitization in ob/ob mice. *Neuron* **41:** 711–722.

169. Chadha, A. *et al.* 2000. The 5HT(1B) receptor agonist, CP-93129, inhibits [(3)H]-GABA release from rat globus pallidus slices and reverses akinesia following intrapallidal injection in the reserpine-treated rat. *Br. J. Pharmacol.* **130:** 1927–1932.

170. Stanford, I.M. & M.G. Lacey. 1996. Differential actions of serotonin, mediated by 5-HT1B and 5-HT2C receptors, on GABA-mediated synaptic input to rat substantia nigra pars reticulata neurons in vitro. *J. Neurosci.* **16:** 7566–7573.

171. Sohn, J.W. *et al.* 2011. Serotonin 2C receptor activates a dinstinct population of arcuate pro-opiomelanocortin neurons via TRPC channels. *Neuron* **71:** 488–497.

Ann. N.Y. Acad. Sci. ISSN 0077-8923

ANNALS OF THE NEW YORK ACADEMY OF SCIENCES

Issue: *The Year in Diabetes and Obesity*

Obesity, leptin, and Alzheimer's disease

Edward B. Lee

Translational Neuropathology Research Laboratory, Division of Neuropathology, Department of Pathology and Laboratory Medicine, Perelman School of Medicine, University of Pennsylvania, Philadelphia, Pennsylvania

Address for correspondence: Edward B. Lee, Translational Neuropathology Research Laboratory, 605B Stellar Chance Laboratories, 422 Curie Blvd, Philadelphia, PA 19104. edward.lee@uphs.upenn.edu

Obesity has various deleterious effects on health largely associated with metabolic abnormalities including abnormal glucose and lipid homeostasis that are associated with vascular injury and known cardiac, renal, and cerebrovascular complications. Advanced age is also associated with increased adiposity, decreased lean mass, and increased risk for obesity-related diseases. Although many of these obesity- and age-related disease processes have long been subsumed to be secondary to metabolic or vascular dysfunction, increasing evidence indicates that obesity also modulates nonvascular diseases such as Alzheimer's disease (AD) dementia. The link between peripheral obesity and neurodegeneration will be explored, using adipokines and AD as a template. After an introduction to the neuropathology of AD, the relationship between body weight, obesity, and dementia will be reviewed. Then, population-based and experimental studies that address whether leptin modulates brain health and mitigates AD pathways will be explored. These studies will serve as a framework for understanding the role of adipokines in brain health.

Keywords: adiponectin; Alzheimer; amyloid; leptin

Introduction

Understanding how obesity adversely affects the aging brain is hindered by the number of metabolic and hormonal pathways that are altered due to both obesity and aging. These changes include alterations in energy expenditure, reduced respiratory quotient, hyperlipidemia, hyperinsulinemia, glucose intolerance, low-grade inflammation, and changes in adipokine levels. Dissecting the relative role of each of these factors remains a challenge. Of the various changes associated with obesity, altered adipokine signaling may be one mechanism whereby obesity affects brain health. Adipokines are known to affect brain physiology and function, and both population and experimental studies suggest that changes in adipokine function may mitigate the pathogenesis of Alzheimer's disease (AD). The interaction between obesity and AD has been explored in several reviews, usually with an emphasis on insulin signaling pathways.[1–4] This review will emphasize the potential role of adipose tissue and adipokines in the pathogenesis of AD with a particular focus on leptin.

Neuropathology of Alzheimer's disease

AD is characterized by an insidious loss of memory and cognition leading to death within 10 years.[5–8] AD brains show neuronal loss and reactive gliosis involving limbic regions (including amygdala and hippocampus) and cerebral cortex with relative sparing of the basal ganglia, cerebellum, brainstem, and spinal cord.[9] Affected brain regions show an abundance of intracellular and extracellular aggregates (Fig. 1). Intraneuronal aggregates called neurofibrillary tangles consist of hyperphosphorylated tau protein in the form of insoluble paired helical filaments.[10] Extracellular deposits called amyloid plaques consist of Aβ peptides in the form of insoluble amyloid fibrils. Many amyloid plaques also contain swollen dystrophic tau-positive neurites and are thus called neuritic plaques. Both plaques and tangles stain avidly using dyes, such as thioflavin S or congo red, that bind to β-pleated sheet structures. Widespread involvement and a high density of plaques and tangles are diagnostic of AD.

Aβ peptides are generated by sequential proteolysis of the amyloid precursor protein (APP) by a

doi: 10.1111/j.1749-6632.2011.06274.x

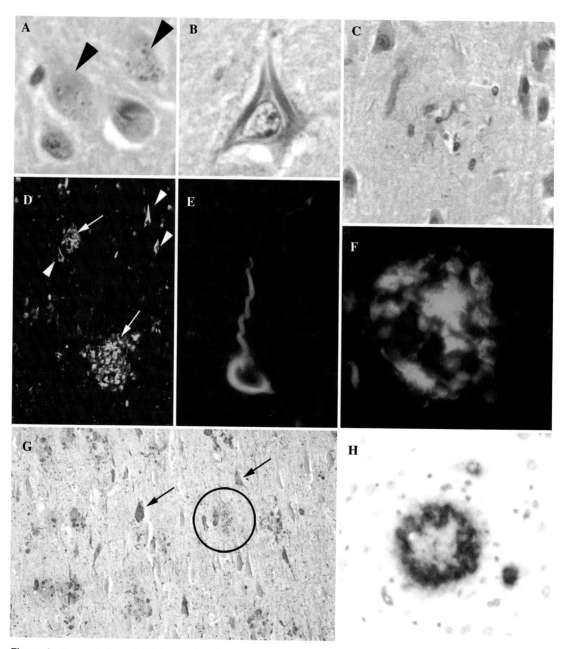

Figure 1. Neuropathology of AD. Images from hematoxylin- and eosin-stained histologic sections (400× magnification) from affected human AD brain show: (A) granulovacuolar degeneration (arrowheads), (B) intracellular neurofibrillary tangles, and (C) waxy extracellular amyloid plaques. As neurofibrillary tangles and amyloid plaques are relatively subtle using routine stains, histologic diagnosis of AD is aided by using dyes that bind to amyloid structures or with antibodies specific for tau or Aβ. (D) Thioflavin S staining (fluorescent green color, 100× magnification) of human AD necortex shows abundant extracellular amyloid plaques (arrows) and intraneuronal neurofibrillary tangles (arrowheads). Higher-power images (400× magnification) show (E) a neurofibrillary tangle and (F) an amyloid plaque. (G) Neurofibrillary tangles (arrows, 100×) are stained with antibodies that recognize phosphorylated tau protein epitopes. Note also the presence of clusters of phospho-tau immunoreactivity (circles) that label dystrophic neurites in association with amyloid plaques. (H) Amyloid plaques form in transgenic mouse overexpressing mutant APP that can be labeled with antibodies against Aβ (400× magnification).

series of endoproteolytic proteases historically called "secretases" prior to their cloning.[9] β-secretase, now known as β-site APP cleaving enzyme (BACE), cleaves at the N-terminus of the Aβ sequence. An alternative cleavage pathway involving α-secretase results in proteolysis within the Aβ domain, precluding the generation of Aβ peptide. After α- or β-cleavage, the remaining C-terminal APP fragments are then cleaved by the γ-secretase enzymatic complex that consists of four proteins (presenilin, Aph1, Pen2, and nicastrin). Importantly, several mutations within the APP or presenilin genes result in autosomal dominant cerebral Aβ amyloidosis. These autosomal dominant amyloidoses usually result in clinical dementia and AD-like neuropathology, although other clinical syndromes and pathologies are observed, such as cerebral amyloid angiopathy, leading to recurrent hemorrhagic strokes. Finally, the vast majority of these mutations result in increased amyloidogenic Aβ peptide generation. Thus, Aβ is central to the pathogenesis of AD dementia.

Tau protein normally functions to bind and stabilize microtubules.[10] Tau is prone to aggregation intracellularly where the protein is ubiquitinated and hyperphosphporylated at multiple sites. Although

tau mutations have not been linked to AD dementia, several tau mutations are causative for other related neurodegenerative dementias indicating that tau dysfunction alone is sufficient for neuronal degeneration. Understanding the processes that influence amyloid plaque or neurofibrillary tangle formation may prove invaluable in mitigating AD and related neurodegenerative diseases.

Recent large-scale studies have been examining the relationship between clinical symptomology, various biomarkers of AD dementia, and brain pathology (Fig. 2).[5–8,11] Biomarkers currently under investigation include cerebrospinal fluid (CSF) Aβ, CSF tau, structural and functional brain imaging using MRI or PET, and synthetic amyloid imaging compounds that detect cerebral amyloid. The clinical spectrum of disease has been expanded in recognition of the fact that AD is likely a protracted and insidious disease. A predementia stage called "mild cognitive impairment" (MCI) can be defined using careful psychometric testing, sometimes coincident with a subjective decline in memory, reasoning, or visual perception that does not reach the diagnostic threshold of dementia.[7] Individuals with MCI are at risk for subsequent dementia. However, even before clinical signs can be detected, abnormal biomarker

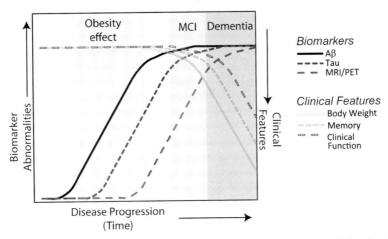

Figure 2. Model of the clinical and biomarker progression of AD. Current efforts are underway to define the relationship between progression of AD (x-axis), various AD biomarkers (left y-axis), and clinical parameters associated with AD (right y-axis). Abnormal biomarker values related to the Aβ peptide (CSF Aβ measurements and/or amyloid dye imaging techniques, black line) indicate that abnormalities related to Aβ can be detected in presymptomatic individuals. Consequently, tau abnormalities and pathology may then develop (blue dotted line), followed by changes in brain structure and function (MRI and PET scans, purple dashed line). The onset of memory decline (empty green dotted line) heralds the clinical designation of "mild cognitive impairment" (MCI), which is typically followed by an overt decline in clinical function (empty red dashed line) and dementia, most commonly diagnosed as AD. Also reflected in this model is the association between obesity and dementia that is thought to occur in the presymptomatic phase of the disease as well as the association between weight loss (empty light blue line) and dementia that typically occurs close to and during the later stages of AD. Adapted and modified from work by Jack et al.[11]

values can be detected in cognitively normal individuals, leading to the concept of preclinical disease characterized by early biological changes including the onset of CNS pathology.[8]

Body weight, obesity, and dementia

With the aging of the Baby Boomers, the number of Americans 65 and older will more than double from 2000 to 2050, and those 85 and older will increase by fivefold.[12−14] Advanced age is the strongest risk factor for AD, and AD is the most common aging-related neurodegenerative disease, with a projected 13 million or more afflicted by 2050 and with a cost of over $1 trillion unless effective interventions are implemented soon.[15−18] Obesity rates have also dramatically increased in the last 25 years such that greater than 1 in 3 adults are obese.[19] Of all the demographic age groups, Baby Boomers have the highest rates of obesity at 40%.[19] These demographics raise the public health concern of increases in aging- and obesity-related diseases.

The relationship between body weight and dementia is complex in that body weight has an age-dependent relationship with dementia (Fig. 2 and Table 1). Individuals with AD have lower body weight,[20] and it is plausible that dementia leads to a negative energy balance secondary to malnutrition. However, reductions in body weight is a harbinger of AD even before clinical symptoms of dementia are detected,[21,22] suggesting that loss of body weight may be a manifestation of early brain dysfunction. Furthermore, lower body mass indexes (BMIs) are associated with abnormal CSF Aβ and tau levels[23] and with increased CNS pathology at autopsy including neurofibrillary tangles and amyloid plaques.[24] Thus, weight loss is a consistent feature of AD dementia and correlates with the presence of abnormal biomarkers and increased brain pathology. However, weight loss associated with AD should be interpreted with caution since dual-energy x-ray absorptiometry studies suggest that weight loss is primarily due to sarcopenia and not loss of fat.[25] Thus total body weight and BMI may not be valid surrogate measures of obesity in the elderly. Given this propensity for weight loss, studies of elderly cohorts examining the relationship between obesity and AD are mixed,[21,22,26−32] perhaps reflecting the difficulties in defining obesity in elderly cohorts based on anthropomorphic measurements such as BMI. For example, using the waist-to-hip ratio as a measure of central obesity reveals that obesity is associated with a significant hazards ratio of 2.5 for the development of AD while BMI in the same elderly cohort was not significantly associated with an increased risk for AD.[31]

Analysis of multiple biomarkers of AD has yielded a model in which AD is a protracted and insidious disease, with pathogenic processes occurring years if not decades prior to clinical symptoms.[11] Keeping this temporal distinction in mind, it is intriguing that mid-life obesity has been found to increase the risk of developing late-life AD (hazards or odds ratios ranging from $\sim$ 1.4 to 3.6; see Table 1).[27,30,33−37] These studies define obesity with different metrics, including BMI, waist circumference, sagittal abdominal diameter, and waist-to-hip ratios. Diabetes mellitus and vascular disease are also associated with dementia.[1] However, in as much as such factors can be treated as separate variables, the risk due to diabetes mellitus and vascular disease appears to be independent of the risk due to obesity. One important caveat to these studies is that most cohorts are clinically defined as having AD dementia without autopsy confirmation. Given the ubiquity of multiple brain pathologies in the elderly including a high prevalence of vascular disease, validation of these findings in autopsy-confirmed cohorts is desirable to define the relative contribution of vascular versus nonvascular pathology.[38,39] Nonetheless, the fact that obesity confers increased risk for AD during the preclinical stage of AD suggests that obesity may modulate biological pathways early in the pathogenesis of AD. Identifying factors that influence brain pathology before the onset of overt neurodegeneration provides an avenue for possible preventative intervention.

Diet and obesity in experimental AD models

Multiple AD mouse models have been generated, most of which overexpress mutant forms of APP and/or tau.[40] In general, expressing APP harboring mutations linked to human disease results in age-dependent accumulation of amyloid plaques and deficits in learning and memory behaviors (Fig. 1H).[41,42] Mutant tau transgenic models develop intracellular tau aggregates that can lead to age-dependent neuronal degeneration.[43] Although these models overexpress high levels of mutant protein and are therefore not entirely physiologic, these mice have proven invaluable in understanding the factors that influence the neuropathology of AD. APP transgenic mice have been fed various diets to determine whether diet can influence cerebral amyloid deposition. Several studies have documented increases in body weight or adiposity in APP transgenic mice in response to high-calorie diets. Diets range from high-fat diets to high-fat and high-cholesterol diets to high-sucrose diets. Remarkably, despite differences in dietary nutrient content, diet-induced obesity is consistently associated with an increase in cerebral amyloid pathology.[44-50] The only exception is a single study in which a Western diet was administered for only four weeks to examine relatively acute changes at an age (one to two months) before amyloid plaque pathology is found.[51] Likewise, several dietary regimens associated with weight loss have been tested, including ketogenic diets and caloric-restriction diets. Again, studies that document weight loss uniformly show a correlation between weight reduction and decreased cerebral amyloid pathology.[52-56] These studies, performed on multiple different APP transgenic strains using a variety of diets from several independent laboratories, provide strong evidence that diet, body weight, and obesity modulate cerebral amyloid pathology.

Leptin and AD dementia

There are many possible factors and mechanisms that may account for this modulation of AD pathology. Indeed, several studies suggest that adipokines, and in particular leptin, may influence the pathogenesis of AD. A prospective study of 785 participants has indicated that higher circulating levels of leptin are associated with a reduction in AD incidence.[57] Higher leptin was associated with a lower incidence of dementia including AD dementia (hazard ratio for AD ~ 0.6), even when correcting for the waist-to-hip ratio, BMI, and vascular risk factors in multivariate statistical models. Higher leptin levels were also associated with higher total cerebral brain volume in the subset of participants who underwent MRI imaging. Since leptin levels are known to fluctuate over time, it is remarkable that a significant association between leptin and AD could be detected using a single leptin measurement. The major determinant of circulating leptin levels is adipose tissue mass, and typically hyperleptinemia is associated with obesity and central leptin resistance.

Thus, it is interesting that there was no association between leptin and AD incidence in the top quartile of participants based on waist-to-hip measurements or in individuals with a BMI > 30. Finally, the mean follow-up time of 8.3 years suggests that many leptin measurements were performed in the preclinical or MCI stages of the disease. This study suggests that leptin during the presymptomatic phase of AD, at least in nonobese individuals, may be neuroprotective and mitigate the progression of AD.

Secreted by adipose tissue, leptin regulates body weight by modulating LR-expressing neurons in the CNS, particularly within the hypothalamus and brainstem.[58-60] However, leptin has pleiotropic metabolic effects, regulating energy expenditure, feeding behavior, locomotor activity, bone mass, growth, thermogenesis, fertility, life span, adrenal function, and thyroid function. Thus, mice with congenital absence of leptin (*ob/ob* mice) or leptin's signaling receptor (*db/db* mice) exhibit a complex phenotype with abnormalities in virtually every organ system. These diverse effects are most congruous with the absence of leptin acting as a signal of starvation, triggering numerous compensatory changes that secondarily lead to obesity.[61] Thus, leptin-deficient models are a complex hybrid of the starvation response and the numerous secondary effects of obesity.

Leptin acts through the longest isoform of leptin receptors (LRb), the only isoform containing the cytoplasmic signaling domain.[58-60] Leptin binding triggers phosphorylation of cytoplasmic tyrosine residues that initiate various signaling pathways including JAK2-STAT3, Erk1/2, and PI3K pathways (Fig. 3). Other signaling molecules may be regulated by leptin, such as AMP kinase (AMPK) and mammalian target of rapamycin complex 1 (mTOR1).[62-65] However, the signaling mechanisms by which leptin affects these molecules are not entirely known, and it is not known whether these pathways result from a direct effect of leptin on LRb.

LRs are present in both hypothalamic and extrahypothalamic neurons, including neurons of the hippocampus and cerebral cortex.[66-74] The major metabolic effects are predominantly due to leptin action on hypothalamic and hindbrain neurons. However, several lines of evidence suggest that leptin has nonmetabolic CNS effects as well. For example, leptin does not exert any metabolic effects

Table 1. Summary of human studies on the relationships between obesity, AD, leptin, and brain function

Reference	Study cohort	Adipokine changes
Stewart et al.[21]	Honolulu–Asia Aging Study (32-year prospective longitudinal study); 1,890 Japanese-American men, of which 112 developed AD	Dementia is associated with weight loss. Weight loss precedes the onset of clinical dementia. Weight loss accelerates by the time of diagnosis.
Ewers et al.[23]	Multicenter cross-sectional study (308 AD, 296 MCI, 147 controls)	Abnormal CSF biomarker signature (tau and β-amyloid) is associated with lower BMI.
Buchman et al.[24]	Religious Order Study (clinical-pathologic study of Catholic clergy); 298 deceased subjects	AD pathology (using a global pathology measure) is associated with lower BMI. Other pathology (infarcts, Lewy bodies) did not correlate with BMI.
Burns et al.[25]	University of Kansas Alzheimer and Memory Program cross-sectional study; of 70 early-stage AD, 70 controls	Lean mass is reduced in early AD individuals compared to non-demented controls. Lean mass is associated with whole-brain volume and white matter volume, and global cognitive performance.
Gustafson et al.[26]	Swedish adults (longitudinal study, 70–88 years old); 392 non-demented individuals, of which 93 developed dementia	Women who developed dementia had higher BMI at age 70, 75, and 79 compared to women who did not develop dementia. No association was observed in men.
Gustafson et al.[27]	Prospective Population Study of Women in Sweden (32-year-longitudinal study); 1,462 women, of which 161 developed dementia	Elevated midlife waist-to-hip ratio increases risk for dementia.
Buchman et al.[28]	Religious Order Study (prospective longitudinal clinical-pathologic study of Catholic clergy, 5.5 years); 918 non-demented individuals, of which 151 developed AD	Declining BMI is associated with increased AD risk.
Hayden et al.[29]	Cache County Study (community-based study in Utah); 3,264 individuals	Obesity (elevated BMI) increases risk of AD in females but not males. Hypertension increases risk of vascular dementia. Diabetes increases risk of vascular dementia in females but not males.
Fitzpatrick et al.[30]	Multisite community-dwelling cohort (prospective longitudinal study, 5.4 years); 2,798 non-demented adults, of which 480 developed dementia (254 AD without vascular dementia and 213 vascular dementia +/− AD)	Midlife obesity (elevated BMI) increases risk for dementia. In late life, low BMI increases risk for dementia and obesity decreases risk for dementia.

Continued

Ann. N.Y. Acad. Sci. 1243 (2011) 15–29 © 2011 New York Academy of Sciences.

Table 1. *Continued*

Reference	Study cohort	Adipokine changes
Luchsinger *et al.*[31]	Washington Heights–Inwood Columbia Aging Project (longitudinal study of randomly recruited community-dwelling cohort in New York City); 1,459 elderly (65+), of which 145 developed AD (5,734 person-years)	Waist-to-hip ratio (but not BMI) is associated with increased AD risk.
Vanhanen *et al.*[32]	Random population study of cardiovascular risk factors and diabetes in Finland (longitudinal study, 3.5 years); 959 subjects (65–74 years old), of which 45 developed probable or possible AD	Metabolic syndrome is associated with AD.
Whitmer *et al.*[33]	Kaiser Permanente Northern California Medical Group (longitudinal study, 27 years) 10,276 individuals of which 713 developed dementia	Individuals who were obese or overweight (elevated BMI) at midlife are at increased risk for dementia.
Whitmer *et al.*[34]	Kaiser Permanente Northern California Medical Group (longitudinal study, 36 years); 10,136 individuals, of which 477 developed AD and 132 developed vascular dementia	Individuals who were obese or overweight (elevated BMI) at midlife are at increased risk for AD and vascular dementia.
Whitmer *et al.*[35]	Kaiser Permanente Northern California Medical Group (longitudinal study, 36 years); 6,583 individuals, of which 1,049 developed dementia	Sagittal abdominal diameter as a measure of central obesity is associated with increased risk for dementia.
Kivipelto *et al.*[36]	Cardiovascular Risk Factors, Aging and Dementia (CAIDE) study (random population-based longitudinal study, 21 years); 1,449 individuals, of which 61 developed dementia and 48 developed AD	Midlife obesity (elevated BMI) is associated with risk of dementia and risk of AD. Additional vascular factors (hypertension, hypercholesterolemia) also increase risk for dementia.
Chiang *et al.*[37]	Nested case–control study of 157 demented and 628 control subjects	Being either underweight or overweight (by BMI) increases risk for dementia, AD, and vascular dementia.
Lieb *et al.*[57]	Framingham study (longitudinal study, 8.3 years); 5,209 individuals, of which 111 developed dementia and 89 developed AD	Higher leptin (single measurement in asymptomatic individuals) is associated with lower risk of dementia and AD. Higher leptin is associated with higher cerebral brain volume by MRI.
Nartia *et al.*[78]	Cross-sectional study of 34 elderly individuals without dementia or metabolic syndrome	Higher leptin is associated with increased gray matter volume in the hippocampus and cerebellum.
Holden *et al.*[79]	Health, Aging and Body Composition (Health ABC) study (prospective longitudinal cohort study, 5 years) of well-functioning community-dwelling elders in Memphis, TN or Pittsburgh, PA	Higher leptin is associated with less cognitive decline as measured by the Modified Mini-Mental State Exam.

Continued

Table 1. *Continued*

Reference	Study cohort	Adipokine changes
Matochik *et al.*[80]	Three human adults with congenital leptin-deficiency treated with leptin; MRI study	Leptin increases gray matter in the anterior cingulate gyrus, inferior parietal lobule, and cerebellum.
Paz-Filho *et al.*[81]	A five-year-old boy with congenital leptin deficiency treated with leptin	Baseline tests showed slow neurocognitive development. After two years of leptin treatment, most neurocognitive domains showed substantial improvement, with some areas exceeding expectations for age.
Baicy *et al.*[81]	Three human adults with congenital leptin deficiency treated with leptin; fMRI study	Leptin reduces brain activation in insular, parietal, and temporal cortex (linked to hunger) and enhances brain activation in prefrontal cortex (linked to inhibition/satiety).
Farooqi *et al.*[83]	Two human individuals with congenital leptin deficiency; fMRI study	Leptin modulates brain activation in ventral striatum and posterolateral ventral striatum (linked to reward/satiety).
Rosenbaum *et al.*[84]	Six obese subjects examined at baseline and after 10% weight loss, then treated with leptin or placebo; fMRI study	Weight loss (a state of relative hypoleptinemia) alters neuronal activity in multiple brain regions. These changes in brain activation could be reversed by leptin treatment.

in mice prior to weaning despite a large postnatal surge, indicative of a function distinct from its role in metabolism.[75,76] The brains of *ob/ob* mice are smaller with reduced levels of synaptic proteins, abnormalities that are partially reversed by leptin treatment.[77] In normal elderly, circulating leptin levels correlate with gray matter volume in various brain regions including the hippocampus,[57,78] and inversely correlates with cognitive decline.[79] Leptin also reverses neurocognitive deficits and structural abnormalities in multiple brain regions in humans with congenital leptin deficiency.[80,81] In leptin-deficient individuals and people with recent weight loss (representing a state of relative leptin deficiency), exogenous leptin alters brain activation in response to food cues.[82–84] These findings indicate that leptin has strong effects on brain structure and function outside the hypothalamus.

A growing literature indicates that leptin is neurotrophic. Leptin promotes dendritic growth cones/filipodia outgrowth in hippocampal and cor-

tical neurons *in vitro*[85,86] and exhibits trophic activity on neurons that regulate feeding behavior *in vivo*.[87,88] Leptin increases adult hippocampal neurogenesis[89] and enhances hippocampal long-term potentiation by enhancing NMDA receptor function in part through MAPK.[90] Indeed, *db/db* mice exhibit defects in hippocampal neuronal morphology and hippocampus-dependent learning and memory behaviors.[91,92] In addition to its neurotrophic role, leptin appears to be neuroprotective,[77] as seen in various models of neuronal injury including injury related to stroke, seizure, neurotrophin withdrawal, excitotoxicity, oxidative damage, apoptosis, 6-hyrdoxydopamine, and tumor necrosis factor-α.[93–99] The pleotropic effects of leptin on neuronal integrity and function makes it possible that leptin may have beneficial effects on the CNS independent of the pathogenic mechanisms of AD.

More relevant to the pathogenesis of AD, leptin reduces Aβ secretion in cultured neuronal cells or organotypic slices,[45,100,101] and chronic leptin

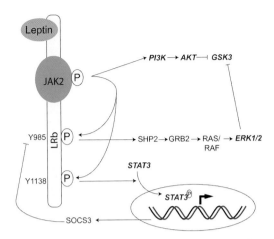

Figure 3. Leptin receptor signaling. LRb is constitutively associated with Janus family of tyrosine kinase 2 (JAK2). Leptin binding to LRb triggers autophosporylation of JAK2[155–157] and subsequent phosphorylation of cytoplasmic LRb tyrosine residues, including Y1138 and Y985. Phosphorylation of Y1138 recruits STAT3, which is then phosphorylated and translocated into the nucleus to alter gene expression, including upregulation of suppressor of cytokine signaling 3 (SOCS3) expression.[142,155] SOCS3 binds to Y985 as a negative feedback regulator of LRb signaling.[141] Y985 serves dual roles in that its phosphorylation promotes binding of the tyrosine phosphatase SHP-2, leading to downstream Erk1/2 phosphorylation/activation.[155,158] In cultured cells, LR activation also triggers phosphoinositide 3-kinase (PI3K)-Akt signaling,[86,89,93,94] although it is unclear whether Akt phosphorylation occurs in vivo.[98,159–161] Both Erk1/2 (via p90RSK) and Akt phosphorylation can lead to downstream GSK3 phsophorylation/inhibition.[86] Signaling molecules that are known to affect APP processing are highlighted in blue italics.

treatment with supraphysiologic doses reduces Aβ levels in brain and serum of APP Tg mice.[45,102] The reduction of Aβ appears to reduce β-secretase expression and/or activity, and the reduction can be blocked by an inhibitor of the AMPK in cultured cells.[45,100,101] Leptin also reduces tau phosphorylation in cultured neuronal cells and organotypic cultures, and this effect was blocked by AMPK and glycogen synthase kinase-3 (GSK3) inhibitors.[100,101,103,104] Several issues remain with regards to the mechanisms whereby leptin may modulate AD pathology. Although activating leptin pathways may influence Aβ or tau pathways, it remains unclear whether altered leptin signaling is physiologically relevant in terms of AD pathogenesis. Toward that end, crossing APP transgenic mice onto a leptin-deficient *ob/ob* background results in worsening of cognitive function, enhancement of cerebrovascular inflammation, and increased cerebral amyloid angiopathy.[105] A fundamental issue with understanding the mechanisms of leptin action *in vivo* is the vast number of metabolic and physiologic parameters that are regulated by leptin. Thus *ob/ob* mice represent an extreme phenotype compared to diet-induced obesity models. Another question that deserves attention reflects the inherent complexity of CNS circuitry, and thus it is unknown whether leptin acts directly on cortical or hippocampal neurons to inhibit amyloid plaque deposition as opposed to an indirect effect via hypothalamic relay neurons. Finally, most cultured cell lines do not express the long LRb isoform of the leptin receptor, and thus it is important to determine whether leptin's effects are mediated through LRb and the known downstream LRb signaling pathways. For example, although it is proposed that leptin modulates Aβ and tau through AMPK, it is unclear how leptin activates AMPK. In skeletal muscle, much of AMPK activation *in vivo* is through autonomic innervation and not a direct effect of leptin binding to LRb.[64] Leptin actually decreases AMPK activity in the hypothalamus and knockout of AMPK in POMC and AgRP expressing hypothalamic neurons has no effect on their leptin responsivity.[63,106]

Many of the other receptor-signaling molecules downstream of LRb are known to affect secretase activity or APP trafficking (Fig. 3, highlighted in blue). First, STAT3 increases BACE expression by binding to its promoter and is also thought to mediate Aβ toxicity.[107–110] Second, Erk1/2 activation increases α-secretase activity, and may inhibit β- and γ-secretase activity.[111–120] PI3K activation increases APP trafficking and the secretion of APP metabolites,[121–124] and constitutively active Akt inhibits APP trafficking by feedback inhibition of PI3K.[125] Finally, inhibition of GSK3 results in an inhibition of γ-secretase.[126,127] Therefore, leptin signaling can potentially intersect with APP processing pathways at multiple levels, and it remains to be determined which pathway mediates leptin's antiamyloidogenic effects *in vivo*.

One additional consideration is the relationship between obesity, aging, and leptin. Circulating leptin levels are high in obese humans and rodents in correlation with adiposity.[60] Aging also results in increased leptin levels and adiposity.[128–130] The maintenance of increased fat despite hyperleptinemia indicates that obesity and aging are both states of leptin resistance. The exact mechanisms of leptin resistance are not completely understood but are in part due to defective leptin transport across the blood–brain barrier and in part are intrinsic to leptin-responsive neurons.[129–140] Intrinsic neuronal leptin resistance has been linked to increased feedback inhibition by SOCS3 and increased protein tyrosine phosphatase 1B (PTP1B) activity, both of which dampen downstream LR signaling pathways.[141–151] This interrelationship between peripheral leptin, central leptin resistance, obesity, and aging should be considered in future clinical and experimental studies on leptin and AD.

Conclusions

Advances in the fields of endocrinology and neuropathology are beginning to reveal a complex relationship between peripheral metabolic factors and brain health. Although obesity increases the risk for AD in humans and diet-induced obesity modulates AD pathology in transgenic mice, the mechanisms that account for these phenomena are not entirely known. In terms of leptin, increased peripheral leptin is associated with reduced incidence of AD in the nonobese elderly, and treating AD transgenic mice with leptin ameliorates AD pathology. It remains to be determined whether central leptin resistance associated with aging and obesity enhances amyloid plaque deposition. Also, the effects of other adipokines, in particular the inflammatory adipokines (e.g., adiponectin, cytokines, and complement), have received little attention with regards to their contribution to AD. Adiponectin is thought to be complementary to the actions of leptin and exhibits anti-inflammatory properties. However, only two small studies have been reported with conflicting results as to whether changes in plasma adiponectin are related to MCI or AD.[152,153] Thus, further studies of the relationship between adipokines and AD are warranted. Finally, despite the emphasis on leptin in this review, several genes associated with lipid homeostasis are thought to influence AD risk including genes encoding apolipoprotein E, apolipoprotein J (clusterin), and sortilin-related receptor.[154] Undoubtedly, multiple metabolic and hormonal changes associated with obesity and aging will prove to influence the brain in health and disease. Together, this burgeoning field is proving that the brain is under the influence of peripheral metabolism and that an integrated physiologic approach to understanding brain health and disease may reveal novel mechanisms that may be amenable to therapeutic intervention.

Acknowledgments

EBL is supported by NIH/NIA K08-AG039510.

Conflicts of interest

The author declares no conflicts of interest.

References

1. Craft, S. 2009. The role of metabolic disorders in Alzheimer disease and vascular dementia: two roads converged. *Arch. Neurol.* **66:** 300–305.
2. Luchsinger, J.A. & R. Mayeux. 2007. Adiposity and Alzheimer's disease. *Curr. Alzheimer Res.* **4:** 127–134.
3. Whitmer, R.A. 2007. The epidemiology of adiposity and dementia. *Curr. Alzheimer Res.* **4:** 117–122.
4. Luchsinger, J.A. & D.R. Gustafson. 2009. Adiposity, type 2 diabetes, and Alzheimer's disease. *J. Alzheimers Dis.* **16:** 693–704.
5. Jack, C.R., Jr., M.S. Albert, D.S. Knopman, *et al.* 2011. Introduction to the recommendations from the National Institute on Aging-Alzheimer's Association workgroups on diagnostic guidelines for Alzheimer's disease. *Alzheimers Dement.* **7:** 257–262.
6. McKhann, G.M., D.S. Knopman, H. Chertkow, *et al.* 2011. The diagnosis of dementia due to Alzheimer's disease: recommendations from the National Institute on Aging-Alzheimer's Association workgroups on diagnostic guidelines for Alzheimer's disease. *Alzheimers Dement.* **7:** 263–269.
7. Albert, M.S., S.T. DeKosky, D. Dickson, *et al.* 2011. The diagnosis of mild cognitive impairment due to Alzheimer's disease: recommendations from the National Institute on Aging-Alzheimer's Association workgroups on diagnostic guidelines for Alzheimer's disease. *Alzheimers Dement.* **7:** 270–279.
8. Sperling, R.A., P.S. Aisen, L.A. Beckett, *et al.* 2011. Toward defining the preclinical stages of Alzheimer's disease: recommendations from the National Institute on Aging-Alzheimer's Association workgroups on diagnostic guidelines for Alzheimer's disease. *Alzheimers Dement.* **7:** 280–292.
9. Lee, E.B. & V.M. Lee. 2007. Biology and molecular neuropathology of beta-amyloid protein. In pages 81–110 of *Neurobiology of Alzheimer's Disease*, 3rd Ed., D. Dawbarn & S.J. Allen, Eds. Oxford. Oxford University Press.
10. Lee, V.M., M. Goedert & J.Q. Trojanowski. 2001. Neurodegenerative tauopathies. *Annu. Rev. Neurosci.* **24:** 1121–1159.
11. Jack, C.R., Jr., D.S. Knopman, W.J. Jagust, *et al.* 2010. Hypothetical model of dynamic biomarkers of the Alzheimer's pathological cascade. *Lancet Neurol.* **9:** 119–128.
12. Hetzel, L. & A. Smith 2001. *The 65 Years and Over Population: 2000.* Census Bureau Brief, C2KBR/01-10, Washington, DC: U.S. Census Bureau.
13. Meyer, J. 2001. *Age: 2000.* Census Bureau Brief C2KBR/01-12, Washington, DC: U.S. Census Bureau.

14. Federal Interagency Forum on Aging-Related Statistics. 2008. *Older Americans 2008: key indicators of well-being.* Washington, DC: U.S. Government Printing Office.

15. The Lewin Group. 2006. Saving lives, saving money: Dividends for Americans investing in Alzheimer research. *Alzheimer's Association Report 2006.*

16. Brookmeyer, R., S. Gray & C. Kawas. 1998. Projections of Alzheimer's disease in the United States and the public health impact of delaying disease onset. *Am. J. Public Health* **88:** 1337–1342.

17. Cogan, J. & O. Mitchell. 2003. Perspectives from the President's Commission on Social Security Reform. *J. Econom. Perspect.* **7:** 149–172.

18. Hebert, L.E., P.A. Scherr, J.L. Bienias, *et al.* 2003. Alzheimer disease in the US population: prevalence estimates using the 2000 census. *Arch. Neurol.* **60:** 1119–1122.

19. Ogden C.L., M.D. Carroll, M.A. McDowell & K.M. Flegal. 2007. Obesity among adults in the United States—no statistically significant change since 2003–2004. NCHS Data Brief No 1. Hyattsville, MD: National Center for Health Statistics.

20. Gillette Guyonnet, S., G. Abellan Van Kan, E. Alix, *et al.* 2007. IANA (International Academy on Nutrition and Aging) Expert group: weight loss and Alzheimer's disease. *J. Nutr. Health Aging* **11:** 38–48.

21. Stewart, R., K. Masaki, Q.L. Xue, *et al.* 2005. A 32-year prospective study of change in body weight and incident dementia: the Honolulu–Asia aging study. *Arch. Neurol.* **62:** 55–60.

22. Barrett-Connor, E., S. Edelstein, *et al.* 1998. Weight loss precedes dementia in community-dwelling older adults. *J. Nutr. Health Aging* **2:** 113–114.

23. Ewers, M., S. Schmitz, O. Hansson, *et al.* 2011. Body mass index is associated with biological CSF markers of core brain pathology of Alzheimer's disease. *Neurobiol. Aging.* [Epub ahead of print]. doi:10.1016/j.neurbiolaging.2011.05.005.

24. Buchman, A.S., J.A. Schneider, R.S. Wilson, *et al.* 2006. Body mass index in older persons is associated with Alzheimer disease pathology. *Neurology* **67:** 1949–1954.

25. Burns, J.M., D.K. Johnson, A. Watts, *et al.* 2010. Reduced lean mass in early Alzheimer disease and its association with brain atrophy. *Arch Neurol.* **67:** 428–433.

26. Gustafson, D., E. Rothenberg, K. Blennow, *et al.* 2003. An 18-year follow-up of overweight and risk of Alzheimer disease. *Arch. Intern. Med.* **163:** 1524–1528.

27. Gustafson, D.R., K. Backman, M. Waern, *et al.* 2009. Adiposity indicators and dementia over 32 years in Sweden. *Neurology* **73:** 1559–1566.

28. Buchman, A.S., R.S. Wilson, J.L. Bienias, *et al.* 2005. Change in body mass index and risk of incident Alzheimer disease. *Neurology* **65:** 892–897.

29. Hayden, K.M., P.P. Zandi, C.G. Lyketsos, *et al.* 2006. Vascular risk factors for incident Alzheimer disease and vascular dementia: the Cache County study. *Alzheimer Dis. Assoc. Disord.* **20:** 93–100.

30. Fitzpatrick, A.L., L.H. Kuller, O.L. Lopez, *et al.* 2009. Midlife and late-life obesity and the risk of dementia: cardiovascular health study. *Arch. Neurol.* **66:** 336–342.

31. Luchsinger, J.A., D. Cheng, M.X. Tang, *et al.* 2011. Central obesity in the elderly is related to late-onset Alzheimer disease. *Alzheimer Dis. Assoc. Disord.* doi:10.1097/WAD.0b013e318222f0d4.

32. Vanhanen, M., K. Koivisto, L. Moilanen, *et al.* 2006. Association of metabolic syndrome with Alzheimer disease: a population-based study. *Neurology* **67:** 843–847.

33. Whitmer, R.A., E.P. Gunderson, E. Barrett-Connor, *et al.* 2005. Obesity in middle age and future risk of dementia: a 27 year longitudinal population based study. *BMJ* **330:** 1360–1362.

34. Whitmer, R.A., E.P. Gunderson, C.P. Quesenberry, Jr., *et al.* 2007. Body mass index in midlife and risk of Alzheimer disease and vascular dementia. *Curr. Alzheimer Res.* **4:** 103–109.

35. Whitmer, R.A., D.R. Gustafson, E. Barrett-Connor, *et al.* 2008. Central obesity and increased risk of dementia more than three decades later. *Neurology* **71:** 1057–1064.

36. Kivipelto, M., T. Ngandu, L. Fratiglioni, *et al.* 2005. Obesity and vascular risk factors at midlife and the risk of dementia and Alzheimer disease. *Arch. Neurol.* **62:** 1556–1560.

37. Chiang, C.J., P.K. Yip, S.C. Wu, *et al.* 2007. Midlife risk factors for subtypes of dementia: a nested case-control study in Taiwan. *Am. J. Geriatr. Psychiatr.* **15:** 762–771.

38. Nelson, P.T., C.D. Smith, E.A. Abner, *et al.* 2009. Human cerebral neuropathology of Type 2 diabetes mellitus. *Biochim. Biophys. Acta* **1792:** 454–469.

39. Sonnen, J.A., E.B. Larson, K. Brickell, *et al.* 2009. Different patterns of cerebral injury in dementia with or without diabetes. *Arch. Neurol.* **66:** 315–322.

40. Duff, K. & F. Suleman. 2004. Transgenic mouse models of Alzheimer's disease: how useful have they been for therapeutic development? *Brief Funct. Genomic Proteomic.* **3:** 47–59.

41. Hsiao, K., P. Chapman, S. Nilsen, *et al.* 1996. Correlative memory deficits, Abeta elevation, and amyloid plaques in transgenic mice. *Science* **274:** 99–102.

42. Games, D., D. Adams, R. Alessandrini, *et al.* 1995. Alzheimer-type neuropathology in transgenic mice overexpressing V717F beta-amyloid precursor protein. *Nature* **373:** 523–527.

43. Ishihara, T., M. Hong, B. Zhang, *et al.* 1999. Age-dependent emergence and progression of a tauopathy in transgenic mice overexpressing the shortest human tau isoform. *Neuron* **24:** 751–762.

44. Cao, D., H. Lu, T.L. Lewis & L. Li. 2007. Intake of sucrose-sweetened water induces insulin resistance and exacerbates memory deficits and amyloidosis in a transgenic mouse model of Alzheimer disease. *J. Biol. Chem.* **282:** 36275–36282.

45. Fewlass, D.C., K. Noboa, F.X. Pi-Sunyer, *et al.* 2004. Obesity-related leptin regulates Alzheimer's Abeta. *FASEB J.* **18:** 1870–1878.

46. Ho, L., W. Qin, P.N. Pompl, *et al.* 2004. Diet-induced insulin resistance promotes amyloidosis in a transgenic mouse model of Alzheimer's disease. *FASEB J.* **18:** 902–904.

47. Julien, C., C. Tremblay, A. Phivilay, *et al.* 2010. High-fat diet aggravates amyloid-beta and tau pathologies in the 3xTg-AD mouse model. *Neurobiol. Aging* **31:** 1516–1531.

48. Levin-Allerhand, J.A., C.E. Lominska & J.D. Smith. 2002. Increased amyloid- levels in APPSWE transgenic mice

treated chronically with a physiological high-fat high-cholesterol diet. *J. Nutr. Health Aging* **6:** 315–319.

49. Pedrini, S., C. Thomas, H. Brautigam, *et al.* 2009. Dietary composition modulates brain mass and solubilizable Abeta levels in a mouse model of aggressive Alzheimer's amyloid pathology. *Mol. Neurodegener.* **4:** 40.

50. Zhao, Z., L. Ho, J. Wang, *et al.* 2005. Connective tissue growth factor (CTGF) expression in the brain is a downstream effector of insulin resistance- associated promotion of Alzheimer's disease beta-amyloid neuropathology. *FASEB J.* **19:** 2081–2082.

51. Studzinski, C.M., F. Li, A.J. Bruce-Keller, *et al.* 2009. Effects of short-term Western diet on cerebral oxidative stress and diabetes related factors in APP x PS1 knock-in mice. *J. Neurochem.* **108:** 860–866.

52. Halagappa, V.K., Z. Guo, M. Pearson, *et al.* 2007. Intermittent fasting and caloric restriction ameliorate age-related behavioral deficits in the triple-transgenic mouse model of Alzheimer's disease. *Neurobiol. Dis.* **26:** 212–220.

53. Mouton, P.R., M.E. Chachich, C. Quigley, *et al.* 2009. Caloric restriction attenuates amyloid deposition in middle-aged dtg APP/PS1 mice. *Neurosci. Lett.* **464:** 184–187.

54. Patel, N.V., M.N. Gordon, K.E. Connor, *et al.* 2005. Caloric restriction attenuates Abeta-deposition in Alzheimer transgenic models. *Neurobiol. Aging* **26:** 995–1000.

55. Van der Auwera, I., S. Wera, *et al.* 2005. A ketogenic diet reduces amyloid beta 40 and 42 in a mouse model of Alzheimer's disease. *Nutr. Metab.* **2:** 28.

56. Wang, J., L. Ho, W. Qin, *et al.* 2005. Caloric restriction attenuates beta-amyloid neuropathology in a mouse model of Alzheimer's disease. *FASEB J.* **19:** 659–661.

57. Lieb, W., A.S. Beiser, R.S. Vasan, *et al.* 2009. Association of plasma leptin levels with incident Alzheimer disease and MRI measures of brain aging. *JAMA* **302:** 2565–2572.

58. Ahima, R.S. & J.S. Flier. 2000. Leptin. *Annu. Rev. Physiol.* **62:** 413–437.

59. Ahima, R.S. & S.Y. Osei. 2004. Leptin signaling. *Physiol. Behav.* **81:** 223–241.

60. Myers, M.G., M.A. Cowley & H. Munzberg. 2008. Mechanisms of leptin action and leptin resistance. *Annu. Rev. Physiol.* **70:** 537–556.

61. Ahima, R.S., D. Prabakaran, C. Mantzoros, *et al.* 1996. Role of leptin in the neuroendocrine response to fasting. *Nature* **382:** 250–252.

62. Andersson, U., K. Filipsson, C.R. Abbott, *et al.* 2004. AMP-activated protein kinase plays a role in the control of food intake. *J. Biol. Chem.* **279:** 12005–12008.

63. Minokoshi, Y., T. Alquier, N. Furukawa, *et al.* 2004. AMP-kinase regulates food intake by responding to hormonal and nutrient signals in the hypothalamus. *Nature* **428:** 569–574.

64. Minokoshi, Y., Y.B. Kim, O.D. Peroni, *et al.* 2002. Leptin stimulates fatty-acid oxidation by activating AMP-activated protein kinase. *Nature* **415:** 339–343.

65. Villanueva, E.C., H. Munzberg, D. Cota, *et al.* 2009. Complex regulation of mammalian target of rapamycin complex 1 in the basomedial hypothalamus by leptin and nutritional status. *Endocrinology* **150:** 4541–4551.

66. Baskin, D.G., M.W. Schwartz, R.J. Seeley, *et al.* 1999. Leptin receptor long-form splice-variant protein expression in neuron cell bodies of the brain and co-localization with neuropeptide Y mRNA in the arcuate nucleus. *J. Histochem. Cytochem.* **47:** 353–362.

67. Burguera, B., M.E. Couce, J. Long, *et al.* 2000. The long form of the leptin receptor (OB-Rb) is widely expressed in the human brain. *Neuroendocrinology* **71:** 187–195.

68. Elmquist, J.K., C. Bjorbaek, R.S. Ahima, *et al.* 1998. Distributions of leptin receptor mRNA isoforms in the rat brain. *J. Comp. Neurol.* **395:** 535–547.

69. Guan, X.M., J.F. Hess, H. Yu, *et al.* 1997. Differential expression of mRNA for leptin receptor isoforms in the rat brain. *Mol. Cell. Endocrinol.* **133:** 1–7.

70. Hakansson, M.L., A.L. Hulting & B. Meister. 1996. Expression of leptin receptor mRNA in the hypothalamic arcuate nucleus—relationship with NPY neurones. *Neuroreport* **7:** 3087–3092.

71. Huang, X.F., I. Koutcherov, S. Lin, *et al.* 1996. Localization of leptin receptor mRNA expression in mouse brain. *Neuroreport* **7:** 2635–2638.

72. Mercer, J.G., K.M. Moar & N. Hoggard. 1998. Localization of leptin receptor (Ob-R) messenger ribonucleic acid in the rodent hindbrain. *Endocrinology* **139:** 29–34.

73. Savioz, A., Y. Charnay, C. Huguenin, *et al.* 1997. Expression of leptin receptor mRNA (long form splice variant) in the human cerebellum. *Neuroreport* **8:** 3123–3126.

74. Scott, M.M., J.L. Lachey, S.M. Sternson, *et al.* 2009. Leptin targets in the mouse brain. *J. Comp. Neurol.* **514:** 518–532.

75. Ahima, R.S. & S.M. Hileman. 2000. Postnatal regulation of hypothalamic neuropeptide expression by leptin: implications for energy balance and body weight regulation. *Regul. Pept.* **92:** 1–7.

76. Ahima, R.S., D. Prabakaran & J.S. Flier. 1998. Postnatal leptin surge and regulation of circadian rhythm of leptin by feeding. Implications for energy homeostasis and neuroendocrine function. *J. Clin. Invest.* **101:** 1020–1027.

77. Ahima, R.S., C. Bjorbaek, S. Osei & J.S. Flier. 1999. Regulation of neuronal and glial proteins by leptin: implications for brain development. *Endocrinology* **140:** 2755–2762.

78. Narita, K., H. Kosaka, H. Okazawa, *et al.* 2009. Relationship between plasma leptin level and brain structure in elderly: a voxel-based morphometric study. *Biol. Psychiatr.* **65:** 992–994.

79. Holden, K.F., K. Lindquist, F.A. Tylavsky, *et al.* 2009. Serum leptin level and cognition in the elderly: findings from the Health ABC Study. *Neurobiol. Aging* **30:** 1483–1489.

80. Matochik, J.A., E.D. London, B.O. Yildiz, *et al.* 2005. Effect of leptin replacement on brain structure in genetically leptin-deficient adults. *J. Clin. Endocrinol. Metab.* **90:** 2851–2854.

81. Paz-Filho, G.J., T. Babikian, R. Asarnow, *et al.* 2008. Leptin replacement improves cognitive development. *PLoS One* **3:** e3098.

82. Baicy, K., E.D. London, J. Monterosso, *et al.* 2007. Leptin replacement alters brain response to food cues in genetically leptin-deficient adults. *Proc. Natl. Acad. Sci. USA* **104:** 18276–18279.

83. Farooqi, I.S., E. Bullmore, J. Keogh, *et al.* 2007. Leptin regulates striatal regions and human eating behavior. *Science* **317:** 1355.

84. Rosenbaum, M., M. Sy, K. Pavlovich, *et al.* 2008. Leptin reverses weight loss-induced changes in regional neural activity responses to visual food stimuli. *J. Clin. Invest.* **118:** 2583–2591.

85. O'Malley, D., N. MacDonald, S. Mizielinska, *et al.* 2007. Leptin promotes rapid dynamic changes in hippocampal dendritic morphology. *Mol. Cell. Neurosci.* **35:** 559–572.

86. Valerio, A., V. Ghisi, M. Dossena, *et al.* 2006. Leptin increases axonal growth cone size in developing mouse cortical neurons by convergent signals inactivating glycogen synthase kinase-3beta. *J. Biol. Chem.* **281:** 12950–12958.

87. Bouret, S.G., S.J. Draper & R.B. Simerly. 2004. Trophic action of leptin on hypothalamic neurons that regulate feeding. *Science* **304:** 108–110.

88. Bouret, S.G., J.N. Gorski, C.M. Patterson, *et al.* 2008. Hypothalamic neural projections are permanently disrupted in diet-induced obese rats. *Cell Metab.* **7:** 179–185.

89. Garza, J.C., M. Guo, W. Zhang & X.Y. Lu. 2008. Leptin increases adult hippocampal neurogenesis in vivo and in vitro. *J. Biol. Chem.* **283:** 18238–18247.

90. Shanley, L.J., A.J. Irving & J. Harvey. 2001. Leptin enhances NMDA receptor function and modulates hippocampal synaptic plasticity. *J. Neurosci.* **21:** RC186.

91. Stranahan, A.M., T.V. Arumugam, R.G. Cutler, *et al.* 2008. Diabetes impairs hippocampal function through glucocorticoid-mediated effects on new and mature neurons. *Nat. Neurosci.* **11:** 309–317.

92. Stranahan, A.M., K. Lee, B. Martin, *et al.* 2009. Voluntary exercise and caloric restriction enhance hippocampal dendritic spine density and BDNF levels in diabetic mice. *Hippocampus* **19:** 951–961.

93. Doherty, G.H., C. Oldreive & J. Harvey. 2008. Neuroprotective actions of leptin on central and peripheral neurons in vitro. *Neuroscience* **154:** 1297–1307.

94. Guo, Z., H. Jiang, X. Xu, *et al.* 2008. Leptin-mediated cell survival signaling in hippocampal neurons mediated by JAK STAT3 and mitochondrial stabilization. *J. Biol. Chem.* **283:** 1754–1763.

95. Shanley, L.J., D. O'Malley, A.J. Irving, *et al.* 2002. Leptin inhibits epileptiform-like activity in rat hippocampal neurones via PI 3-kinase-driven activation of BK channels. *J. Physiol.* **545:** 933–944.

96. Valerio, A., M. Dossena, P. Bertolotti, *et al.* 2009. Leptin is induced in the ischemic cerebral cortex and exerts neuroprotection through NF-kappaB/c-Rel-dependent transcription. *Stroke* **40:** 610–617.

97. Weng, Z., A.P. Signore, Y. Gao, *et al.* 2007. Leptin protects against 6-hydroxydopamine-induced dopaminergic cell death via mitogen-activated protein kinase signaling. *J. Biol. Chem.* **282:** 34479–34491.

98. Zhang, F. & J. Chen. 2008. Leptin protects hippocampal CA1 neurons against ischemic injury. *J. Neurochem.* **107:** 578–587.

99. Zhang, F., S. Wang, A.P. Signore & J. Chen. 2007. Neuroprotective effects of leptin against ischemic injury induced by oxygen-glucose deprivation and transient cerebral ischemia. *Stroke* **38:** 2329–2336.

100. Greco, S.J., S. Sarkar, J.M. Johnston & N. Tezapsidis. 2009. Leptin regulates tau phosphorylation and amyloid through AMPK in neuronal cells. *Biochem. Biophys. Res. Commun.* **380:** 98–104.

101. Marwarha, G., B. Dasari, J.R. Prasanthi, *et al.* 2010. Leptin reduces the accumulation of Abeta and phosphorylated tau induced by 27-hydroxycholesterol in rabbit organotypic slices. *J. Alzheimers Dis.* **19:** 1007–1019.

102. Greco, S.J., K.J. Bryan, S. Sarkar, *et al.* 2010. Leptin reduces pathology and improves memory in a transgenic mouse model of Alzheimer's disease. *J. Alzheimers Dis.* **19:** 1155–1167.

103. Greco, S.J., S. Sarkar, G. Casadesus, *et al.* 2009. Leptin inhibits glycogen synthase kinase-3beta to prevent tau phosphorylation in neuronal cells. *Neurosci. Lett.* **455:** 191–194.

104. Greco, S.J., S. Sarkar, J.M. Johnston, *et al.* 2008. Leptin reduces Alzheimer's disease-related tau phosphorylation in neuronal cells. *Biochem. Biophys. Res. Commun.* **376:** 536–541.

105. Takeda, S., N. Sato, K. Uchio-Yamada, *et al.* 2010. Diabetes-accelerated memory dysfunction via cerebrovascular inflammation and Abeta deposition in an Alzheimer mouse model with diabetes. *Proc. Natl. Acad. Sci. USA* **107:** 7036–7041.

106. Claret, M., M.A. Smith, R.L. Batterham, *et al.* 2007. AMPK is essential for energy homeostasis regulation and glucose sensing by POMC and AgRP neurons. *J. Clin. Invest.* **117:** 2325–2336.

107. Wan, J., A.K. Fu, F.C. Ip, *et al.* 2010. Tyk2/STAT3 signaling mediates beta-amyloid-induced neuronal cell death: implications in Alzheimer's disease. *J. Neurosci.* **30:** 6873–6881.

108. Sambamurti, K., R. Kinsey, B. Maloney, *et al.* 2004. Gene structure and organization of the human beta-secretase (BACE) promoter. *FASEB J.* **18:** 1034–1036.

109. Tamagno, E., M. Parola, P. Bardini, *et al.* 2005. Beta-site APP cleaving enzyme up-regulation induced by 4-hydroxynonenal is mediated by stress-activated protein kinases pathways. *J. Neurochem.* **92:** 628–636.

110. Wen, Y., W.H. Yu, B. Maloney, *et al.* 2008. Transcriptional regulation of beta-secretase by p25/cdk5 leads to enhanced amyloidogenic processing. *Neuron* **57:** 680–690.

111. Mills, J., D. Laurent Charest, F. Lam, *et al.* 1997. Regulation of amyloid precursor protein catabolism involves the mitogen-activated protein kinase signal transduction pathway. *J. Neurosci.* **17:** 9415–9422.

112. Avramovich, Y., T. Amit & M.B. Youdim. 2002. Non-steroidal anti-inflammatory drugs stimulate secretion of non-amyloidogenic precursor protein. *J. Biol. Chem.* **277:** 31466–31473.

113. Liu, F., Y. Su, B. Li & B. Ni. 2003. Regulation of amyloid precursor protein expression and secretion via activation of ERK1/2 by hepatocyte growth factor in HEK293 cells transfected with APP751. *Exp. Cell Res.* **287:** 387–396.

114. Manthey, D., S. Heck, S. Engert & C. Behl. 2001. Estrogen induces a rapid secretion of amyloid beta precursor protein via the mitogen-activated protein kinase pathway. *Eur. J. Biochem.* **268:** 4285–4291.

115. Canet-Aviles, R.M., M. Anderton, N.M. Hooper, *et al.* 2002. Muscarine enhances soluble amyloid precursor protein secretion in human neuroblastoma SH-SY5Y by a pathway dependent on protein kinase C(alpha), src-tyrosine kinase and extracellular signal-regulated kinase but not phospholipase C. *Brain Res. Mol. Brain Res.* **102:** 62–72.

116. Tamagno, E., M. Guglielmotto, L. Giliberto, *et al.* 2009. JNK and ERK1/2 pathways have a dual opposite effect on the expression of BACE1. *Neurobiol. Aging* **30:** 1563–1573.

117. Kim, S.K., H.J. Park, H.S. Hong, *et al.* 2006. ERK1/2 is an endogenous negative regulator of the gamma-secretase activity. *FASEB J.* **20:** 157–159.

118. Kojro, E., R. Postina, C. Buro, *et al.* 2006. The neuropeptide PACAP promotes the alpha-secretase pathway for processing the Alzheimer amyloid precursor protein. *FASEB J.* **20:** 512–514.

119. Bandyopadhyay, S., D.M. Hartley, C.M. Cahill, *et al.* 2006. Interleukin-1alpha stimulates non-amyloidogenic pathway by alpha-secretase (ADAM-10 and ADAM-17) cleavage of APP in human astrocytic cells involving p38 MAP kinase. *J. Neurosci. Res.* **84:** 106–118.

120. Zhu, X., H.G. Lee, A.K. Raina, *et al.* 2002. The role of mitogen-activated protein kinase pathways in Alzheimer's disease. *Neurosignals* **11:** 270–281.

121. Adlerz, L., S. Holback, G. Multhaup & K. Iverfeldt. 2007. IGF-1-induced processing of the amyloid precursor protein family is mediated by different signaling pathways. *J. Biol. Chem.* **282:** 10203–10209.

122. Gasparini, L., G.K. Gouras, R. Wang, *et al.* 2001. Stimulation of beta-amyloid precursor protein trafficking by insulin reduces intraneuronal beta-amyloid and requires mitogen-activated protein kinase signaling. *J. Neurosci.* **21:** 2561–2570.

123. Petanceska, S.S. & S. Gandy. 1999. The phosphatidylinositol 3-kinase inhibitor wortmannin alters the metabolism of the Alzheimer's amyloid precursor protein. *J. Neurochem.* **73:** 2316–2320.

124. Solano, D.C., M. Sironi, C. Bonfini, *et al.* 2000. Insulin regulates soluble amyloid precursor protein release via phosphatidyl inositol 3 kinase-dependent pathway. *FASEB J.* **14:** 1015–1022.

125. Shineman, D.W., A.S. Dain, M.L. Kim & V.M. Lee. 2009. Constitutively active Akt inhibits trafficking of amyloid precursor protein and amyloid precursor protein metabolites through feedback inhibition of phosphoinositide 3-kinase. *Biochemistry* **48:** 3787–3794.

126. Phiel, C.J., C.A. Wilson, V.M. Lee & P.S. Klein. 2003. GSK-3alpha regulates production of Alzheimer's disease amyloid-beta peptides. *Nature* **423:** 435–439.

127. Su, Y., J. Ryder, B. Li, *et al.* 2004. Lithium, a common drug for bipolar disorder treatment, regulates amyloid-beta precursor protein processing. *Biochemistry* **43:** 6899–6908.

128. Ahren, B., S. Mansson, R.L. Gingerich & P.J. Havel. 1997. Regulation of plasma leptin in mice: influence of age, high-fat diet, and fasting. *Am. J. Physiol.* **273:** R113–120.

129. Li, H., M. Matheny, M. Nicolson, *et al.* 1997. Leptin gene expression increases with age independent of increasing adiposity in rats. *Diabetes* **46:** 2035–2039.

130. Scarpace, P.J., M. Matheny, R.L. Moore & N. Tumer. 2000.

Impaired leptin responsiveness in aged rats. *Diabetes* **49:** 431–435.

131. Carrascosa, J.M., M. Ros, A. Andres, *et al.* 2009. Changes in the neuroendocrine control of energy homeostasis by adiposity signals during aging. *Exp. Gerontol.* **44:** 20–25.

132. Gabriely, I., X.H. Ma, X.M. Yang, *et al.* 2002. Leptin resistance during aging is independent of fat mass. *Diabetes* **51:** 1016–1021.

133. Ma, X.H., R. Muzumdar, X.M. Yang, *et al.* 2002. Aging is associated with resistance to effects of leptin on fat distribution and insulin action. *J. Gerontol. A Biol. Sci. Med. Sci.* **57:** B225–231.

134. Muzumdar, R.H., X. Ma, X. Yang, *et al.* 2006. Central resistance to the inhibitory effects of leptin on stimulated insulin secretion with aging. *Neurobiol. Aging* **27:** 1308–1314.

135. Qian, H., M.J. Azain, D.L. Hartzell & C.A. Baile. 1998. Increased leptin resistance as rats grow to maturity. *Proc. Soc. Exp. Biol. Med.* **219:** 160–165.

136. Scarpace, P.J., M. Matheny & N. Tumer. 2001. Hypothalamic leptin resistance is associated with impaired leptin signal transduction in aged obese rats. *Neuroscience* **104:** 1111–1117.

137. Shek, E.W. & P.J. Scarpace. 2000. Resistance to the anorexic and thermogenic effects of centrally administered leptin in obese aged rats. *Regul. Pept.* **92:** 65–71.

138. Zhang, Y., M. Matheny, N. Tumer & P.J. Scarpace. 2004. Aged-obese rats exhibit robust responses to a melanocortin agonist and antagonist despite leptin resistance. *Neurobiol. Aging* **25:** 1349–1360.

139. El-Haschimi, K., D.D. Pierroz, S.M. Hileman, *et al.* 2000. Two defects contribute to hypothalamic leptin resistance in mice with diet-induced obesity. *J. Clin. Invest.* **105:** 1827–1832.

140. Fernandez-Galaz, C., T. Fernandez-Agullo, F. Campoy, *et al.* 2001. Decreased leptin uptake in hypothalamic nuclei with ageing in Wistar rats. *J. Endocrinol.* **171:** 23–32.

141. Bjorbak, C., H.J. Lavery, S.H. Bates, *et al.* 2000. SOCS3 mediates feedback inhibition of the leptin receptor via Tyr985. *J. Biol. Chem.* **275:** 40649–40657.

142. Dunn, S.L., M. Bjornholm, S.H. Bates, *et al.* 2005. Feedback inhibition of leptin receptor/Jak2 signaling via Tyr1138 of the leptin receptor and suppressor of cytokine signaling 3. *Mol. Endocrinol.* **19:** 925–938.

143. Bjorbaek, C., J.K. Elmquist, J.D. Frantz, *et al.* 1998. Identification of SOCS-3 as a potential mediator of central leptin resistance. *Mol. Cell.* **1:** 619–625.

144. Peralta, S., J.M. Carrascosa, N. Gallardo, *et al.* 2002. Ageing increases SOCS-3 expression in rat hypothalamus: effects of food restriction. *Biochem. Biophys. Res. Commun.* **296:** 425–428.

145. Wang, Z.W., W.T. Pan, Y. Lee, *et al.* 2001. The role of leptin resistance in the lipid abnormalities of aging. *FASEB J.* **15:** 108–114.

146. Bence, K.K., M. Delibegovic, B. Xue, *et al.* 2006. Neuronal PTP1B regulates body weight, adiposity and leptin action. *Nat. Med.* **12:** 917–924.

147. Cheng, A., N. Uetani, P.D. Simoncic, *et al.* 2002. Attenuation of leptin action and regulation of obesity by protein tyrosine phosphatase 1B. *Dev. Cell.* **2:** 497–503.

148. Morrison, C.D., C.L. White, Z. Wang, *et al.* 2007. Increased hypothalamic protein tyrosine phosphatase 1B contributes to leptin resistance with age. *Endocrinology* **148:** 433–440.

149. White, C.L., A. Whittington, M.J. Barnes, *et al.* 2009. HF diets increase hypothalamic PTP1B and induce leptin resistance through both leptin-dependent and -independent mechanisms. *Am. J. Physiol. Endocrinol. Metab.* **296:** E291–E299.

150. Zabolotny, J.M., K.K. Bence-Hanulec, A. Stricker-Krongrad, *et al.* 2002. PTP1B regulates leptin signal transduction in vivo. *Dev. Cell.* **2:** 489–495.

151. Zabolotny, J.M., Y.B. Kim, L.A. Welsh, *et al.* 2008. Protein-tyrosine phosphatase 1B expression is induced by inflammation in vivo. *J. Biol. Chem.* **283:** 14230–14241.

152. Une, K., Y.A. Takei, N. Tomita, *et al.* 2011. Adiponectin in plasma and cerebrospinal fluid in MCI and Alzheimer's disease. *Eur. J. Neurol.* **18:** 1006–1009.

153. Bigalke, B., B. Schreitmuller, K. Sopova, *et al.* 2011. Adipocytokines and CD34 progenitor cells in Alzheimer's disease. *PLoS One* **6:** e20286.

154. Bertram, L., C.M. Lill & R.E. Tanzi. 2010. The genetics of Alzheimer disease: back to the future. *Neuron* **68:** 270–281.

155. Banks, A.S., S.M. Davis, S.H. Bates & M.G. Myers, Jr. 2000. Activation of downstream signals by the long form of the leptin receptor. *J. Biol. Chem.* **275:** 14563–14572.

156. Kloek, C., A.K. Haq, S.L. Dunn, *et al.* 2002. Regulation of Jak kinases by intracellular leptin receptor sequences. *J. Biol. Chem.* **277:** 41547–41555.

157. Li, C. & J.M. Friedman. 1999. Leptin receptor activation of SH2 domain containing protein tyrosine phosphatase 2 modulates Ob receptor signal transduction. *Proc. Natl. Acad. Sci. USA* **96:** 9677–9682.

158. Bjorbaek, C., R.M. Buchholz, S.M. Davis, *et al.* 2001. Divergent roles of SHP-2 in ERK activation by leptin receptors. *J. Biol. Chem.* **276:** 4747–4755.

159. Carvalheira, J.B., M.A. Torsoni, M. Ueno, *et al.* 2005. Cross-talk between the insulin and leptin signaling systems in rat hypothalamus. *Obes. Res.* **13:** 48–57.

160. Morton, G.J., R.W. Gelling, K.D. Niswender, *et al.* 2005. Leptin regulates insulin sensitivity via phosphatidylinositol-3-OH kinase signaling in mediobasal hypothalamic neurons. *Cell Metab.* **2:** 411–420.

161. Zhao, A.Z., J.N. Huan, S. Gupta, *et al.* 2002. A phosphatidylinositol 3-kinase phosphodiesterase 3B-cyclic AMP pathway in hypothalamic action of leptin on feeding. *Nat. Neurosci.* **5:** 727–728.

Ann. N.Y. Acad. Sci. ISSN 0077-8923

ANNALS OF THE NEW YORK ACADEMY OF SCIENCES
Issue: *The Year in Diabetes and Obesity*

Interactions between metabolism and circadian clocks: reciprocal disturbances

Julien Delezie and Etienne Challet

Department of Neurobiology of Rhythms, Institute of Cellular and Integrative Neurosciences, Centre National de la Recherche Scientifique, UPR3212 associated with University of Strasbourg, Strasbourg, France

Address for correspondence: Etienne Challet, CNRS and University of Strasbourg, Institute of Cellular and Integrative Neurosciences, 5 rue Blaise Pascal, Strasbourg, FR 67000, France. challet@inci-cnrs.unistra.fr

Obesity is a medical condition of excess body fat, recognized as a global epidemic. Besides genetic factors, overconsumption of high-energy food and a sedentary lifestyle are major obesogenic causes. A newly identified determinant is altered circadian rhythmicity. To anticipate and adapt to daily changes in the environment, organisms have developed an endogenous circadian timing system, comprising a main circadian clock, located in the suprachiasmatic nucleus (SCN) of the hypothalamus, principally synchronized to the light–dark cycle. Secondary peripheral clocks are found in various tissues, such as the liver, pancreas, and adipose tissue. These clocks control the rhythmic patterns of myriad metabolic processes. We will review the evidence that metabolic dysfunction is associated with circadian disturbances at both central and peripheral levels and, conversely, that disruption of circadian clock functioning can lead to obesity. The roots of these reciprocal interactions will be illustrated by transcriptional crosstalk between metabolic and circadian systems. Chronotherapeutic approaches of dieting to maintain or restore a proper circadian alignment could be useful to limit the magnitude of metabolic risks.

Keywords: circadian rhythm; clock gene; metabolism; obesity; feeding

Introduction

Over recent decades, obesity has become a major health problem, while at the same time being one of the leading preventable causes of death in the world.[1] Obesity is a pathological condition defined as excessive fat accumulation and is associated with major complications, such as diabetes, hypertension, and cardiovascular diseases. Besides a few genetic factors, the main contributor to obesity is an overconsumption of food that is high in calories and saturated fat. In addition to high-fat, hypercaloric diets, sedentary lifestyles have supplanted regular physical activity, resulting in a positive energy balance (more energy intake, less energy expenditure) and obesity.[2]

Along with these factors, timing aspects of food intake and metabolic regulation have to be taken into consideration. In living organisms, most essential biological functions show a rhythmic pattern close to 24 hours. These endogenous daily variations, called circadian rhythms (from the latin: *circa* meaning about and *dies* meaning day), allow organisms to anticipate and prepare for periodic changes in the environment (e.g., light–dark cycle or food availability). The timing and duration of many physiological, metabolic, and behavioral processes are therefore dictated by a circadian timing system in coordination with the environment.

After a brief introduction of the circadian timing system, we will review the literature showing that the occurrence of obesity and/or diabetes is associated with circadian disturbances. Next, we will present laboratory studies demonstrating that direct circadian disruptions can have a broad impact on metabolism. We will also highlight the fact that irregular mealtimes and/or unusual lighting conditions are major contributors of circadian misalignment, perturbing both clock rhythmicity and metabolic homeostasis. By a reinforcing effect, circadian misalignment, resulting from inappropriate timing of food intake and/or exposure to

doi: 10.1111/j.1749-6632.2011.06246.x

Ann. N.Y. Acad. Sci. 1243 (2011) 30–46 © 2011 New York Academy of Sciences.

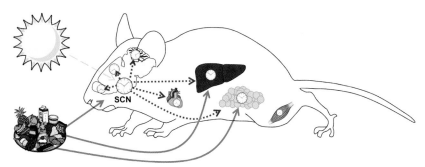

Figure 1. Organization of the circadian timing system. The master clock, located in the suprachiamatic nuclei (SCN) of the hypothalamus, adjusts the timing of many secondary clocks/oscillators in the brain and peripheral organs, in part via nervous pathways (dotted red lines). Light perceived by the retina is the most potent synchronizer of the SCN clock (dashed yellow arrow), while meal time can synchronize peripheral clocks (blue arrows).

unusual sleep/wake cycles, increases the likelihood of metabolic risk factors, and can even lead to metabolic disruptions. Finally, we will illustrate the transcriptional interactions between metabolism and the circadian system, and their importance in the development of overweight.

The circadian metabolism

The circadian timing system: an overview

In mammals, the circadian timing system is composed of several endogenous clocks, allowing biological functions to oscillate and be in phase with daily changes in the environment. The main circadian clock is located in the SCN of the anterior hypothalamus. The SCN is composed of multiple coupled cellular clocks that can generate circadian oscillations.[3] For a proper phase adjustment of the circadian timing system to the external environment, SCN neurons receive direct input from the retina in order to be synchronized (i.e., reset) to the 24-h light–dark cycle.[4] When light activates photoreceptors, in particular the intrinsically photosensitive retinal ganglion cells, nerve impulses are conducted directly through the retinohypothalamic tract to the SCN.[5] As a result, the synchronized SCN orchestrates the rhythmicity of many aspects of metabolism, physiology, and behavior via neuronal connections and humoral factors, with a 24-h period (Fig. 1).

The functioning of a circadian clock is dependent on a core clock mechanism involving specific genes called "clock genes." Among them period homolog 1–3 (*Per1, Per2, Per3*), cryptochrome 1,2 (*Cry1, Cry2*), circadian locomotor output cycles kaput (*Clock*) or its analog neuronal PAS do-

main protein 2 (*Npas2*), brain and muscle Arnt-like 1 (*Bmal1*), reverse viral erythroblastis oncogene products (*Rev-erba* and *Rev-erbb*), and retinoic acid-related orphan receptors (*Rora, Rorb, Rorg*) are essential.[6] Clock genes are coexpressed (in virtually all tissues) and their products reciprocally interact at the transcriptional/translational levels to generate circadian oscillations. At least three autoregulatory feedback loops are interconnected: one positive in which CLOCK and BMAL1 dimerize to activate the E-box-mediated transcription of *Per* and *Cry* genes; one negative whereby upon reaching a critical concentration, PER and CRY proteins enter into the nucleus to inhibit the transactivation mediated by CLOCK:BMAL1, therefore inhibiting their own transcription; and an interconnecting loop, in which *Rors* can activate the transcription of *Bmal1* and *Npas2*, whereas *Rev-erbs* can repress *Bmal1, Clock,* and *Npas2*, via retinoic acid-related orphan receptor response element (RORE) (Fig. 2).[7–10] This loop ensures the fine tuning of circadian rhythms. In addition, posttranslational mechanisms such as protein phosphorylation, affect stabilization, degradation, and subcellular localization of clock proteins, thus contributing to the molecular clockwork.[11]

Circadian control of metabolic functions

A few hypothalamic nuclei, including the paraventricular nucleus, receive direct neuronal connections from the SCN[12,13] and project to peripheral tissues, such as the liver,[14,15] pancreas,[16] or adipose tissue[17] via autonomic output pathways. Considerable experimental work has highlighted the important role of hypothalamic nuclei in the control of feeding and energy metabolism. The ventromedial

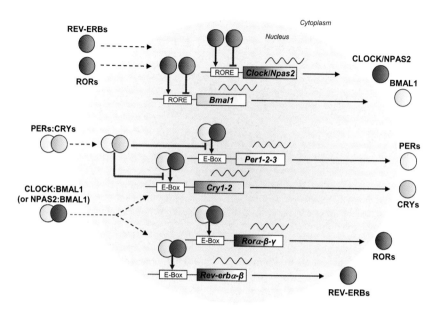

Figure 2. Simplified cellular model of the mammalian molecular clockwork. Circadian rhythms are generated by transcriptional/translational feedback regulatory loops of core clock genes. CLOCK (or NPAS2) and BMAL1 can dimerize to rhythmically transactivate genes containing a specific DNA sequence (E-box) in their promoter region. As a result, the transcriptional activity of *Pers, Crys, Rors,* and *Rev-erbs* is enhanced, and their products from translational activity are cyclically released in the cytoplasm. Then, when PERs and CRYs proteins reach a critical concentration, they form heterodimers that translocate into the nucleus to repress transcriptional activity induced by CLOCK (NPAS2):BMAL1, leading to their own repression. An additional loop involves the nuclear receptors *Rev-erbs* and *Rors,* which can translocate into the nucleus to modulate *Bmal1, Clock,* and *Npas2* transcription via opposite action on a RORE sequence located in their promoter.

hypothalamic nucleus, lateral hypothalamus, and arcuate nucleus (ARC) contain glucose-sensing neurons and receive nutritional information from blood-borne signals and neuronal messages from brainstem nuclei, including parabrachial nucleus and nucleus of the solitary tract (NTS). Among the key hormones that modulate feeding via hypothalamic activity, leptin synthesized by adipocytes acts on ARC, in particular, to inhibit appetite and stimulate energy expenditure.[18] Insulin, released from the β cells of the pancreas, also has anorexigenic effects on the metabolic hypothalamus.[19] On the other hand, ghrelin, released by the stomach, activates neuropeptide Y/Agouti-related peptide-containing neurons in the ARC to increase appetite and decrease energy expenditure.[20] An important role of the SCN is to orchestrate the internal ticking of different central and peripheral tissues. Therefore, 24-h rhythmic patterns can be observed for a plethora of metabolic functions, such as glucose,[21,22] nonesterified fatty acids (NEFA), insulin,[22] and leptin levels.[23]

The clock genes mentioned above are not only expressed in the SCN, but also in other brain regions and peripheral tissues.[24–26] In the liver, clock genes show a robust circadian pattern of expression.[25] In rats, destruction of the SCN abolishes the circadian rhythm of food intake.[27] SCN lesions do not abolish *Per2* rhythms in peripheral tissues, but produce internal desynchrony.[28] Microarray analysis of the mouse liver transcriptome showed that 9% of more than 2,000 genes studied oscillate in a circadian manner and may be under the control of the SCN.[29] Thus, it is likely that the SCN modulates both behavior and metabolism by adjusting the phase of peripheral oscillators. Recent genome-wide transcriptome analyses performed in the SCN, liver, and adrenal glands of mice, revealed that around 10% of transcripts are regulated in a circadian manner.[30–35] Of the 49 nuclear receptors that are key actors of metabolic regulations (see below), approximately 40% were cyclic in the liver or white adipose tissue (WAT).[36] Liver posttranscriptional and translational mechanisms contribute as well to circadian coordination.[37] While the master clock in the SCN is mainly synchronized by light, clock gene oscillations in peripheral tissues can be shifted by feeding time (Fig. 1).[25,38,39] In contrast, the SCN clock is relatively impervious to the synchronizing effect of meal time, provided that the animals are exposed to a light–dark cycle and ingest enough daily energy. Under severe food restriction (i.e., caloric restriction), however, the phase of the SCN and its synchronization to light are modified.[40] Expression in the SCN of receptors to metabolic hormones (i.e., insulin, ghrelin, and leptin) raises the possibility that peripheral hormonal signals can feed back to the SCN.[41–43]

Therefore, the whole circadian system participates in the daily variation of metabolism. Several biological approaches and genetic models have given further insight into the maintenance of metabolic homeostasis and the crosstalk between the circadian system and metabolism, as will be further discussed below.

Metabolic diseases are associated with circadian disturbances

Genetic obesity and diabetes

Monogenic causes of obesity and diabetes are relatively rare, especially in humans. For instance, early-onset obesity has been associated with a mutation in the leptin receptor in humans.[44] In rodents, however, genetic syndromes of obesity and diabetes mellitus offer models of choice to analyze circadian disturbances associated with metabolic physiopathology.

In obese Zucker rats, which carry a mutation (i.e., *fa*) in the leptin receptor gene, daily rhythms of locomotor activity, body temperature, and feeding are phase advanced (i.e., the active phase starts in the afternoon in contrast to the nocturnal onset in *+/?* littermates) and their day–night amplitude is generally reduced.[45–47] Increased daytime feeding is also observed in obese mice carrying the null mutation of a receptor to prostaglandin E2 (i.e., EP3 subtype).[48] As a rule, the amplitude of the sleep–wake cycle and activity–rest rhythm is dampened in genetically obese rats and mice, diabetic or not, due in part to increased wake/activity during daytime and increased sleep at night.[49–54]

The molecular clockwork in peripheral tissues is consistently disrupted in genetically obese, diabetic or not, mice. More precisely, in obese *ob/ob* and KK mice as well as in obese and diabetic KK-A[Y] mice, the amplitude of daily profiles of clock gene expression in the liver or white adipose tissue is generally reduced, if not barely sizeable.[55,56] In the liver of obese and diabetic *db/db* mice, the molecular clockwork is differentially modified according to the clock gene considered.[51]

Of interest, in *ob/ob* mice, alterations in peripheral clocks occur earlier than metabolic symptoms, such as morbid obesity and hyperinsulinemia, thus suggesting that altered clockwork can play a role in obesity in addition to the specific deficiency of leptin.[55] Within the central nervous system of *ob/ob* or KK-A[Y] mice, clock gene oscillations have been studied in the NTS. The most salient changes concern *Bmal1* and *Rev-erba*, whose daily expression is up- and downregulated, respectively.[57] Moreover, the molecular clockwork of the SCN is not markedly affected in leptin-deficient, obese (i.e., *ob/ob*) mice.[55] Unexpectedly in view of the severe dampening of overt rhythmicity in *db/db* mice, the amplitude of SCN molecular oscillations is significantly increased in these mice compared to *db/+* littermates.[51] Finally, it is worth mentioning that *ob/ob* mice show increased photic resetting of the master clock.[54]

Diet-induced obesity

In nature, species are not often confronted with food abundance. On the contrary, food can be rare for most animals and foraging is a key for survival (thus contributing to energy expenditure). Consequently, obese animals in the wild are uncommon, except for some species in which overweighting is important to support long periods of fasting (e.g., penguins, bears), and those species living in proximity to humans and consuming greasy food that is discarded by people. Most laboratory-based research on obesity is carried out in rodents.[58] Control animals usually have an *ad libitum* access to a normocaloric chow diet. Despite this free access, most rodents regulate their consumption and the time when they eat and do not become obese.

Obesity can be induced by feeding rodents on an *ad libitum* basis with a high-fat diet (HFD, more than 50% of metabolizable energy derived from fat). Both the amount and dietary fat type alter body mass and composition.[59] Short-term high-fat feeding reduces circadian variations of leptin levels in rats[60] and humans,[61] thus suggesting that dampened circulating leptin could contribute to the development of obesity. In mice, high-fat feeding attenuates the daily pattern of food intake, with a higher consumption during the day and a concomitant decrease during the active period, before significant mass gain. In WAT of mice fed with HDF, expression of metabolic genes can be downregulated at night, such as sterol regulatory element-binding protein 1c (*Srebp-1c*) or fatty-acid binding protein 4 (*Fabp4*), while expression of others is barely affected, like acetyl-CoA carboxylase (*Acc*) and fatty acid synthase (*Fas*). Other transcriptional changes are detected in the liver of these mice: expression of *Acc*, *Fas*, and *Fabp1* is upregulated, while the nighttime peak of *Srebp-1c* is phase-advanced to the afternoon. Moreover, changes in the concentration and temporal pattern of expression of glucose, insulin, leptin, and NEFA are also observed.[62] High-fat feeding also leads to difficulties in maintaining wakefulness during the active period and increases nonrapid eye movement sleep in mice[63] as well as postprandial sleepiness in humans,[64] suggesting that the metabolic state affects neural structures regulating sleep. Equally interesting, HFD seems to have a direct effect on the main circadian clock. In mice, HFD lengthens the free-running period[62] and disrupts photic synchronization of the SCN to light, as shown by slower re-entrainment to shifted light–dark cycle and reduction in light-induced phase shifts.[65] There is also a clear change in neuropeptide expression in the mediobasal hypothalamus, despite no major modification of the core clock machinery in that region.[62] In the brainstem, more precisely in the NTS, mice fed with HFD display altered daily patterns of clock gene expression, including downregulated *Rev-erbα*, and upregulated *Bmal1* and *Clock* mRNA levels.[57] Taken together, these results suggest that central dysfunctions may contribute to the development of obesity.

Oscillations of clock genes have been found in human WAT,[66] but no difference has been detected in the characteristics of these oscillations between lean, overweight, and diabetic individuals.[67] By contrast, the circadian timing of peripheral tissues is markedly modified by fat overload in rodents. HFD alters the diurnal variation in glucose tolerance, and insulin sensitivity by influencing clock functioning.[68] In the liver, changes are seen in the level as well as the rhythmic pattern of major components of lipid homeostasis and adiponectin metabolic pathway, with parallel modifications in clock gene ex-

pression.[62,69] In HFD-fed animals, expression of metabolic actors is asynchronous in liver and adipose tissue, suggesting the importance of temporal coordination among metabolic tissues. Furthermore, HFD also attenuates the amplitude of *Clock*, *Bmal1,* and *Per2* in adipose tissue.[62] Hence, altered circadian clock function within adipose tissue may promote excess fat storage (especially intra-abdominal fat). However, it is important to note that HFD-induced changes in clock gene expression could be gender specific, since a recent study in female mice did not obtain the same results. Indeed, eight weeks of HFD had only mild effects on clock gene profiles in the liver and adipose tissue, in spite of the presence of hyperlipidemia, hyperglycemia, and overweight.[70] Moreover, the time and duration of feeding are also important. Four or eight weeks of HFD failed to alter peripheral clocks, whereas 11 weeks did.[70,71] The differences between strains, gender, starting age of HFD feeding, and its duration, add a level of complexity to the comprehension of the risk factors that trigger obesity in rodents.

In summary, impairment of clock gene oscillations and metabolic pathways may explain the altered coordination of metabolic functions and clock-controlled output signaling, contributing to obesity and associated disorders (e.g., diabetes, sleep disturbances). Recent evidence also demonstrates that disruption of the circadian timing system solely, has various consequences on metabolism.

Circadian disruption is associated with metabolic dysfunctions

Altered endogenous clockwork

As aforementioned, clock genes are expressed in virtually all tissues and circadian clocks participate in the daily regulation of metabolic functions such as glucose and lipid metabolism.[22,68]

One of the first clock genes studied was *Clock*. Homozygous C57BL/6J *Clock* mutant mice are hyperphagic, show a dampened feeding pattern, with increased food intake during the rest period, and attenuated energy expenditure at night, thus contributing to fat excess. *Clock* mutant mice display severe metabolic alterations, including hypercholesteronemia, hypertriglyceridemia, hepatic steatosis, and hyperglycemia. In addition, *Clock* mutation leads to day–night changes in the expression of hypothalamic neuropeptides, like CART (Cocaine and amphetamine regulated transcript) and orexin mRNA, which play a role in central circuits controlling feeding and arousal.[72] Furthermore, *Clock* mutation induces profound changes in glucose homeostasis, such as increased insulin sensitivity and altered gluconeogenesis.[68] Of interest, in the liver, *Clock* has been shown to directly drive the expression of glycogen synthase 2 gene via E-boxes.[73] In *Clock* mutant mice generated on a CBA/6CaH background (which synthesize melatonin contrary to the C57BL/6J strain), impairments in glucose tolerance, insulin secretion, liver *Pepck* mRNA expression, and increased insulin sensitivity are also observed, although these mice do not become spontaneously obese unlike C57BL/6J *Clock* mutants.[74] Moreover, *Clock* (Jcl:ICR) mutant mice display levels of triglycerides and NEFA lower than control mice, and cholesterol and glucose levels do not differ. Due to reduced lipid absorption and hepatic lipogenesis, these mice challenged with HFD show reduced body mass elevation, leptin, and insulin levels.[75,76] In spite of these discrepancies, due notably to strain-related differences, mutation of the *Clock* gene clearly has an impact on lipid metabolism, since *Clock* has been shown to participate in liver cholesterol accumulation[77] and to amplify obesity in *ob/ob* mice.[78]

Bmal1, a close partner of *Clock*, has been shown to participate in adipocyte differentiation and lipogenesis.[79] Sensitivity to exogenous insulin is increased by deletion of *Bmal1*, while gluconeogenesis is suppressed.[68] Liver-specific deletion of *Bmal1* in mice nicely confirmed its strong involvement in glucose metabolism. *L-Bmal1*$^{-/-}$ mice have impaired expression of clock-related genes involved in hepatic glucose regulation such as genes encoding glucose transporter 2, glucokinase, or pyruvate kinase. *L-Bmal1*$^{-/-}$ mice were hypoglycemic during the resting period, were more glucose tolerant, had normal insulin sensitivity and production, and normal total body fat content compared to wild-type mice.[80] Altogether, these results demonstrate that *Clock* and *Bmal1* modulate hepatic function to regulate glucose and fatty acid homeostasis. Interestingly, two *Bmal1* haplotypes have been associated with diabetes in humans[81] as well as *Clock* polymorphisms and related haplotypes that may play a role in the development of obesity.[82,83]

Recent elegant studies have explored the role of *Clock* and *Bmal1* in the pancreatic islets, demonstrating that the pancreas harbors a functional circadian oscillator.[84,85] They showed that pancreas-specific *Bmal1* mutant mice have higher blood glucose levels during the whole 24-h cycle, impaired glucose tolerance, and reduced insulin secretion. Moreover, pancreatic islets of these mutant mice have altered development and produced less insulin, suggesting that intact clock functioning in the pancreas is essential for normal insulin secretion.[85] This study establishes clearly that circadian components can regulate local metabolism.

Mutation of the core clock gene *Per2* can also lead to abnormal conditions. In *Per2*$^{-/-}$ (*Per2tm1Brd*) mice, daily corticosterone rhythm is markedly attenuated. Of interest, when fed with HFD, these mice eat more during the rest period compared to wild-type mice and develop obesity.[86] Moreover, the rhythmic pattern in *Per2*$^{-/-}$ mice of alpha-melanocyte-stimulating hormone (α-MSH), a powerful appetite suppressing peptide, is disrupted and peripheral injection of α-MSH induces weight loss.[86] Interestingly, the circadian rhythm of *Per2* was dampened in the mediobasal hypothalamus of *Clock* mutant mice that are obese.[72] In mice in which *Per2* is fully ablated, lipid metabolism was altered with decreases in both plasma NEFA and total triacylglycerol (TAG), and TAG contents in the WAT.[87] In *Per2*$^{-/-}$ mice, and to a lesser extent in *Per1*$^{-/-}$ mice, glucose tolerance was increased (i.e., improved) compared to wild-type animals.[88] By contrast, in *Per1*$^{-/-}$ and *Per2*$^{-/-}$ double-mutant mice (129/sv background), glucose tolerance and insulin sensitivity were both attenuated.[80] Triple-mutant mice for *Per1-Per2-Per3* gain more body mass on HFD than wild-type mice, similar to *Per3* single-mutant mice, thus indicating that the *Per3* mutation alone accounts for the obese phenotype.[89]

Along with core clock components, secondary actors of circadian oscillations take part in metabolic functions. *Rora*, activator of *Bmal1* transcription, has been shown to participate in the regulation of apolipoprotein C-III (*Apo C-III*) gene involved in triglyceride metabolism,[90] and lipid homeostasis in skeletal muscle.[91] *Rev-erba*, repressor of *Bmal1*, is involved in adipocyte differentiation[92,93] and rhythmic bile and lipid homeostasis.[94] *Rev-erba*$^{-/-}$ mice displayed elevated serum Apo C-III and triglycerides levels.[95] Moreover, although the deletion of *Rev-erba* alone has only a minor effect on hepatic glucose regulation,[94] the alterations are more pronounced with concomitant mutation of *Per2*.[96] Indeed, the expression of key enzymes of glucose metabolism, such as glucose-6-phosphatase or glucokinase, was more affected in the liver of *Rev-erba$^{-/-}$/Per2* mutant mice.

From all these results, it is tempting to think that studying the effects of clock gene disruption could shed light on the incapacity of physiological control mechanisms to cope with adverse consequences, for instance of overweight. However, the effects of a mutation in the Nocturnin gene, which encodes a circadian deadenylase important for posttranscriptional regulation of circadian-related genes,[97] do not fit with this thought. *Nocturnin* knockout mice exhibit no change in circadian rhythm of locomotor activity and liver clock gene expression, although they have altered expression of metabolic genes, reduced lipid absorption, and are resistant to diet-induced obesity. This study indicates that circadian metabolism can be disrupted without noteworthy modification in core clock functioning while a specific subset of circadian downstream targets involved in lipid metabolism is affected.[98] Ongoing research into the complex crosstalk between components of the circadian system and metabolism may lead to prevention and improve treatment of metabolic disorders in the future.

Altered rhythmic "environment"

There are two main external causes of disruption in circadian rhythmicity. The first one concerns chronic changes in timing of light–dark cycles, such as chronic jet lag. The second way relates to behavioral activity (e.g., physical activity, feeding) occurring during the usual resting period (nighttime in humans, daytime in nocturnal rodents) with long-term shifts, such as during night work (also called permanent shift work), or short-term shifts, like rotating shift work. As detailed below, these desynchronizing situations have deleterious consequences on circadian organization and metabolic health.

Housing mice in light–dark cycles that are too short (i.e., 20 h) for enabling daily synchronization of their master clock leads to larger body mass gain and increased insulin/glucose ratio, indicative in the fasted state of insulin resistance.[99] The same paradigm has also been shown to aggravate cardiovascular disease in mice.[100] In human subjects exposed to controlled 28-h sleep–wake cycles under dim light (so-called "forced desynchronization" protocol), circadian misalignment impairs glucose tolerance and reduces sensitivity to insulin.[101] Additionally, constant exposure of mice to bright or dim light leads to increased body mass and reduced glucose tolerance compared to mice housed under a regular light–dark cycle.[102]

Repeated weekly shifts of 24-h light–dark cycle in rats fed with regular chow diet lead to chronic desynchronization and trigger higher body mass gain[103] as well as impaired insulin regulation.[104] Interestingly, expression of FABP4 is upregulated in WAT of rats exposed to repeated light–dark shifts.[105] A number of epidemiological studies in different countries have highlighted increased metabolic risks for cardio-metabolic syndrome, including increased disturbances in lipid metabolism (e.g., high levels of cholesterol and triglycerides),[106–110] glucose metabolism (e.g., high fasting insulin and glucose),[108,111] increased concentration of leucocytes, reflecting systemic inflammation,[108] and hypertension.[106,110]

Chronic sleep disturbance or sleep restriction under a regular light–dark cycle alters glucose homeostasis in rats.[112] In humans, recurrent sleep debt is a newly identified risk factor for obesity and diabetes,[113,114] indicating that it is likely an aggravating factor for metabolic disturbances in night workers.

Being nocturnal animals, laboratory rats and mice exposed to a light–dark cycle consume most of their daily food during the night period. In rodents, daytime feeding is a potent synchronizer of peripheral clocks.[25,38,39,115] Access to food restricted to a few hours during the light phase usually leads to mild body mass loss or no change at all.[38,116,117] In more rare cases, food-restricted rats with chow diet available only for a few hours can increase their body mass.[118] A clear contribution of circadian timing of food intake in body mass gain has been shown in Zucker rats (Fig. 3).[46] As mentioned above, *fa/fa* rats ingest a larger proportion of food during the usual resting phase (i.e., light phase) than control animals. This study was the first to demonstrate that by limiting food access to the normal period of activity and feeding (i.e., nighttime in nocturnal rats), Zucker rats gained less body mass compared to free-fed animals, in spite of similar amounts of food intake between both groups.[46] More recent

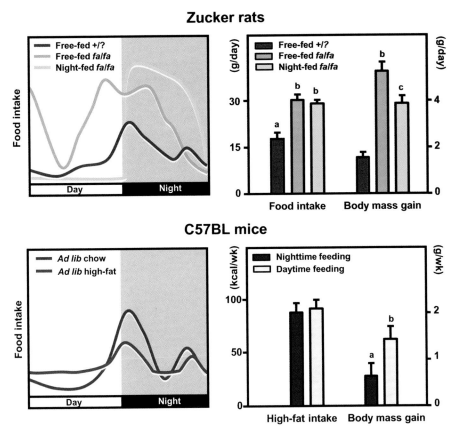

Figure 3. Importance of feeding time in genetic or diet-induced obesity. In Zucker rats (upper panels), obese individuals (i.e., *fa/fa*; blue lines and bars) eat more during daytime than control littermates (+/?; red lines and bars). When food access is limited to nighttime (orange lines and bars), *fa/fa* rats gain less body mass in spite of similar whole energy intake compared to free-fed individuals (modified with permission from Ref. 46). In C57BL6 mice (lower panels), free access to a high-fat diet is associated with an increase in daytime feeding (purple line), while chow feeding is mostly nocturnal (red line). If high-fat feeding is restricted to daytime or nighttime hours (light and dark purple bars, respectively), body mass gain is larger in the former, despite comparable energy intake (drawn from data in Refs. 62 and 118).

observations confirm nicely the metabolic consequences of unusual timing of feeding. Mice fed *ad libitum* with HFD display a rapid increase in daytime feeding that takes place weeks before the obese phenotype is detectable.[62] Furthermore, when HFD was restricted to the light phase, mice gained more body mass than those on the same diet but with access limited to the dark phase (Fig. 3).[119]

Another paradigm used to awaken rodents during their resting period (i.e., daytime) is forced activity that leads to internal desynchronization.[120] Keeping food intake to the normal feeding period (i.e., night) in spite of diurnal forced activity prevents body mass and metabolic changes.[121] Considering that exposure to bright light at night is an aggravating factor

for the occurrence of pathologies in human night workers,[122] it may be clinically relevant to develop shift-work models in day-active animals.

In humans, night-eating syndrome (NES) is characterized by a delayed pattern of calorie intake (i.e., lack of appetite in the morning and evening or nocturnal hyperphagia). In contrast to this delayed meal timing, the daily rhythm of plasma ghrelin is largely phase advanced, while the rhythm in plasma glucose is phase opposed in patients with NES compared to those in control subjects.[123] Elevated nocturnal, but not "evening," feeding has been correlated with an increased risk of overweight in some,[124,125] but not all epidemiological studies.[126]

Transcriptional networks connecting molecular clockwork and metabolic pathways

As aforementioned, a set of clock genes is responsible for the generation of circadian oscillations. From genetic strategies allowing modifications of the genome in mice, it has been discussed above that most, if not all, clock gene deletions lead to a broad range of metabolic diseases. In addition, we have introduced the effects of unhealthy food and incorrect timing of food intake on metabolic regulatory centers and the core clock machinery. In this last section, we will give an overview of the emergent understanding of the communication within the circadian clock circuitry. We will illustrate the different molecular pathways by which clock-related nuclear receptors are involved in metabolism and the effects of nutrient "sensors" on core clock components (Fig. 4).

The nuclear receptors' dynamic network

Transcriptomal analyses have demonstrated that a large number of nuclear receptors are expressed in a circadian manner.[36] Among them, *Rors, Rev-erbs,* and peroxisome proliferator-activated receptor (*Ppars*) genes appear to be pivotal players at the interface between the circadian system and metabolism.[127]

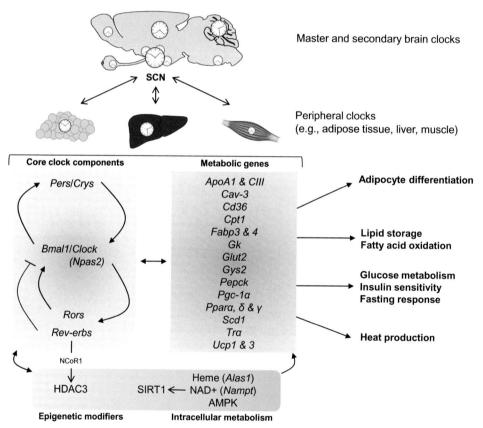

Figure 4. A schematic illustration of the cross-talk between circadian components and metabolic regulators. The master clock housed in the SCN is connected to several brain and peripheral clocks to orchestrate rhythmic activities. All clocks share a common molecular mechanism in which the clock genes are coexpressed, and the generation of circadian oscillations is made from transcriptional/translational interactions (represented in the gray box; for more details, see Fig. 2). Clock genes can influence, directly or indirectly, the rhythmic expression of many metabolic genes (listed in the blue box). Clock components can also control rate-limiting enzymes in the NAD$^+$ salvage pathway (i.e., *Nampt*) and heme biosynthesis (i.e., *Alas1*). Intracellular metabolism through the action of SIRT1, AMPK, and heme can impinge both metabolic genes and core clock machinery. In addition, epigenetic modifiers, such as HDAC3 recruited by REV-ERBα via NCoR1, modulate clock and metabolic gene transcription (orange box).

As introduced above, RORs and REV-ERBs compete for binding RORE in clock gene promoters.[7–10] Interestingly, *Rev-erba* can repress its own transcription on a functional REV-ERBα binding site (RevDR2) located in its promoter.[128] RORα being able to bind to this site participates in the control of *Rev-erba* transcription.[129] Hence, genes containing either RORE or RevDR2 in their promoter are activated by RORα and repressed by REV-ERBα. This highlights the occurrence of dynamic interactions within the core clock machinery. In skeletal muscle, *Rora* directly regulates the mouse caveolin-3 (*Cav-3*) and carnitine palmitoyltransferase-1 (*Cpt1*) genes, involved in fatty acid metabolism.[91] *Rora* also enhances activity of the human Apo C-III gene promoter[90] and binds to the rodent apolipoprotein A-I (*ApoA1*) RORE.[130] Additional evidence for a role of *Rora* in metabolism is provided by the fact that cholesterol is a putative ligand of RORα.[131]

Numerous studies have shown that REV-ERBs also influence lipid and energy homeostasis. The expression of a dominant negative version of *Rev-erbb* in transfected cell lines attenuates expression of genes involved in lipid metabolism, such as *Fabp3-4*, cluster of differentiation 36 (*Cd36*), stearoyl-coenzyme A desaturase 1 (*Scd1*), and cellular energy balance (e.g., uncoupling protein 3, *Ucp3*). Similarly to *Rora*, *Rev-erba* can bind directly to the human Apo C-III promoter[95] and the rat Apoa-I promoter RORE.[132] For the repressive action on *Bmal1* transcription, *Rev-erba* has been shown to recruit the nuclear receptor corepressor (NCoR)/histone deacetylase 3 (HDAC3) complex.[133] Of interest, genetic disruption of NCoR1-HDAC3 interaction in mice induces changes in *Bmal1* expression and circadian behavior with concomitant effects on metabolism (e.g., increased insulin sensitivity, altered expression of metabolic genes). Surprisingly, loss of a functional NCoR1-HDAC3 complex also protects mice from diet-induced obesity.[134] On the other hand, a recent study has explored the role of the circadian genomic recruitment of HDAC3 in the mouse liver. They showed that REV-ERBα controls the circadian expression of lipid metabolism genes by recruiting the repressive chromatin modifier HDAC3 (and NCoR) to the genome during the light period, therefore preventing lipogenesis at a time when animals are resting. In addition, deletion of either *Hdac3* or *Rev-erba* results in hepatic steatosis indicating steady lipogenesis.[135] These findings

demonstrate that the circadian control of epigenetic modifiers by clock components is critical for normal metabolic processing. Additional evidence of the involvement of *Rev-erbs* in metabolism is provided by studies on heme, which has diverse biological functions, including oxygen sensing, cell respiration, and metabolism.[136] Heme, whose expression occurs in a circadian manner,[137] can bind to both REV-ERBs.[138] Heme binding to REV-ERBs facilitates recruitment of the nuclear corepressor NCoR.[133,138] The rate-limiting enzyme in heme biosynthesis, aminolevulinate synthase 1 (*Alas1*), is directly controlled by the clock.[139] Heme biosynthesis is also influenced by the nutritional status through the regulation of *Alas1* by the PPARγ coactivator 1α (PGC-1α).[140] This nuclear receptor coactivator is induced by fasting[140] and participates in a variety of metabolic pathways such as glucose and lipid regulation.[141] Moreover, both PGC-1α and heme are able to modulate the expression of circadian genes.[137,142,143] These results illustrate how REV-ERBs can sense dynamic metabolic changes and transmit them to the core clock machinery.

PPARs are members of the nuclear hormone receptor superfamily of ligand-activated transcription factors. The three PPARs (α, δ, γ) have been shown to regulate carbohydrate, lipid, lipoprotein, and energy metabolism.[144,145] *Ppara* is rhythmically expressed in tissues with high fatty acid catabolism rates such as the liver and adipose tissue. *Pparg* is rhythmically expressed in liver and WAT, while *Ppard* expression oscillates in liver and brown adipose tissue (BAT).[36] PPARα is likely to play a role in connecting circadian physiology to metabolism. Pparα-deficient mice (*Ppara*$^{-/-}$) have normal rhythmic behavior and clock gene expression in the SCN, but PPARα deficiency alters *Bmal1* and *Per3* expression in the liver. Moreover, *Ppara* deficiency leads to disrupted phase resetting of *Bmal1* when food is provided during the light period, indicating that PPARα may control *Bmal1*. Indeed, PPARα directly regulates hepatic *Bmal1* expression through a response element located in its promoter.[146] Besides, it has been shown that *Ppara* is a clock-controlled gene[147] and daytime feeding inverts its circadian expression pattern in the liver.[146] Interestingly, PPARα is also connected to the nuclear receptor *Rev-erba* because the PPARα agonists (fibrates) induce liver expression of *Rev-erba*. In addition, PPARα (as well as PPARγ) can directly transactivate *Rev-erbα* via RevDR2 located in its promoter.[92,132,148] Clearly, all these data demonstrate that the metabolic sensor PPARα may play a prominent role in circadian functioning. Other results indicate that PER2 has the capacity to recruit PPARα or REV-ERBα for the modulation of *Bmal1* expression,[96] again showing intimate interactions between clock and metabolic components in the clock circuitry.

PPARγ and PPARδ are both involved in energy homeostasis. A recent study reveals that PER2 can interact directly with PPARγ to repress its transcriptional activity. Ablation of *Per2* in cell culture increased induction of adipogenic genes, while deletion of *Per2* in mice results in slight changes in circadian expression of PPARγ target genes in WAT.[87] These results demonstrate that the control of PPARγ by a circadian actor is essential for normal lipid metabolism. Interestingly, PGC-1 (PPARγ coactivator 1, as introduced above), which is involved in thermogenesis and associated metabolic responses,[142,149] is rhythmically expressed in phase with *Pparg*, *Ppard*, and thermogenic genes, such as *Ucp1* and thyroid receptor α (*Tra*), in BAT.[36] Furthermore, PGC-1 can specifically bind PPARγ,[149] whereas the latter can also interact with the *Ucp1* promoter.[150] All these data suggest that PPARs could transmit (diurnal) changes in heat dissipation to the circadian system.

These data suggest that nuclear receptors are controlling an amazing array of metabolic functions and are capable of communicating the body's metabolic state to the core clock machinery. Incidentally, other nuclear receptor subgroups also participate in the interplay between metabolic and circadian physiology (e.g., retinoid X receptor, liver X receptor, and estrogen-related receptor).[36,127,151]

Nutrient sensors interact with clock components

The tight connection between the circadian timing system and metabolism is also underscored by the role of nutrient sensors. Clock adaptation to metabolic reactions is likely to be achieved also by direct input of nutrient sensing regulators to the intrinsic clock machinery. However, we are aware that the subdivision between nuclear receptors presented above and metabolic sensors that we will introduce in this section may appear rather arbitrary.

Recent evidence has demonstrated that local changes in cellular energy, such as redox reactions (portmanteau for reduction-oxidation), can influence the circadian expression of core clock genes and clock-related nuclear receptors. Nicotinamide adenine dinucleotide (NAD^+) and its reduced form NADH are coenzymes found in all living cells. NAD^+ also exists in a phosphorylated form $NADP^+$ and can be reduced to NADPH. $NAD(P)^+$ and $NAD(P)H$ are involved in cellular redox reactions. Interestingly, CLOCK:BMAL1 and NPAS2:BMAL1 heterodimers can sense intracellular redox status. The DNA-binding activities of these dimers are influenced by both reduced and oxidized forms of NAD(H) and NADP(H) in an opposing manner. The reduced forms (NADH and NADPH) activate DNA binding of CLOCK:BMAL1 and NPAS2:BMAL1, whereas the oxidized forms (NAD^+ and $NADP^+$) inhibit it, consistent with a role as redox sensors.[152] These results raise the possibility that cell energy metabolism can influence circadian rhythmicity. For example, these clock protein sensors might participate in the rhythm imposed by the alternation of fasting and feeding. Indeed, NAD:NADH ratio is modified under fasting and feeding conditions since starvation lowers NADP:NADPH (i.e., shift toward a reduced state) in both rat liver mitochondria and cytoplasm.[153] Thus, for feeding synchronization, it is plausible that the cellular redox status could transmit changes in energy metabolism directly to the clock architecture. In this context, it is tempting to think that irregular mealtimes could also contribute to circadian misalignment by subtle perturbations of local circadian oscillator functioning.

Sirtuin 1 (SIRT1), another energy sensor, has recently been found to link circadian to metabolic physiology. SIRT1 is a NAD-dependent histone deacetylase that contributes to epigenetic gene silencing and a plethora of biological processes ranging from gluconeogenesis, insulin secretion and sensitivity, lipid regulation, mitochondrial activity, thermogenesis, adipogenesis and adipocyte differentiation, and apoptosis. SIRT1 also plays a crucial role in the caloric restriction-dependent life span extension.[154–156] SIRT1, whose expression occurs in a circadian manner, has been shown to influence circadian transcription of several clock genes (e.g., *Per2*, *Cry1*, *Bmal1*, and *Rora*).[157] Moreover, SIRT1 can directly bind CLOCK:BMAL1 heterodimers and promote deacetylation of PER2,[157] BMAL1, and histone H3.[158] Interestingly, SIRT1 can also affect expression of metabolic regulatory transcription factors. It can interact with and deacetylate PGC-1α to control the expression of gluconeogenic and glycolytic genes.[159] In addition, hepatic SIRT1 is able to modulate the expression of PPARα.[160] Importantly, SIRT1 can also repress the fat regulator PPARγ and it is activated during fasting to promote fat mobilization in WAT, again demonstrating its clear implication in lipid homeostasis.[161] Furthermore, SIRT1 has been shown to be decreased in adipose tissue endothelial cells from obese human subjects.[162] Of interest, since fat accumulation is associated with several adverse complications, such as diabetes and hypertension, caloric restriction (and consequent fat depletion) that has multiple biological and life-extending benefits[163] may be used to prevent or treat metabolic disruptions.

In addition to NAD(P)$^+$ and SIRT1, AMP-activated protein kinase (AMPK) is a further important nutrient sensor. AMPK is sensitive to fluctuations in the cellular AMP:ATP ratio and can be activated by various factors such as exercise, glucose deprivation, or leptin treatment. The functions of AMPK cover the whole-body energy balance (e.g., food intake, body mass, lipid and glucose homeostasis, cholesterol and triglyceride synthesis, energy expenditure).[164] In mouse skeletal muscle and cultured myotubes, AMPK has been demonstrated to regulate genes involved in energy metabolism by acting in coordination with SIRT1. Interestingly, AMPK activation increases NAD$^+$ levels, which in turn enhance SIRT1 activity, resulting in the deacetylation and activation of the downstream SIRT1 target PGC-1α.[165] Deletion of the AMPKγ3 subunit in mice leads to impaired expression profiles of clock genes in skeletal muscle in response to the AMPK activator AICAR (5-amino-4-imidazole-carboxamide riboside), and attenuated daily variations of the respiratory exchange ratio.[166] AMPK also has direct actions on the clock machinery. AMPK phosphorylates and destabilizes CRY1.[167] Casein kinase Iε, an important regulator of PER proteins stability, is also phosphorylated by AMPK that induces subsequent degradation of PER2 and phase shifts of peripheral oscillators.[168] Recently, it has been demonstrated that mice deficient for either AMPKα1 or AMPKα2 have altered circadian feeding behavior and free-running periods.[169] Surprisingly, the rhythmic gene expression of leptin, PGC-1α and nicotinamide phosphoryl-transferase (NAMPT), a rate-limiting enzyme in the NAD$^+$ salvage pathway regulated by CLOCK:BMAL1,[170,171] was abolished in AMPK-deficient mice.[169] This study reveals that AMPK is to some extent involved in the cycling of the NAMPT-(NAD$^+$)-SIRT1-PGC-1α pathway. In addition, prolonged activation of SIRT1 by its agonist SRT1720 causes an indirect activation of AMPK, and both SIRT1 and AMPK respond to low-energy levels.[164,172] Therefore, SIRT1 and AMPK may have overlapping functions to ensure the fine tuning of metabolic and clock regulations. Consequently, if a drug exerts effects on these actors, it is advisable to also explore its influence on the core clock machinery.

Finally, it is important to mention that the mammalian molecular circadian clockwork (based on transcriptional–translational events) overviewed in this section is not a unique cellular clock model. Indeed, circadian redox rhythms of peroxiredoxins, which are antioxidant enzymes, can occur independently of transcription, thus defining a metabolic nontranscriptional oscillator.[173]

Conclusion

At the molecular/cellular levels, the recent findings cited above highlight multiple transcriptional crossroads between circadian and metabolic pathways in organs involved in metabolism, namely liver, adipose tissue, pancreas, and muscle. Nuclear receptors such as *Rors* and *Rev-erbs* are well situated to receive metabolic signals and integrate them into the core clock architecture. In addition, we show that fluctuations in cellular metabolism can directly influence the transcriptional activity of core clock components such as *Cry1, Per2, Clock,* and *Bmal1.*

At the level of the organism, the circadian timing system provides internal temporal organization controlled locally by peripheral clocks/oscillators reset by feeding time, and supervised by the master SCN clock mainly reset by ambient light. Impairment of this internal timing due to altered endogenous clockwork or misalignment with external cues, light, and/or mealtime, has a deleterious impact on metabolic health.

Overconsumption of "junk" (most often hyper-caloric) food is a well-acknowledged causal factor of obesity. In addition to the type and quantity of food eaten, we have reviewed here the importance of the hour of the day when food is eaten. In short, it seems that the recommendation of "doing the right thing at the right time" is relevant for the relation between food intake and circadian rhythmicity, in that significant amounts of ingested fuels at the wrong circadian time (i.e., resting period) can predispose to increased adiposity and other metabolic risks. This link, together with the putative obesogenic property of repeated light–dark shifts or chronic shift work, leads to the concept that we called "chronobesity".[65] Furthermore, metabolic diseases are associated with circadian disturbances in behavior and physiology, not only in peripheral organs but also in the brain. Together, these findings suggest that management of circadian disorders is especially important in obese and diabetic people to prevent a kind of vicious circle that could amplify health problems.

We propose that dietary strategies for limiting, or preventing, overweight and obesity could be further optimized by taking into account circadian rhythmicity to maintain (or restore) normal temporal organization and synchronization to local time, that is, by developing chronotherapeutic approaches of dieting.

Acknowledgments

Due to space limitations, we apologize for not citing additional pertinent references. We are grateful to Dr. David Hicks for helpful comments on the manuscript. J.D. is supported by a doctoral fellowship from the French Ministry of National Education and Research, and E.C. is supported by Centre National de Recherche Scientifique, Université de Strasbourg and Agence Nationale pour la Recherche "Jeunes chercheurs/jeunes chercheuses" ANR-07-JCJC-0111.

Conflicts of interest

The authors declare no conflicts of interest.

References

1. Barness, L.A., J.M. Opitz & E. Gilbert-Barness. 2007. Obesity: genetic, molecular, and environmental aspects. *Am. J. Med. Genet. A* **143A:** 3016–3034.
2. Tataranni, P.A. & E. Ravussin. 1997. Effect of fat intake on energy balance. *Ann. N.Y. Acad. Sci.* **819:** 37–43.
3. Welsh, D.K. *et al.* 1995. Individual neurons dissociated from rat suprachiasmatic nucleus express independently phased circadian firing rhythms. *Neuron.* **14:** 697–706.
4. Meijer, J.H. & W.J. Schwartz. 2003. In search of the pathways for light-induced pacemaker resetting in the suprachiasmatic nucleus. *J. Biol. Rhythms* **18:** 235–249.
5. Hattar, S. *et al.* 2002. Melanopsin-containing retinal ganglion cells: architecture, projections, and intrinsic photosensitivity. *Science* **295:** 1065–1070.
6. Ko, C.H. & J.S. Takahashi. 2006. Molecular components of the mammalian circadian clock. *Hum. Mol. Genet.* **15:** R271–R277.
7. Preitner, N. *et al.* 2002. The orphan nuclear receptor REV-ERBalpha controls circadian transcription within the positive limb of the mammalian circadian oscillator. *Cell* **110:** 251–260.
8. Guillaumond, F. *et al.* 2005. Differential control of Bmal1 circadian transcription by REV-ERB and ROR nuclear receptors. *J. Biol. Rhythms* **20:** 391–403.
9. Crumbley, C. *et al.* 2010. Characterization of the core mammalian clock component, NPAS2, as a REV-ERBalpha/RORalpha target gene. *J. Biol. Chem.* **285:** 35386–35392.
10. Crumbley, C. & T.P. Burris. 2011. Direct regulation of Clock expression by REV-ERB. *PLoS One* **6:** e17290.
11. Lee, C. *et al.* 2001. Posttranslational mechanisms regulate the mammalian circadian clock. *Cell* **107:** 855–867.
12. Dibner, C., U. Schibler & U. Albrecht. 2010. The mammalian circadian timing system: organization and coordination of central and peripheral clocks. *Annu. Rev. Physiol.* **72:** 517–549.
13. Watts, A.G. & L.W. Swanson. 1987. Efferent projections of the suprachiasmatic nucleus: II. Studies using retrograde transport of fluorescent dyes and simultaneous peptide immunohistochemistry in the rat. *J. Comp. Neurol.* **258:** 230–252.
14. la Fleur, S.E. *et al.* 2000. Polysynaptic neural pathways between the hypothalamus, including the suprachiasmatic nucleus, and the liver. *Brain Res.* **871:** 50–56.
15. Shibata, S. 2004. Neural regulation of the hepatic circadian rhythm. *Anat. Rec. A Discov. Mol. Cell. Evol. Biol.* **280:** 901–909.
16. Buijs, R.M. *et al.* 2001. Parasympathetic and sympathetic control of the pancreas: a role for the suprachiasmatic nucleus and other hypothalamic centers that are involved in the regulation of food intake. *J. Comp. Neurol.* **431:** 405–423.
17. Kreier, F. *et al.* 2002. Selective parasympathetic innervation of subcutaneous and intra-abdominal fat–functional implications. *J. Clin. Invest.* **110:** 1243–1250.
18. Ahima, R.S. & M.A. Lazar. 2008. Adipokines and the peripheral and neural control of energy balance. *Mol. Endocrinol.* **22:** 1023–1031.
19. Gerozissis, K. 2008. Brain insulin, energy and glucose homeostasis; genes, environment and metabolic pathologies. *Eur. J. Pharmacol.* **585:** 38–49.
20. Nogueiras, R., M.H. Tschop & J.M. Zigman. 2008. Central nervous system regulation of energy metabolism: ghrelin versus leptin. *Ann. N.Y. Acad. Sci.* **1126:** 14–19.
21. La Fleur, S.E. *et al.* 1999. A suprachiasmatic nucleus generated rhythm in basal glucose concentrations. *J. Neuroendocrinol.* **11:** 643–652.

22. Yamamoto, H., K. Nagai & H. Nakagawa. 1987. Role of SCN in daily rhythms of plasma glucose, FFA, insulin and glucagon. *Chronobiol. Int.* **4:** 483–491.

23. Kalsbeek, A. *et al.* 2001. The suprachiasmatic nucleus generates the diurnal changes in plasma leptin levels. *Endocrinology* **142:** 2677–2685.

24. Tei, H. *et al.* 1997. Circadian oscillation of a mammalian homologue of the Drosophila period gene. *Nature* **389:** 512–516.

25. Damiola, F. *et al.* 2000. Restricted feeding uncouples circadian oscillators in peripheral tissues from the central pacemaker in the suprachiasmatic nucleus. *Genes Dev.* **14:** 2950–2961.

26. Abe, M. *et al.* 2002. Circadian rhythms in isolated brain regions. *J. Neurosci.* **22:** 350–356.

27. Nagai, K. *et al.* 1978. Effect of bilateral lesions of the suprachiasmatic nuclei on the circadian rhythm of food-intake. *Brain Res.* **142:** 384–389.

28. Yoo, S.H. *et al.* 2004. PERIOD2:LUCIFERASE real-time reporting of circadian dynamics reveals persistent circadian oscillations in mouse peripheral tissues. *Proc. Natl. Acad. Sci. USA* **101:** 5339–5346.

29. Akhtar, R.A. *et al.* 2002. Circadian cycling of the mouse liver transcriptome, as revealed by cDNA microarray, is driven by the suprachiasmatic nucleus. *Curr. Biol.* **12:** 540–550.

30. Hughes, M.E. *et al.* 2009. Harmonics of circadian gene transcription in mammals. *PLoS Genet.* **5:** e1000442.

31. Miller, B.H. *et al.* 2007. Circadian and CLOCK-controlled regulation of the mouse transcriptome and cell proliferation. *Proc. Natl. Acad. Sci. USA* **104:** 3342–3347.

32. Oishi, K. *et al.* 2003. Genome-wide expression analysis of mouse liver reveals CLOCK-regulated circadian output genes. *J. Biol. Chem.* **278:** 41519–41527.

33. Oishi, K. *et al.* 2005. Genome-wide expression analysis reveals 100 adrenal gland-dependent circadian genes in the mouse liver. *DNA Res.* **12:** 191–202.

34. Ueda, H.R. *et al.* 2002. A transcription factor response element for gene expression during circadian night. *Nature* **418:** 534–539.

35. Lowrey, P.L. & J.S. Takahashi. 2004. Mammalian circadian biology: elucidating genome-wide levels of temporal organization. *Annu. Rev. Genomics Hum. Genet.* **5:** 407–441.

36. Yang, X. *et al.* 2006. Nuclear receptor expression links the circadian clock to metabolism. *Cell* **126:** 801–810.

37. Reddy, A.B. *et al.* 2006. Circadian orchestration of the hepatic proteome. *Curr. Biol.* **16:** 1107–1115.

38. Feillet, C.A. *et al.* 2006. Lack of food anticipation in Per2 mutant mice. *Curr. Biol.* **16:** 2016–2022.

39. Stokkan, K.A. *et al.* 2001. Entrainment of the circadian clock in the liver by feeding. *Science* **291:** 490–493.

40. Challet, E. 2010. Interactions between light, mealtime and calorie restriction to control daily timing in mammals. *J. Comp. Physiol. B* **180:** 631–644.

41. Unger, J. *et al.* 1989. Distribution of insulin receptor-like immunoreactivity in the rat forebrain. *Neuroscience* **31:** 143–157.

42. Zigman, J.M. *et al.* 2006. Expression of ghrelin receptor mRNA in the rat and the mouse brain. *J. Comp. Neurol.* **494:** 528–548.

43. Hakansson, M.L. *et al.* 1998. Leptin receptor immunoreac-

tivity in chemically defined target neurons of the hypothalamus. *J. Neurosci.* **18:** 559–572.

44. Clement, K. *et al.* 1998. A mutation in the human leptin receptor gene causes obesity and pituitary dysfunction. *Nature* **392:** 398–401.

45. Fukagawa, K. *et al.* 1992. Advance shift of feeding circadian rhythm induced by obesity progression in Zucker rats. *Am. J. Physiol.* **263:** R1169–R1175.

46. Mistlberger, R.E., H. Lukman & B.G. Nadeau. 1998. Circadian rhythms in the Zucker obese rat: assessment and intervention. *Appetite* **30:** 255–267.

47. Murakami, D.M., B.A. Horwitz & C.A. Fuller. 1995. Circadian rhythms of temperature and activity in obese and lean Zucker rats. *Am. J. Physiol.* **269:** R1038–R1043.

48. Sanchez-Alavez, M. *et al.* 2007. Night eating and obesity in the EP3R-deficient mouse. *Proc. Natl. Acad. Sci. USA* **104:** 3009–3014.

49. Danguir, J. 1989. Sleep patterns in the genetically obese Zucker rat: effect of acarbose treatment. *Am. J. Physiol.* **256:** R281–R283.

50. Megirian, D., J. Dmochowski & G.A. Farkas. 1998. Mechanism controlling sleep organization of the obese Zucker rats. *J. Appl. Physiol.* **84:** 253–256.

51. Kudo, T. *et al.* 2004. Night-time restricted feeding normalises clock genes and Pai-1 gene expression in the db/db mouse liver. *Diabetologia* **47:** 1425–1436.

52. Laposky, A.D. *et al.* 2006. Altered sleep regulation in leptin-deficient mice. *Am. J. Physiol. Regul. Integr. Comp. Physiol.* **290:** R894–R903.

53. Laposky, A.D. *et al.* 2008. Sleep-wake regulation is altered in leptin-resistant (db/db) genetically obese and diabetic mice. *Am. J. Physiol. Regul. Integr. Comp. Physiol.* **295:** R2059–R2066.

54. Sans-Fuentes, M.A., A. Diez-Noguera & T. Cambras. 2010. Light responses of the circadian system in leptin deficient mice. *Physiol. Behav.* **99:** 487–494.

55. Ando, H. *et al.* 2011. Impairment of peripheral circadian clocks precedes metabolic abnormalities in ob/ob mice. *Endocrinology* **152:** 1347–1354.

56. Ando, H. *et al.* 2005. Rhythmic messenger ribonucleic acid expression of clock genes and adipocytokines in mouse visceral adipose tissue. *Endocrinology* **146:** 5631–5636.

57. Kaneko, K. *et al.* 2009. Obesity alters circadian expressions of molecular clock genes in the brainstem. *Brain Res.* **1263:** 58–68.

58. West, D.B. & B. York. 1998. Dietary fat, genetic predisposition, and obesity: lessons from animal models. *Am. J. Clin. Nutr.* **67:** 505S–512S.

59. Hill, J.O. *et al.* 1992. Development of dietary obesity in rats: influence of amount and composition of dietary fat. *Int. J. Obes. Relat. Metab. Disord.* **16:** 321–333.

60. Cha, M.C., C.J. Chou & C.N. Boozer. 2000. High-fat diet feeding reduces the diurnal variation of plasma leptin concentration in rats. *Metabolism* **49:** 503–507.

61. Havel, P.J. *et al.* 1999. High-fat meals reduce 24-h circulating leptin concentrations in women. *Diabetes* **48:** 334–341.

62. Kohsaka, A. *et al.* 2007. High-fat diet disrupts behavioral and molecular circadian rhythms in mice. *Cell Metab.* **6:** 414–421.

63. Jenkins, J.B. *et al.* 2006. Sleep is increased in mice with obesity induced by high-fat food. *Physiol. Behav.* **87:** 255–262.

64. Wells, A.S. *et al.* 1997. Influences of fat and carbohydrate on postprandial sleepiness, mood, and hormones. *Physiol. Behav.* **61:** 679–686.

65. Mendoza, J., P. Pevet & E. Challet. 2008. High-fat feeding alters the clock synchronization to light. *J. Physiol.* **586:** 5901–5910.

66. Garaulet, M. *et al.* 2011. An approximation to the temporal order in endogenous circadian rhythms of genes implicated in human adipose tissue metabolism. *J. Cell Physiol.* **226:** 2075–2080.

67. Otway, D.T. *et al.* 2011. Rhythmic diurnal gene expression in human adipose tissue from individuals who are lean, overweight, and type 2 diabetic. *Diabetes* **60:** 1577–1581.

68. Rudic, R.D. *et al.* 2004. BMAL1 and CLOCK, two essential components of the circadian clock, are involved in glucose homeostasis. *PLoS Biol.* **2:** e377.

69. Barnea, M., Z. Madar & O. Froy. 2009. High-fat diet delays and fasting advances the circadian expression of adiponectin signaling components in mouse liver. *Endocrinology* **150:** 161–168.

70. Yanagihara, H. *et al.* 2006. High-fat feeding exerts minimal effects on rhythmic mRNA expression of clock genes in mouse peripheral tissues. *Chronobiol. Int.* **23:** 905–914.

71. Hsieh, M.C. *et al.* 2010. Abnormal expressions of circadian-clock and circadian clock-controlled genes in the livers and kidneys of long-term, high-fat-diet-treated mice. *Int. J. Obes. (Lond)* **34:** 227–239.

72. Turek, F.W. *et al.* 2005. Obesity and metabolic syndrome in circadian Clock mutant mice. *Science* **308:** 1043–1045.

73. Doi, R., K. Oishi & N. Ishida. 2010. CLOCK regulates circadian rhythms of hepatic glycogen synthesis through transcriptional activation of Gys2. *J. Biol. Chem.* **285:** 22114–22121.

74. Kennaway, D.J. *et al.* 2007. Metabolic homeostasis in mice with disrupted Clock gene expression in peripheral tissues. *Am. J. Physiol. Regul. Integr. Comp. Physiol.* **293:** R1528–R1537.

75. Oishi, K. *et al.* 2006. Disrupted fat absorption attenuates obesity induced by a high-fat diet in Clock mutant mice. *FEBS Lett.* **580:** 127–130.

76. Kudo, T. *et al.* 2007. Attenuating effect of clock mutation on triglyceride contents in the ICR mouse liver under a high-fat diet. *J. Biol. Rhythms* **22:** 312–323.

77. Kudo, T. *et al.* 2008. Clock mutation facilitates accumulation of cholesterol in the liver of mice fed a cholesterol and/or cholic acid diet. *Am. J. Physiol. Endocrinol. Metab.* **294:** E120–130.

78. Oishi, K. *et al.* 2006. CLOCK is involved in obesity-induced disordered fibrinolysis in ob/ob mice by regulating PAI-1 gene expression. *J. Thromb. Haemost.* **4:** 1774–1780.

79. Shimba, S. *et al.* 2005. Brain and muscle Arnt-like protein-1 (BMAL1), a component of the molecular clock, regulates adipogenesis. *Proc. Natl. Acad. Sci. USA* **102:** 12071–12076.

80. Lamia, K.A., K.F. Storch & C.J. Weitz. 2008. Physiological significance of a peripheral tissue circadian clock. *Proc. Natl. Acad. Sci. USA* **105:** 15172–15177.

81. Woon, P.Y. *et al.* 2007. Aryl hydrocarbon receptor nuclear translocator-like (BMAL1) is associated with susceptibility to hypertension and type 2 diabetes. *Proc. Natl. Acad. Sci. USA* **104:** 14412–14417.

82. Scott, E.M., A.M. Carter & P.J. Grant. 2008. Association between polymorphisms in the Clock gene, obesity and the metabolic syndrome in man. *Int. J. Obes. (Lond)* **32:** 658–662.

83. Sookoian, S. *et al.* 2008. Genetic variants of Clock transcription factor are associated with individual susceptibility to obesity. *Am. J. Clin. Nutr.* **87:** 1606–1615.

84. Sadacca, L.A. *et al.* 2011. An intrinsic circadian clock of the pancreas is required for normal insulin release and glucose homeostasis in mice. *Diabetologia* **54:** 120–124.

85. Marcheva, B. *et al.* 2010. Disruption of the clock components CLOCK and BMAL1 leads to hypoinsulinaemia and diabetes. *Nature* **466:** 627–631.

86. Yang, S. *et al.* 2009. The role of mPer2 clock gene in glucocorticoid and feeding rhythms. *Endocrinology* **150:** 2153–2160.

87. Grimaldi, B. *et al.* 2010. PER2 controls lipid metabolism by direct regulation of PPARgamma. *Cell Metab.* **12:** 509–520.

88. Dallmann, R. *et al.* 2006. Impaired daily glucocorticoid rhythm in Per1 (Brd) mice. *J. Comp. Physiol. A* **192:** 769–775.

89. Dallmann, R. & D.R. Weaver. 2010. Altered body mass regulation in male mPeriod mutant mice on high-fat diet. *Chronobiol. Int.* **27:** 1317–1328.

90. Raspe, E. *et al.* 2001. Transcriptional regulation of apolipoprotein C-III gene expression by the orphan nuclear receptor RORalpha. *J. Biol. Chem.* **276:** 2865–2871.

91. Lau, P. *et al.* 2004. RORalpha regulates the expression of genes involved in lipid homeostasis in skeletal muscle cells: caveolin-3 and CPT-1 are direct targets of ROR. *J. Biol. Chem.* **279:** 36828–36840.

92. Fontaine, C. *et al.* 2003. The orphan nuclear receptor Rev-Erbalpha is a peroxisome proliferator-activated receptor (PPAR) gamma target gene and promotes PPARgamma-induced adipocyte differentiation. *J. Biol. Chem.* **278:** 37672–37680.

93. Wang, J. & M.A. Lazar. 2008. Bifunctional role of Rev-erbalpha in adipocyte differentiation. *Mol. Cell. Biol.* **28:** 2213–2220.

94. Le Martelot, G. *et al.* 2009. REV-ERBalpha participates in circadian SREBP signaling and bile acid homeostasis. *PLoS Biol.* **7:** e1000181.

95. Raspe, E. *et al.* 2002. Identification of Rev-erbalpha as a physiological repressor of apoC-III gene transcription. *J. Lipid Res.* **43:** 2172–2179.

96. Schmutz, I. *et al.* 2010. The mammalian clock component PERIOD2 coordinates circadian output by interaction with nuclear receptors. *Genes Dev.* **24:** 345–357.

97. Baggs, J.E. & C.B. Green. 2003. Nocturnin, a deadenylase in Xenopus laevis retina: a mechanism for posttranscriptional control of circadian-related mRNA. *Curr. Biol.* **13:** 189–198.

98. Green, C.B. *et al.* 2007. Loss of Nocturnin, a circadian deadenylase, confers resistance to hepatic steatosis and diet-induced obesity. *Proc. Natl. Acad. Sci. USA* **104:** 9888–9893.

99. Karatsoreos, I.N. *et al.* 2011. Disruption of circadian clocks has ramifications for metabolism, brain, and behavior. *Proc. Natl. Acad. Sci. USA* **108:** 1657–1662.

100. Martino, T.A. *et al.* 2007. Disturbed diurnal rhythm alters gene expression and exacerbates cardiovascular disease with rescue by resynchronization. *Hypertension* **49:** 1104–1113.

101. Scheer, F.A. *et al.* 2009. Adverse metabolic and cardiovascular consequences of circadian misalignment. *Proc. Natl. Acad. Sci. USA* **106:** 4453–4458.

102. Fonken, L.K. *et al.* 2010. Light at night increases body mass by shifting the time of food intake. *Proc. Natl. Acad. Sci. USA* **107:** 18664–18669.

103. Tsai, L.L. *et al.* 2005. Repeated light-dark shifts speed up body weight gain in male F344 rats. *Am. J. Physiol. Endocrinol. Metab.* **289:** E212–E217.

104. Bartol-Munier, I. *et al.* 2006. Combined effects of high-fat feeding and circadian desynchronization. *Int. J. Obes. (Lond)* **30:** 60–67.

105. Mishra, A. *et al.* 2009. Proteomic changes in the hypothalamus and retroperitoneal fat from male F344 rats subjected to repeated light-dark shifts. *Proteomics* **9:** 4017–4028.

106. Nakamura, K. *et al.* 1997. Shift work and risk factors for coronary heart disease in Japanese blue-collar workers: serum lipids and anthropometric characteristics. *Occup. Med. (Lond)* **47:** 142–146.

107. Karlsson, B.H. *et al.* 2003. Metabolic disturbances in male workers with rotating three-shift work. Results of the WOLF study. *Int. Arch. Occup. Environ. Health* **76:** 424–430.

108. Sookoian, S. *et al.* 2007. Effects of rotating shift work on biomarkers of metabolic syndrome and inflammation. *J. Intern. Med.* **261:** 285–292.

109. Dochi, M. *et al.* 2009. Shift work is a risk factor for increased total cholesterol level: a 14-year prospective cohort study in 6886 male workers. *Occup. Environ. Med.* **66:** 592–597.

110. Di Lorenzo, L. *et al.* 2003. Effect of shift work on body mass index: results of a study performed in 319 glucose-tolerant men working in a Southern Italian industry. *Int. J. Obes. Relat. Metab. Disord.* **27:** 1353–1358.

111. Suwazono, Y. *et al.* 2006. Long-term longitudinal study on the relationship between alternating shift work and the onset of diabetes mellitus in male Japanese workers. *J. Occup. Environ. Med.* **48:** 455–461.

112. Barf, R.P., P. Meerlo & A.J. Scheurink. 2010. Chronic sleep disturbance impairs glucose homeostasis in rats. *Int. J. Endocrinol.* **2010:** 819414.

113. Spiegel, K. *et al.* 2009. Effects of poor and short sleep on glucose metabolism and obesity risk. *Nat. Rev. Endocrinol.* **5:** 253–261.

114. Nedeltcheva, A.V. *et al.* 2009. Exposure to recurrent sleep restriction in the setting of high caloric intake and physical inactivity results in increased insulin resistance and reduced glucose tolerance. *J. Clin. Endocrinol. Metab.* **94:** 3242–3250.

115. Hara, R. *et al.* 2001. Restricted feeding entrains liver clock without participation of the suprachiasmatic nucleus. *Genes Cells* **6:** 269–278.

116. Sutton, G.M. *et al.* 2008. The melanocortin-3 receptor is required for entrainment to meal intake. *J. Neurosci.* **28:** 12946–12955.

117. Castillo, M.R. *et al.* 2004. Entrainment of the master circadian clock by scheduled feeding. *Am. J. Physiol. Regul. Integr. Comp. Physiol.* **287:** R551–R555.

118. Martinez-Merlos, M.T. *et al.* 2004. Dissociation between adipose tissue signals, behavior and the food-entrained oscillator. *J. Endocrinol.* **181:** 53–63.

119. Arble, D.M. *et al.* 2009. Circadian timing of food intake contributes to weight gain. *Obesity* **17:** 2100–2102.

120. Salgado-Delgado, R. *et al.* 2008. Internal desynchronization in a model of night-work by forced activity in rats. *Neuroscience* **154:** 922–931.

121. Salgado-Delgado, R. *et al.* 2010. Food intake during the normal activity phase prevents obesity and circadian desynchrony in a rat model of night work. *Endocrinology* **151:** 1019–1029.

122. Arendt, J. 2010. Shift work: coping with the biological clock. *Occup. Med. (Lond)* **60:** 10–20.

123. Goel, N. *et al.* 2009. Circadian rhythm profiles in women with night eating syndrome. *J. Biol. Rhythms* **24:** 85–94.

124. Colles, S.L., J.B. Dixon & P.E. O'Brien. 2007. Night eating syndrome and nocturnal snacking: association with obesity, binge eating and psychological distress. *Int. J. Obes. (Lond)* **31:** 1722–1730.

125. Lundgren, J.D. *et al.* 2010. The relationship of night eating to oral health and obesity in community dental clinic patients. *Gen. Dent.* **58:** e134–e139.

126. Striegel-Moore, R.H. *et al.* 2010. Nocturnal eating: association with binge eating, obesity, and psychological distress. *Int. J. Eat. Disord.* **43:** 520–526.

127. Teboul, M. *et al.* 2008. The nuclear hormone receptor family round the clock. *Mol. Endocrinol.* **22:** 2573–2582.

128. Adelmant, G. *et al.* 1996. A functional Rev-erb alpha responsive element located in the human Rev-erb alpha promoter mediates a repressing activity. *Proc. Natl. Acad. Sci. USA* **93:** 3553–3558.

129. Raspe, E. *et al.* 2002. Transcriptional regulation of human Rev-erbalpha gene expression by the orphan nuclear receptor retinoic acid-related orphan receptor alpha. *J. Biol. Chem.* **277:** 49275–49281.

130. Vu-Dac, N. *et al.* 1997. Transcriptional regulation of apolipoprotein A-I gene expression by the nuclear receptor RORalpha. *J. Biol. Chem.* **272:** 22401–22404.

131. Kallen, J. *et al.* 2004. Crystal structure of the human RORalpha Ligand binding domain in complex with cholesterol sulfate at 2.2 A. *J. Biol. Chem.* **279:** 14033–14038.

132. Vu-Dac, N. *et al.* 1998. The nuclear receptors peroxisome proliferator-activated receptor alpha and Rev-erbalpha mediate the species-specific regulation of apolipoprotein A-I expression by fibrates. *J. Biol. Chem.* **273:** 25713–25720.

133. Yin, L. & M.A. Lazar. 2005. The orphan nuclear receptor Rev-erbalpha recruits the N-CoR/histone deacetylase 3 corepressor to regulate the circadian Bmal1 gene. *Mol. Endocrinol.* **19:** 1452–1459.

134. Alenghat, T. *et al.* 2008. Nuclear receptor corepressor and histone deacetylase 3 govern circadian metabolic physiology. *Nature* **456:** 997–1000.

135. Feng, D. *et al.* 2011. A circadian rhythm orchestrated by histone deacetylase 3 controls hepatic lipid metabolism. *Science* **331:** 1315–1319.

136. Tsiftsoglou, A.S., A.I. Tsamadou & L.C. Papadopoulou. 2006. Heme as key regulator of major mammalian cellular functions: molecular, cellular, and pharmacological aspects. *Pharmacol. Ther.* **111:** 327–345.

137. Kaasik, K. & C.C. Lee. 2004. Reciprocal regulation of haem biosynthesis and the circadian clock in mammals. *Nature* **430:** 467–471.

138. Raghuram, S. *et al.* 2007. Identification of heme as the ligand for the orphan nuclear receptors REV-ERBalpha and REV-ERBbeta. *Nat. Struct. Mol. Biol.* **14:** 1207–1213.

139. Zheng, B. *et al.* 2001. Nonredundant roles of the mPer1 and mPer2 genes in the mammalian circadian clock. *Cell* **105:** 683–694.

140. Handschin, C. *et al.* 2005. Nutritional regulation of hepatic heme biosynthesis and porphyria through PGC-1alpha. *Cell* **122:** 505–515.

141. Lin, J., C. Handschin & B.M. Spiegelman. 2005. Metabolic control through the PGC-1 family of transcription coactivators. *Cell Metab.* **1:** 361–370.

142. Liu, C. *et al.* 2007. Transcriptional coactivator PGC-1alpha integrates the mammalian clock and energy metabolism. *Nature* **447:** 477–481.

143. Dioum, E.M. *et al.* 2002. NPAS2: a gas-responsive transcription factor. *Science* **298:** 2385–2387.

144. Gervois, P. *et al.* 2000. Regulation of lipid and lipoprotein metabolism by PPAR activators. *Clin. Chem. Lab. Med.* **38:** 3–11.

145. Yoon, M. 2009. The role of PPARalpha in lipid metabolism and obesity: focusing on the effects of estrogen on PPARalpha actions. *Pharmacol. Res.* **60:** 151–159.

146. Canaple, L. *et al.* 2006. Reciprocal regulation of brain and muscle Arnt-like protein 1 and peroxisome proliferator-activated receptor alpha defines a novel positive feedback loop in the rodent liver circadian clock. *Mol. Endocrinol.* **20:** 1715–1727.

147. Oishi, K., H. Shirai & N. Ishida. 2005. CLOCK is involved in the circadian transactivation of peroxisome-proliferator-activated receptor alpha (PPARalpha) in mice. *Biochem. J.* **386:** 575–581.

148. Gervois, P. *et al.* 1999. Fibrates increase human REV-ERBalpha expression in liver via a novel peroxisome proliferator-activated receptor response element. *Mol. Endocrinol.* **13:** 400–409.

149. Puigserver, P. *et al.* 1998. A cold-inducible coactivator of nuclear receptors linked to adaptive thermogenesis. *Cell* **92:** 829–839.

150. Sears, I.B. *et al.* 1996. Differentiation-dependent expression of the brown adipocyte uncoupling protein gene: regulation by peroxisome proliferator-activated receptor gamma. *Mol. Cell. Biol.* **16:** 3410–3419.

151. Asher, G. & U. Schibler. 2011. Crosstalk between components of circadian and metabolic cycles in mammals. *Cell Metab.* **13:** 125–137.

152. Rutter, J. *et al.* 2001. Regulation of clock and NPAS2 DNA binding by the redox state of NAD cofactors. *Science* **293:** 510–514.

153. Williamson, D.H., P. Lund & H.A. Krebs. 1967. The redox state of free nicotinamide-adenine dinucleotide in the cytoplasm and mitochondria of rat liver. *Biochem. J.* **103:** 514–527.

154. Yu, J. & J. Auwerx. 2009. The role of sirtuins in the control of metabolic homeostasis. *Ann. N.Y. Acad. Sci.* **1173**(Suppl 1): E10–E19.

155. Dali-Youcef, N. *et al.* 2007. Sirtuins: the 'magnificent seven', function, metabolism and longevity. *Ann. Med.* **39:** 335–345.

156. Blander, G. & L. Guarente. 2004. The Sir2 family of protein deacetylases. *Annu. Rev. Biochem.* **73:** 417–435.

157. Asher, G. *et al.* 2008. SIRT1 regulates circadian clock gene expression through PER2 deacetylation. *Cell* **134:** 317–328.

158. Nakahata, Y. *et al.* 2008. The NAD+-dependent deacetylase SIRT1 modulates CLOCK-mediated chromatin remodeling and circadian control. *Cell* **134:** 329–340.

159. Rodgers, J.T. *et al.* 2005. Nutrient control of glucose homeostasis through a complex of PGC-1alpha and SIRT1. *Nature* **434:** 113–118.

160. Purushotham, A. *et al.* 2009. Hepatocyte-specific deletion of SIRT1 alters fatty acid metabolism and results in hepatic steatosis and inflammation. *Cell Metab.* **9:** 327–338.

161. Picard, F. *et al.* 2004. Sirt1 promotes fat mobilization in white adipocytes by repressing PPAR-gamma. *Nature* **429:** 771–776.

162. Villaret, A. *et al.* 2010. Adipose tissue endothelial cells from obese human subjects: differences among depots in angiogenic, metabolic, and inflammatory gene expression and cellular senescence. *Diabetes* **59:** 2755–2763.

163. Barzilai, N. & I. Gabriely. 2001. The role of fat depletion in the biological benefits of caloric restriction. *J. Nutr.* **131:** 903S–906S.

164. Kahn, B.B. *et al.* 2005. AMP-activated protein kinase: ancient energy gauge provides clues to modern understanding of metabolism. *Cell Metab.* **1:** 15–25.

165. Canto, C. *et al.* 2009. AMPK regulates energy expenditure by modulating NAD+ metabolism and SIRT1 activity. *Nature* **458:** 1056–1060.

166. Vieira, E. *et al.* 2008. Relationship between AMPK and the transcriptional balance of clock-related genes in skeletal muscle. *Am. J. Physiol. Endocrinol. Metab.* **295:** E1032–E1037.

167. Lamia, K.A. *et al.* 2009. AMPK regulates the circadian clock by cryptochrome phosphorylation and degradation. *Science* **326:** 437–440.

168. Um, J.H. *et al.* 2007. Activation of 5'-AMP-activated kinase with diabetes drug metformin induces casein kinase Iepsilon (CKIepsilon)-dependent degradation of clock protein mPer2. *J. Biol. Chem.* **282:** 20794–20798.

169. Um, J.H. *et al.* 2011. AMPK regulates circadian rhythms in a tissue- and isoform-specific manner. *PLoS One* **6:** e18450.

170. Ramsey, K.M. *et al.* 2009. Circadian clock feedback cycle through NAMPT-mediated NAD+ biosynthesis. *Science* **324:** 651–654.

171. Nakahata, Y. *et al.* 2009. Circadian control of the NAD+ salvage pathway by CLOCK-SIRT1. *Science* **324:** 654–657.

172. Bordone, L. & L. Guarente. 2005. Calorie restriction, SIRT1 and metabolism: understanding longevity. *Nat. Rev. Mol. Cell. Biol.* **6:** 298–305.

173. O'Neill, J.S. & A.B. Reddy. 2011. Circadian clocks in human red blood cells. *Nature* **469:** 498–503.

Ann. N.Y. Acad. Sci. ISSN 0077-8923

ANNALS OF THE NEW YORK ACADEMY OF SCIENCES
Issue: *The Year in Diabetes and Obesity*

The role of stearoyl-CoA desaturase in obesity, insulin resistance, and inflammation

Harini Sampath[1] and James M. Ntambi[2]

[1]Center for Research on Occupational and Environmental Toxicology, Oregon Health & Science University, Portland, Oregon.
[2]Departments of Biochemistry and Nutritional Sciences, University of Wisconsin-Madison, Madison, Wisconsin

Address for correspondence: James M. Ntambi, Department of Biochemistry, University of Wisconsin, 433 Babcock Drive, Madison, WI 53706. ntambi@biochem.wisc.edu

Stearoyl-CoA desaturase 1 (SCD1) is an essential lipogenic enzyme that has been shown to play an intrinsic role in the development of obesity and related conditions, such as insulin resistance. Through the generation of various mouse models of SCD1 deficiency, we have come to understand that SCD1 plays a role, directly or indirectly, in diverse metabolic processes, including lipogenesis, fatty acid oxidation, insulin signaling, thermogenesis, and inflammation. This review will address recent advances in our understanding of this key regulator of cellular metabolic processes, including the role of SCD1 in maintaining skin barrier integrity and the role of skin SCD1 in the metabolic phenotype elicited by global SCD1 deficiency.

Keywords: lipogenesis; fatty acid oxidation; skin barrier; thermogenesis; leptin resistance

Introduction

Stearoyl-CoA desaturase (SCD) is a membrane-bound delta-9 desaturase that catalyzes the insertion of the first cis-double bond at the delta-9 position of 12–19 carbon saturated fatty acids, thereby converting them to monounsaturated fatty acids (MUFAs). The degree of unsaturation of cellular lipids plays a role in cell signaling and membrane fluidity. In addition, the monounsaturated products of SCD are the major substrates for synthesis of complex lipids such as diacylglycerols, phospholipids, triglycerides (TGs), wax esters, and cholesterol esters. Therefore, SCD is a highly regulated and conserved enzyme with multiple isoforms having overlapping but distinct tissue distribution and substrate specificity.[1,2] Like other desaturases, SCD is a nonheme iron-containing enzyme and requires molecular oxygen, NADH, as well as cytochrome b5 and cytochrome b5 reductase, or an alternate electron transport system for catalytic activity. The SCD protein is anchored in the ER membrane via four transmembrane domains with both N- and C-termini facing the cytosol, and three conserved and catalytically important his-box motifs.[3,4]

There are four known isoforms of SCD (SCD1–4) in the mouse,[5–10] all located within a 200-kb region on chromosome 19 and encoding 350–360 amino acid proteins with >80% amino acid sequence identity. Differences in the 5'-flanking region confer some divergence in tissue-specificity among the isoforms. *Scd2* shares significant sequence homology with *Scd1* and is ubiquitously expressed but is especially high in the murine brain, particularly during the neonatal myelination period.[6,7] In the mouse, SCD2 appears to play an important role during development and is required for the formation of an intact skin barrier in the neonate.[7] SCD3 is expressed in the Harderian gland and skin of the mouse, albeit at significantly lower levels than SCD1, and shows a preference for palmitoyl-CoA over stearoyl-CoA.[5,9,11] SCD4 is mainly expressed in the heart and is greatly induced in the heart of $Scd1^{-/-}$ mice.[8,12]

The remainder of this review will focus on SCD1, the best-characterized isoform of SCD, and its role in obesity and related pathologies. The majority of what we know regarding the role of SCD1 in obesity and related conditions comes from studies conducted in mice with either a naturally occurring mutation of the *Scd1* gene (asebia mice) or mice with a targeted deletion of the enzyme. Tissue-specific roles of SCD1 are also being delineated, largely because of the creation of conditional knockout mouse models and transient knock-down models using antisense oligonucleotides (ASO). There is also significant interest in understanding the potential role of SCD1 in human disease; this topic has been recently reviewed elsewhere.[13]

SCD1: expression and regulation

The mouse SCD1 isoform has been very well characterized for both its systemic roles as well as tissue-specific contributions. It is expressed ubiquitously and is significantly induced in liver in response to high-carbohydrate feeding and saturated fat feeding.[14–17] In addition, it is expressed in the undifferentiated cells of the sebaceous gland in the skin, where it plays a critical role in maintenance of sebocyte development and skin lipid composition.[10,18,19] It prefers palmitate and stearate as substrates, converting them to palmitoleate and oleate, respectively. Despite the relative abundance of these MUFA products in both our diets and tissues, SCD1 is a highly regulated enzyme, suggesting that the endogenous synthesis of MUFAs may play a distinct role in cell signaling as compared to MUFAs derived from the diet.

The *Scd1* gene is induced by glucose, fructose, saturated fatty acids, and insulin, as well as by the actions of the lipogenic transcription factor sterol regulatory element binding protein-1c (SREBP-1c) and the nuclear receptor, LXR.[2,20] Conversely, the adipokine leptin, as well as polyunsaturated fatty acids, are known repressors of *Scd1* gene expression.[2,20] The SCD1 protein is also regulated post-translationally. SCD1 is rapidly degraded in microsomal fractions with a half-life of three to four hours at 37 °C via a microsomal protease that has been identified as a plasminogen-like protease.[21–23] In addition, SCD1 is also known to be degraded via the proteasomal pathway, which requires a 66-residue N-terminal segment of the protein containing PEST sequences.[24] Mainly through studies using various rodent models of SCD1 deficiency, SCD1 has been shown to play a critical role in the development of metabolic diseases, including diet and leptin-deficiency or leptin-resistance induced obesity, hepatic steatosis, insulin resistance, and atherosclerosis, as well as diverse metabolic processes including

maintenance of skin barrier integrity and nonshivering thermogenesis.[10,12,14–18,25–36]

Role of SCD1 in hepatic lipogenesis and atherosclerosis

The SCD1 enzyme plays a central role in the *de novo* lipogenic pathway, by catalyzing the further processing of fats synthesized by fatty acid synthase into products that are primed for incorporation into storage lipids, such as TGs. Furthermore, given its upregulation by prolipogenic hormones and transcription factors such as insulin and SREBP-1c, it has become clear that SCD1 plays a vital role in *de novo* lipogenesis. Indeed, mice deficient in SCD1 because of a targeted whole-body deletion of the enzyme are extremely resistant to a high-carbohydrate diet-induced obesity and hepatic steatosis.[14–16] A large part of this protection from glucose- and fructose-induced pathologies appears to be due to reductions in hepatic lipogenesis, since liver-specific deletion of SCD1 in a conditional knockout confers the same protection from carbohydrate-induced obesity and hepatic steatosis as whole body deletion of SCD1.[15]

Interestingly, not only are *Scd1*$^{-/-}$ mice protected from carbohydrate-induced obesity, but also from many of the deleterious effects of saturated fats, including increased hepatic lipogenesis, hypertriglyceridemia, weight gain, and insulin resistance.[15,17,32] Both whole-body and liver-specific SCD1 knockouts are resistant to saturated fat induced increases in *de novo* lipogenesis.[15,17] Furthermore, concurrent transient knockdown of SCD1 in liver, adipose, and macrophages via ASO confers a similar protection from saturated fat–induced hepatic steatosis and obesity.[32]

Interestingly, transient knockdown of hepatic and adipose SCD1 by ASO does not seem to confer protection against atherosclerosis, despite reductions in hepatic lipogenesis and circulating lipids.[32] In fact, SCD1-knockdown mice developed greater atherosclerotic lesions, especially in the abdominal aorta, compared to control mice, with a significant enrichment of circulating lipoproteins and macrophages with saturated fatty acids.[32] This study also reported a hypersensitivity to toll-like receptor-4 agonists in macrophages derived from SCD1-knockdown animals, suggesting that increased inflammatory cytokine release from SCD1-knockdown macrophages may mediate the increased incidence of atherosclerosis in these mice.[32]

Although these phenotypes were not reversed by supplementing the diet of SCD1-knockdown animals with MUFAs, feeding n-3 PUFAs derived from fish oil in a subsequent report appeared to abolish the atherosclerosis associated with SCD1-knockdown.[37] Another study using the naturally occurring global SCD1-deletion strain ab[J] in the hypercholesterolemic LDL-receptor deficient background reported similar increases in atherosclerosis, despite reductions in hepatic steatosis and circulating lipids in SCD1-deficient mice.[31] However, this study did not find an altered macrophage inflammatory response in macrophages derived from SCD1-deficient mice nor indeed any effect of SCD1 deficiency on macrophage function.[31] Therefore, the role of SCD1 in macrophages and associated inflammation is as yet unclear. To further complicate the story, another study[38] reported that chronic intermittent hypoxia (CIH), which is associated with atherosclerosis, was accompanied, in human subjects, with increased hepatic SCD1 levels. Conversely, ASO inhibition of SCD1 in a murine model of CIH resulted in significantly reduced rates of both dyslipidemia and atherosclerosis.[38] Therefore, further studies are certainly warranted in establishing either a pro- or antiatherosclerotic role for SCD1 and examining adjuvant therapies to combat any undesirable proatherosclerotic side effects of pharmacological inhibition of SCD1.

Role of SCD1 in fatty acid oxidation and thermogenesis

Although the essential role of SCD1 in lipogenesis elucidated via these animal studies is not entirely surprising, a unique feature of the SCD1-deficient mouse model is the observed increase in lipid oxidation. This increase in fat oxidation greatly contributes to their protection from diet-induced obesity, especially in the face of diets containing high amounts of MUFAs.[10,17,35,36,39,40] After a four-hour fast, levels of β-hydroxybutyrate were significantly higher in $Scd1^{-/-}$ mice, relative to WT controls, indicating increased fatty acid oxidation in these mice.[10] It has since been shown that indeed, fatty acid oxidation is significantly increased in liver, brown adipose tissue (BAT), and skeletal muscle of mice with a global SCD1 deficiency.[35,39,40] This increase in fatty acid oxidation is mediated, at least partly, by induction of the AMP-activated protein

kinase (AMPK), resulting in phosphorylation and inactivation of acetyl-CoA carboxylase (ACC), and a consequent derepression of the carnitine palmitoyl transferase-1 (CPT-1) enzyme responsible for transport of fatty acids into the mitochondria for β-oxidation.[40] In addition, as the product of ACC, malonyl-CoA can act as a repressor of CPT-1, the reduction in gene expression of Acc in $Scd1^{-/-}$ mice[14–17] likely plays a role in the robust upregulation in fatty acid oxidation observed in these mice. In addition, genes of fatty acid oxidation, including $Cpt-1$, acyl CoA oxidase, and very long-chain acyl-CoA dehydrogenase are also upregulated in $Scd1^{-/-}$ mice.[10] Although the nuclear receptor peroxisome proliferator activated receptor-alpha (PPARα) is a major player in transcriptional regulation of fatty acid oxidation,[20] it does not appear to be required for the induction of oxidative genes because of SCD1 deficiency, because deletion of SCD1 in a PPARα-null mouse model does not abolish the effects of SCD1 deletion of fatty acid oxidation.[41] In addition to fatty acid oxidation, whole body thermogenesis is also significantly upregulated in $Scd1^{-/-}$ mice. Increased signaling through the β3-adrenergic receptor pathway in BAT of $Scd1^{-/-}$ mice results in activation of the peroxisome proliferator-activated receptor-gamma coactivator-1alpha and increased uncoupling via uncoupling protein-1, thereby increasing the rate of basal thermogenesis and consequently, whole body energy expenditure, in $Scd1^{-/-}$ mice.[35]

Although global deletion of SCD1 upregulates systemic fatty acid oxidation and protects animals from high-fat diet induced weight gain, liver-specific deletion of SCD1 does not confer the same protection from high-fat diet (HFD)-induced obesity, or upregulate fatty acid oxidation, or thermogenesis.[15] In addition to the metabolic role of SCD1, one of the first observations in mice lacking SCD1 was the development of severe alopecia and sebocyte hypoplasia, leading to dry skin with altered lipid composition. Given these cutaneous abnormalities in SCD1-deficient mice, a skin-specific model of SCD1-ablation was developed.[18] Interestingly, deletion of SCD1 in the skin not only recapitulated all the cutaneous phenotypes observed in $Scd1^{-/-}$ mice, but also induced genes of fatty acid oxidation and thermogenesis, and increased whole body energy expenditure in animals, thereby protecting them from

HFD-induced weight gain.[18] Interestingly, however, maintaining skin-specific $Scd1^{-/-}$ mice in a thermoneutral environment did not abolish their protection from diet-induced obesity.[42] Skin-specific deletion of SCD1, unlike global SCD1 deletion, did not protect mice from fasting–refeeding induced hepatic lipogenesis.[18] Therefore, although some of the favorable metabolic features of global SCD1 deletion may be explained by increased energy demands because of heat loss in the $Scd1^{-/-}$ mouse, the insights gained from liver and skin-specific SCD1 deletion have helped to uncouple the effects of SCD1 deletion on hepatic lipogenesis, specifically, from those on whole body energy expenditure, thermogenesis, and lipid oxidation. Furthermore, these studies in the skin-specific $Scd1^{-/-}$ mice underscore the need for similar studies in mouse models such as the $Dgat1^{-/-}$ mouse, which also displays protection from diet-induced obesity and cutaneous abnormalities.[43–45] For a more detailed review on the consideration of nonshivering thermogenesis in metabolic studies, the reader is directed to recent review on the topic.[46]

The role of SCD1 in insulin sensitivity

In addition to resistance to obesity and hepatic steatosis, $Scd1^{-/-}$ mice are also protected from the pathological decline in insulin sensitivity that often accompanies obesity and fatty liver.[28–30] Despite having lower fasting plasma insulin levels, $Scd1^{-/-}$ mice have increased insulin signaling through increased insulin receptor tyrosine phosphorylation and reduced Ser/Thr phosphorylation of IRS-1 in multiple tissues, including skeletal muscle, liver, adipose tissue, and heart.[12,27–30,35] In addition, levels of protein tyrosine phosphatase-1B, which has been shown to attenuate insulin signaling,[47,48] are reduced in skeletal muscle and BAT of $Scd1^{-/-}$ mice.[29,30] Furthermore, as mentioned above, AMPK activation and fatty acid oxidation are significantly increased in liver, muscle, and BAT, and ceramide synthesis and content is significantly reduced in muscle of $Scd1^{-/-}$ mice.[35,39,40] Because ceramides are thought to mediate lipid-induced aberrations in insulin signaling,[49–51] the reductions in ceramide synthesis and increased fat oxidation in $Scd1^{-/-}$ mice may also contribute to their increased insulin sensitivity.

SCD1 deficiency has been shown to significantly improve insulin signaling in both a high-fat-diet–induced model of obesity, as well as in the leptin-resistant agouti obese mouse.[28] Transient knockdown of hepatic and adipose SCD1 by ASO treatment has also been shown to attenuate diet-induced obesity and improve hepatic insulin signaling,[52,53] although similar effects were not observed in liver-specific $Scd1^{-/-}$ mice.[15] It has been recently reported that skin-specific deletion of SCD1 also completely protects mice against diet-induced insulin resistance, likely because of a protection from diet-induced obesity and hepatic steatosis.[18] A recent study also showed that inhibition of SCD1 in 3T3-L1 adipocytes stimulated basal glucose uptake via an upregulation of GLUT-1, without any changes in GLUT-4 levels.[54] However, adipose-specific deletion of SCD1, although resulting in increased GLUT-1 levels, did not confer increased insulin sensitivity in mice.[54]

Although SCD1 deficiency attenuates obesity to a significant extent in several mouse models of obesity, including the leptin-resistant ob/ob mouse, insulin signaling parameters are not improved by SCD1 deficiency in this background.[27,28] In fact, in the context of a diabetes-prone BtBr mouse strain, SCD1 deficiency appears to exacerbate the diabetic phenotype of leptin-deficient ob/ob mice, by impairing islet function.[27] In the more widely studied C57Bl/6 strain, however, SCD1 deficiency does not cause reduced insulin levels in ob/ob mice, arguing against an islet defect in this background.[28] However, regardless of the underlying mechanism, it appears that the increased insulin signaling observed upon global SCD1 inhibition requires the presence of leptin.[28]

SCD1 in inflammation and cancer

Obesity is generally accompanied by chronic inflammation, which plays a role in many of the secondary pathologies associated with obesity. Therefore, SCD1 inhibition, which is associated with reduced obesity, but may result in increased saturated fat accumulation, is of particular interest in studying the link between obesity and inflammation. The tissue-specific roles of SCD1 in inflammation have been recently reviewed in detail elsewhere.[55] In brief, the few studies to date examining the role of SCD1 in various types of inflammation have not yielded consistent support for either a pro- or anti-inflammatory role for SCD1. For instance, as discussed above, studies on the role of SCD1 in atherosclerosis and insulin signaling have suggested a potential macrophage inflammation phenotype and β cell dysfunction, as well as increased systemic inflammation associated with SCD1 deletion.[27,31,32] However, other studies have also suggested that macrophage inflammation is unaffected by SCD1 inhibition.[31,56] Similarly, although SCD1 inhibition has been shown to reduce adipose inflammation,[56] adipose-specific inhibition of SCD1 results in slightly increased expression of the proinflammatory cytokine tumor necrosis factor α and reduced levels of circulating adiponectin.[54] In addition to these organ systems, SCD1 also appears to play a role in ulcerative colitis,[57,58] cutaneous inflammation,[42,59,60] and myocyte[61] and endothelial dysfunction.[62,63] Although the role of SCD1 on inflammation appears to vary somewhat by tissue-type, it is interesting to note that in so many instances, inhibition of SCD1 causes increased inflammation, despite amelioration of metabolic disease, which is generally associated with an improvement of inflammation. Given this dichotomy, it becomes particularly interesting to examine the role of SCD1 in the development of cancer, which has been associated with both obesity and lipid accumulation, as well as inflammation.[64–66] Since the hyperproliferative nature of cancer cells places a greater demand for synthesis of lipids for cellular constituents and energy demands, it follows that increased SCD1 activity may be required to meet this demand. Indeed, as has been reviewed extensively elsewhere, SCD1 has been reported to be induced in many cancers, including esophageal and colonic carcinomas and hepatic adenomas.[67] Furthermore, SCD1 inhibition appears to have an antiproliferative effect on many neoplastic cell types including lung, prostate, colon, and breast cancer cells,[68–73] leading to suggestions that SCD1 may be a druggable target in the fight against cancer.[73,74] In contrast, a study has reported a consistent reduction in SCD1 activity in prostate carcinomas,[75] suggesting that the role of SCD1 in tumorigenesis may not be generalized across cancer types. Furthermore, given that particular cancers, such as hepatocellular carcinomas (HCCs), are known to be affected by both severity of hepatic steatosis as well as by downstream inflammation,[64] it will be interesting to see if the divergence of metabolic symptoms and inflammatory markers in the $Scd1^{-/-}$ mouse model can be exploited to understand the mechanisms leading to the development of cancers such as HCCs.

SCD1: a double-edged sword

Initially identified from a model of alopecia and sebocyte atrophy, a compelling role for SCD1 in the development of obesity, hepatic steatosis, and obesity-associated insulin and leptin resistance has been established. Emerging evidence suggests that unqualified inhibition of SCD1, whether systemic or restricted to specific organ systems, may not be desirable as it may result in an increased propensity to cellular inflammation. Furthermore, any consideration of SCD1 as a pharmaceutical target will have to differentiate between metabolic phenotypes elicited by local SCD1 inhibition in tissues such as liver versus indirect effects of SCD1 inhibition in peripheral tissues such as skin. Nevertheless, the multiple rodent models that have been developed, as well as several pharmacological inhibitors that are currently available, will likely increase our understanding of this enzyme that appears to have a dual role in mediating the progression of obesity and related pathologies.

Conflicts of interest

The authors declare no conflicts of interest.

References

1. Nakamura, M.T. & T.Y. Nara. 2004. Structure, function, and dietary regulation of delta6, delta5, and delta9 desaturases. *Annu. Rev. Nutr.* **24:** 345–376.
2. Sampath, H. & J.M. Ntambi. 2006. Stearoyl-coenzyme A desaturase 1, sterol regulatory element binding protein-1c and peroxisome proliferator-activated receptor-alpha: independent and interactive roles in the regulation of lipid metabolism. *Curr. Opin. Clin. Nutr. Metab. Care* **9:** 84–88.
3. Man, W.C. *et al.* 2006. Membrane topology of mouse stearoyl-CoA desaturase 1. *J. Biol. Chem.* **281:** 1251–1260.
4. Shanklin, J. & E.B. Cahoon. 1998. Desaturation and related modifications of fatty acids. *Annu. Rev. Plant Physiol. Plant Mol. Biol.* **49:** 611–641.
5. Miyazaki, M., S.M. Bruggink & J.M. Ntambi. 2006. Identification of mouse palmitoyl-coenzyme A Delta9-desaturase. *J. Lipid Res.* **47:** 700–704.
6. Kaestner, K.H. *et al.* 1989. Differentiation-induced gene expression in 3T3-L1 preadipocytes. A second differentially expressed gene encoding stearoyl-CoA desaturase. *J. Biol. Chem.* **264:** 14755–14761.
7. Miyazaki, M. *et al.* 2005. Stearoyl-CoA desaturase-2 gene expression is required for lipid synthesis during early skin and liver development. *Proc. Natl. Acad. Sci. USA* **102:** 12501–12506.

8. Miyazaki, M. *et al.* 2003. Identification and characterization of murine SCD4, a novel heart-specific stearoyl-CoA desaturase isoform regulated by leptin and dietary factors. *J. Biol. Chem.* **278:** 33904–33911.

9. Zheng, Y. *et al.* 2001. Scd3–a novel gene of the stearoyl-CoA desaturase family with restricted expression in skin. *Genomics* **71:** 182–191.

10. Ntambi, J.M. *et al.* 2002. Loss of stearoyl-CoA desaturase-1 function protects mice against adiposity. *Proc. Natl. Acad. Sci. USA* **99:** 11482–11486.

11. Miyazaki, M. *et al.* 2001. Oleoyl-CoA is the major de novo product of stearoyl-CoA desaturase 1 gene isoform and substrate for the biosynthesis of the Harderian gland 1-alkyl-2,3-diacylglycerol. *J. Biol. Chem.* **276:** 39455–39461.

12. Dobrzyn, P. *et al.* 2008. Loss of stearoyl-CoA desaturase 1 inhibits fatty acid oxidation and increases glucose utilization in the heart. *Am. J. Physiol. Endocrinol. Metab.* **294:** E357–E364.

13. Sampath, H.N. & M. James. 2008. Role of stearoyl-CoA desaturase in human metabolic disease. *Future Lipidology* **3:** 163–173.

14. Miyazaki, M. *et al.* 2004. Stearoyl-CoA desaturase 1 gene expression is necessary for fructose-mediated induction of lipogenic gene expression by sterol regulatory element-binding protein-1c-dependent and -independent mechanisms. *J. Biol. Chem.* **279:** 25164–25171.

15. Miyazaki, M. *et al.* 2007. Hepatic stearoyl-CoA desaturase-1 deficiency protects mice from carbohydrate-induced adiposity and hepatic steatosis. *Cell. Metab.* **6:** 484–496.

16. Miyazaki, M., Y.C. Kim & J.M. Ntambi. 2001. A lipogenic diet in mice with a disruption of the stearoyl-CoA desaturase 1 gene reveals a stringent requirement of endogenous monounsaturated fatty acids for triglyceride synthesis. *J. Lipid Res.* **42:** 1018–1024.

17. Sampath, H. *et al.* 2007. Stearoyl-CoA desaturase-1 mediates the pro-lipogenic effects of dietary saturated fat. *J. Biol. Chem.* **282:** 2483–2493.

18. Sampath, H. *et al.* 2009. Skin-specific deletion of stearoyl-CoA desaturase-1 alters skin lipid composition and protects mice from high fat diet-induced obesity. *J. Biol. Chem.* **284:** 19961–19973.

19. Sundberg, J.P. *et al.* 2000. Asebia-2J (Scd1(ab2J)): a new allele and a model for scarring alopecia. *Am. J. Pathol.* **156:** 2067–2075.

20. Sampath, H. & J.M. Ntambi. 2005. Polyunsaturated fatty acid regulation of genes of lipid metabolism. *Annu. Rev. Nutr.* **25:** 317–340.

21. Heinemann, F.S., G. Korza & J. Ozols. 2003. A plasminogen-like protein selectively degrades stearoyl-CoA desaturase in liver microsomes. *J. Biol. Chem.* **278:** 42966–42975.

22. Heinemann, F.S. *et al.* 2003. A microsomal endopeptidase from liver that preferentially degrades stearoyl-CoA desaturase. *Biochemistry* **42:** 6929–6937.

23. Heinemann, F.S. & J. Ozols. 1998. Degradation of stearoyl-coenzyme A desaturase: endoproteolytic cleavage by an integral membrane protease. *Mol. Biol. Cell* **9:** 3445–3453.

24. Kato, H., K. Sakaki & K. Mihara. 2006. Ubiquitin-proteasome-dependent degradation of mammalian ER stearoyl-CoA desaturase. *J. Cell Sci.* **119:** 2342–2353.

25. Biddinger, S.B. *et al.* 2006. Leptin suppresses stearoyl-CoA desaturase 1 by mechanisms independent of insulin and sterol regulatory element-binding protein-1c. *Diabetes* **55:** 2032–2041.

26. Dobrzyn, P. *et al.* 2010. Loss of stearoyl-CoA desaturase 1 rescues cardiac function in obese leptin-deficient mice. *J. Lipid Res.* **51:** 2202–2210.

27. Flowers, J.B. *et al.* 2007. Loss of stearoyl-CoA desaturase-1 improves insulin sensitivity in lean mice but worsens diabetes in leptin-deficient obese mice. *Diabetes* **56:** 1228–1239.

28. Miyazaki, M. *et al.* 2009. Stearoyl-CoA desaturase-1 deficiency attenuates obesity and insulin resistance in leptin-resistant obese mice. *Biochem. Biophys. Res. Commun.* **380:** 818–822.

29. Rahman, S.M. *et al.* 2003. Stearoyl-CoA desaturase 1 deficiency elevates insulin-signaling components and down-regulates protein-tyrosine phosphatase 1B in muscle. *Proc. Natl. Acad. Sci. USA* **100:** 11110–11115.

30. Rahman, S.M. *et al.* 2005. Stearoyl-CoA desaturase 1 deficiency increases insulin signaling and glycogen accumulation in brown adipose tissue. *Am. J. Physiol. Endocrinol. Metab.* **288:** E381–E387.

31. MacDonald, M.L. *et al.* 2009. Despite antiatherogenic metabolic characteristics, SCD1-deficient mice have increased inflammation and atherosclerosis. *Arterioscler. Thromb Vasc. Biol.* **29:** 341–347.

32. Brown, J.M. *et al.* 2008. Inhibition of stearoyl-coenzyme A desaturase 1 dissociates insulin resistance and obesity from atherosclerosis. *Circulation* **118:** 1467–1475.

33. Feingold, K.R. 2009. The outer frontier: the importance of lipid metabolism in the skin. *J. Lipid Res.* **50 Suppl:** S417–S422.

34. Fluhr, J.W. *et al.* 2003. Glycerol regulates stratum corneum hydration in sebaceous gland deficient (asebia) mice. *J. Invest. Dermatol.* **120:** 728–737.

35. Lee, S.H. *et al.* 2004. Lack of stearoyl-CoA desaturase 1 upregulates basal thermogenesis but causes hypothermia in a cold environment. *J. Lipid Res.* **45:** 1674–1682.

36. Cohen, P. *et al.* 2002. Role for stearoyl-CoA desaturase-1 in leptin-mediated weight loss. *Science* **297:** 240–243.

37. Brown, J.M. *et al.* 2010. Combined therapy of dietary fish oil and stearoyl-CoA desaturase 1 inhibition prevents the metabolic syndrome and atherosclerosis. *Arterioscler. Thromb Vasc. Biol.* **30:** 24–30.

38. Savransky, V. *et al.* 2008. Dyslipidemia and atherosclerosis induced by chronic intermittent hypoxia are attenuated by deficiency of stearoyl coenzyme A desaturase. *Circ. Res.* **103:** 1173–1180.

39. Dobrzyn, A. *et al.* 2005. Stearoyl-CoA desaturase-1 deficiency reduces ceramide synthesis by downregulating serine palmitoyltransferase and increasing beta-oxidation in skeletal muscle. *Am. J. Physiol. Endocrinol. Metab.* **288:** E599–E607.

40. Dobrzyn, P. *et al.* 2004. Stearoyl-CoA desaturase 1 deficiency increases fatty acid oxidation by activating AMP-activated protein kinase in liver. *Proc. Natl. Acad. Sci. USA* **101:** 6409–6414.

41. Miyazaki, M. *et al.* 2004. Reduced adiposity and liver steatosis by stearoyl-CoA desaturase deficiency are independent

of peroxisome proliferator-activated receptor-alpha. *J. Biol. Chem.* **279:** 35017–35024.

42. Flowers, M.T. *et al.* 2011. Metabolic changes in skin caused by Scd1 deficiency: a focus on retinol metabolism. *PLoS One* **6:** e19734.

43. Smith, S.J. *et al.* 2000. Obesity resistance and multiple mechanisms of triglyceride synthesis in mice lacking Dgat. *Nat. Genet.* **25:** 87–90.

44. Chen, H.C. *et al.* 2003. Analysis of energy expenditure at different ambient temperatures in mice lacking DGAT1. *Am. J. Physiol. Endocrinol. Metab.* **284:** E213–E218.

45. Shih, M.Y. *et al.* 2009. Retinol esterification by DGAT1 is essential for retinoid homeostasis in murine skin. *J. Biol. Chem.* **284:** 4292–4299.

46. Cannon, B. & J. Nedergaard. 2011. Nonshivering thermogenesis and its adequate measurement in metabolic studies. *J. Exp. Biol.* **214:** 242–253.

47. Ahmad, F. *et al.* 1997. Alterations in skeletal muscle protein-tyrosine phosphatase activity and expression in insulin-resistant human obesity and diabetes. *J. Clin. Invest.* **100:** 449–458.

48. Kenner, K.A. *et al.* 1993. Regulation of protein tyrosine phosphatases by insulin and insulin-like growth factor I. *J. Biol. Chem.* **268:** 25455–25462.

49. Summers, S.A. *et al.* 1998. Regulation of insulin-stimulated glucose transporter GLUT4 translocation and Akt kinase activity by ceramide. *Mol. Cell. Biol.* **18:** 5457–5464.

50. Chavez, J.A. *et al.* 2005. Acid ceramidase overexpression prevents the inhibitory effects of saturated fatty acids on insulin signaling. *J. Biol. Chem.* **280:** 20148–20153.

51. Bruce, C.R. *et al.* 2006. Endurance training in obese humans improves glucose tolerance and mitochondrial fatty acid oxidation and alters muscle lipid content. *Am. J. Physiol. Endocrinol. Metab.* **291:** E99–E107.

52. Gutierrez-Juarez, R. *et al.* 2006. Critical role of stearoyl-CoA desaturase-1 (SCD1) in the onset of diet-induced hepatic insulin resistance. *J. Clin. Invest.* **116:** 1686–1695.

53. Jiang, G. *et al.* 2005. Prevention of obesity in mice by antisense oligonucleotide inhibitors of stearoyl-CoA desaturase-1. *J. Clin. Invest.* **115:** 1030–1038.

54. Hyun, C.K. *et al.* 2010. Adipose-specific deletion of stearoyl-CoA desaturase 1 up-regulates the glucose transporter GLUT1 in adipose tissue. *Biochem. Biophys. Res. Commun.* **399:** 480–486.

55. Liu, X., M.S. Strable & J.M. Ntambi. 2011. Stearoyl CoA desaturase 1: role in cellular inflammation and stress. *Adv. Nutr.* **2:** 15–22.

56. Liu, X. *et al.* 2010. Loss of stearoyl-CoA desaturase-1 attenuates adipocyte inflammation. *Arterioscler. Thromb Vasc. Biol.* **30:** 31–38.

57. Chen, C. *et al.* 2008. Metabolomics reveals that hepatic stearoyl-CoA desaturase 1 downregulation exacerbates inflammation and acute colitis. *Cell. Metab.* **7:** 135–147.

58. MacDonald, M.L. *et al.* 2009. Absence of stearoyl-CoA desaturase-1 does not promote DSS-induced acute colitis. *Biochim. Biophys. Acta* **1791:** 1166–1172.

59. Brown, W.R. & M.H. Hardy. 1988. A hypothesis on the cause of chronic epidermal hyperproliferation in asebia mice. *Clin. Exp. Dermatol.* **13:** 74–77.

60. Oran, A. *et al.* 1997. Cyclosporin inhibits intercellular adhesion molecule-1 expression and reduces mast cell numbers in the asebia mouse model of chronic skin inflammation. *Br. J. Dermatol.* **136:** 519–526.

61. Peter, A. *et al.* 2009. Individual stearoyl-coa desaturase 1 expression modulates endoplasmic reticulum stress and inflammation in human myotubes and is associated with skeletal muscle lipid storage and insulin sensitivity in vivo. *Diabetes* **58:** 1757–1765.

62. Peter, A. *et al.* 2008. Induction of stearoyl-CoA desaturase protects human arterial endothelial cells against lipotoxicity. *Am. J. Physiol. Endocrinol. Metab.* **295:** E339–E349.

63. Qin, X. *et al.* 2007. Laminar shear stress up-regulates the expression of stearoyl-CoA desaturase-1 in vascular endothelial cells. *Cardiovasc. Res.* **74:** 506–514.

64. Park, E.J. *et al.* 2010. Dietary and genetic obesity promote liver inflammation and tumorigenesis by enhancing IL-6 and TNF expression. *Cell* **140:** 197–208.

65. Li, N., S.I. Grivennikov & M. Karin. 2011. The unholy trinity: inflammation, cytokines, and STAT3 shape the cancer microenvironment. *Cancer Cell* **19:** 429–431.

66. Calle, E.E. & R. Kaaks. 2004. Overweight, obesity and cancer: epidemiological evidence and proposed mechanisms. *Nat. Rev. Cancer* **4:** 579–591.

67. Igal, R.A. 2010. Stearoyl-CoA desaturase-1: a novel key player in the mechanisms of cell proliferation, programmed cell death and transformation to cancer. *Carcinogenesis* **31:** 1509–1515.

68. Scaglia, N., J.M. Caviglia & R.A. Igal. 2005. High stearoyl-CoA desaturase protein and activity levels in simian virus 40 transformed-human lung fibroblasts. *Biochim. Biophys. Acta* **1687:** 141–151.

69. Scaglia, N. & R.A. Igal. 2005. Stearoyl-CoA desaturase is involved in the control of proliferation, anchorage-independent growth, and survival in human transformed cells. *J. Biol. Chem.* **280:** 25339–25349.

70. Scaglia, N., J.W. Chisholm & R.A. Igal. 2009. Inhibition of stearoylCoA desaturase-1 inactivates acetyl-CoA carboxylase and impairs proliferation in cancer cells: role of AMPK. *PLoS One* **4:** e6812.

71. Hess, D., J.W. Chisholm & R.A. Igal. 2010. Inhibition of stearoylCoA desaturase activity blocks cell cycle progression and induces programmed cell death in lung cancer cells. *PLoS One* **5:** e11394.

72. Fritz, V. *et al.* 2010. Abrogation of de novo lipogenesis by stearoyl-CoA desaturase 1 inhibition interferes with oncogenic signaling and blocks prostate cancer progression in mice. *Mol. Cancer Ther.* **9:** 1740–1754.

73. Morgan-Lappe, S.E. *et al.* 2007. Identification of Ras-related nuclear protein, targeting protein for xenopus kinesin-like protein 2, and stearoyl-CoA desaturase 1 as promising cancer targets from an RNAi-based screen. *Cancer Res.* **67:** 4390–4398.

74. Brown, J.M. & L.L. Rudel. 2010. Stearoyl-coenzyme A desaturase 1 inhibition and the metabolic syndrome: considerations for future drug discovery. *Curr. Opin. Lipidol.* **21:** 192–197.

75. Moore, S. *et al.* 2005. Loss of stearoyl-CoA desaturase expression is a frequent event in prostate carcinoma. *Int. J. Cancer* **114:** 563–571.

Ann. N.Y. Acad. Sci. ISSN 0077-8923

ANNALS OF THE NEW YORK ACADEMY OF SCIENCES

Issue: *The Year in Diabetes and Obesity*

Diabetes, cancer, and metformin: connections of metabolism and cell proliferation

Emily Jane Gallagher and Derek LeRoith

Division of Endocrinology, Diabetes and Bone Diseases, Department of Medicine, Mount Sinai Medical Center, New York, New York

Address for correspondence: Derek LeRoith, Mount Sinai Medical Center, Box 1055, One Gustave L. Levy Place, New York, NY 10029. Derek.LeRoith@mssm.edu

Diabetes is associated with an increased risk of developing and dying from cancer. This increased risk may be due to hyperglycemia, hyperinsulinemia, and insulin resistance or other factors. Metformin has recently gained much attention as it appears to reduce cancer incidence and improve prognosis of patients with diabetes. *In vitro* data and animal studies support these findings from human epidemiological studies. Metformin has multiple potential mechanisms by which it inhibits cancer development and growth. For example, metaformin inhibits hepatic gluconeogenesis, thus decreasing circulating glucose levels, and it increases insulin sensitivity, thus reducing circulating insulin levels. Intracellularly, metformin activates AMPK, which decreases protein synthesis and cell proliferation. Metaformin also reduces aromatase activity in the stromal cells of the mammary gland. Finally, metformin may diminish the recurrence and aggressiveness of tumors by reducing the stem cell population and inhibiting epithelial to mesenchymal transition. Here, we discuss the metabolic abnormalities that occur in tumor development and some of the mechanisms through which metformin may alter these pathways and reduce tumor growth.

Keywords: diabetes; insulin resistance; cancer; metformin

Introduction

For over a century, an association between diabetes and cancer has been recognized.[1] Initially, many were skeptical that the association was real, including the statistician Karl Pearson, who wrote: "I must frankly admit that at first I viewed Dr. Maynard's conclusion as in some-way based on disregarded spurious correlation, and due to non-allowance for population, age or general unhealthiness factors. But I have been gradually forced by the pressure of these statistical results to consider it something very real."[2] Decades of epidemiological evidence have now accumulated, supporting the link between diabetes and an increased incidence of certain cancers in different populations, after adjusting for age and other confounding factors such as obesity. In addition, epidemiological studies report that those with diabetes who develop cancer have a worse prognosis after treatment with chemotherapy or surgery and have a greater mortality than those without diabetes.[3–5]

Meta-analyses have pooled data from case-control and cohort studies to examine the association between diabetes and cancer at specific sites. These studies have demonstrated that having diabetes increases the risk of pancreatic, hepatocellular, and endometrial cancer to approximately twice that of the nondiabetic population.[6–9] Some studies have reported a similar increase in the risk of bladder cancer, although others have reported a more modest increase in risk of approximately 20%.[10,11] The risk of kidney cancer is reported to be approximately 40% higher, and colorectal cancer approximately 30% higher, in diabetic individuals compared to those without diabetes.[12,13] Diabetes is associated with a 20% increased risk of breast cancer;[14] those with diabetes are more likely to present with advanced stage breast cancer and are more likely than those without diabetes to die from breast cancer.[4,15] Notably, epidemiological studies have reported that the risk of developing prostate cancer is lower in those with diabetes, although in men who develop prostate cancer, diabetes is associated with

doi: 10.1111/j.1749-6632.2011.06285.x

 Ann. N.Y. Acad. Sci. 1243 (2011) 54–68 © 2011 New York Academy of Sciences.

a greater risk of mortality, recurrence, and treatment failure.[16,17] Across all cancers, it remains to be determined whether diabetes is truly associated with greater cancer mortality. Having diabetes almost doubles the age-adjusted mortality in the general population without cancer; therefore, the data reporting that diabetes is associated with increased cancer mortality could simply be a reflection of the increased mortality related to having diabetes, rather than a specific increase related to having diabetes and cancer.[18] Furthermore, although the body of epidemiological evidence supporting the association between diabetes and certain cancers is substantial, the data from these studies merely demonstrate that diabetes and certain cancers are associated, not that there is a causal link between the two conditions. To further understand the connection between the two conditions and to determine whether a causal relationship between diabetes and cancer development is plausible, some of the biological factors that are common to the two conditions have been identified and studied in humans, as well as in animals and *in vitro* systems.

In 2010, 100 years after the first publications on the subject of diabetes and cancer by Maynard and Pearson, a consensus report was published by the American Diabetes Association (ADA) and the American Cancer Society (ACS) to (1) review the scientific knowledge regarding the association between diabetes and cancer; (2) explore the risk factors common to both conditions; (3) examine their possible biological links; and (4) determine whether treatments for diabetes influence cancer risk or prognosis. The report acknowledged that for more common cancers, diabetes is associated with an increased risk, but there is less evidence for less common cancers; therefore, it calls for more research to determine whether there is an association between diabetes and less common tumors. The risk factors cited as common to both conditions and the proposed biological links are outlined in Table 1; they include nonmodifiable (age, sex, and race/ethnicity) and modifiable (overweight/obesity, smoking, alcohol intake, physical activity level, and diet) risk factors. The prevalence of most cancers increases with age, with 78% of newly diagnosed cancers occurring in those over 55 years of age. Similarly, the prevalence of diabetes increases with age, from 10.8% in those aged 40–59 years up to 23.8% in those aged 60 years or more. Apart from tumors that are sex-

Table 1. The risk factors and biological links between diabetes and cancer as outlined in the American Diabetes Association/American Cancer Society Consensus Report, 2010

Factors linking diabetes and cancer from the American Diabetes Association/American Cancer Society consensus report 2010		
Nonmodifiable risk factors	Modifiable risk factors	Biological links
Age	Overweight/ obesity	Hyperglycemia
Sex	Physical activity	Insulin
Race/ethnicity	Diet	IGF-1
		Estrogen and androgen bioavailability
		Cytokines

specific or almost completely sex-specific (prostate, testicular, cervical, endometrial, and breast cancers), men are more likely than women to develop cancer and men also have a slightly higher risk of developing diabetes. Cancer and diabetes risks are also different in different ethnic groups. African Americans are more likely to develop and die from cancer and are also more likely to develop diabetes than other ethnic groups. Highlighting these risk factors can identify individuals at greater risk of developing diabetes and cancer and direct efforts toward reducing their modifiable risk factors; however, it does not answer the question of whether diabetes and cancer are more likely to occur in an individual because of risk factors common to both conditions, or if having the metabolic disturbances that occur in diabetes increase the risk of cancer.[19]

Type 2 diabetes (T2DM) is characterized by insulin resistance and endogenous hyperinsulinemia, before the eventual development of the frank hyperglycemia by which we define the condition.[20,21] Both hyperglycemia and hyperinsulinemia have been cited as possible mechanisms through which diabetes may stimulate tumor growth.[19] Obesity has been known for many years to increase the risk of T2DM and is itself associated with an increased risk of cancer.[22,23] Obesity potentially contributes to tumor progression through the effects of hyperinsulinemia, increased circulating estrogen, and chronic inflammation with altered regulation of cytokines and adipokines such as tumor necrosis factor alpha (TNF-α), interleukin-6 (IL-6), fatty acid synthase, resistin, leptin, and adiponectin.[24,25] Therefore, in many individuals with diabetes and obesity there are multiple physiological elements that may contribute to tumor development. Diabetes treatments may also influence the risk of developing cancer. Recent population-based cohort studies have reported that insulin secretagogues and insulin analogs may increase the risk of developing cancer, whereas metformin treatment may decrease the risk.[26–30] None of these studies are randomized controlled trials and there are multiple factors that may be confounding the data, such as comorbidities, duration of diabetes, glycemic control, and preexisting undiagnosed tumors. In view of these potential confounding factors, the ADA/ACS have concluded that the data on these medications is inconclusive and further studies need to be conducted to investigate these potential links.[19]

In this review, we will examine the clinical and scientific studies that explore the roles of hyperglycemia and hyperinsulinemia in cancer development as well as those that are investigating whether metformin reduces cancer development and progression. There are many factors apart from hyperinsulinemia and hyperglycemia that are important in the relationship between diabetes and cancer metabolism, including oncogenes and tumor suppressor genes, glutamine metabolism, inflammation, and obesity; these have recently been reviewed elsewhere.[25,31–34]

Hyperinsulinemia, hyperglycemia, and cancer

Insulin

Insulin resistance and hyperinsulinemia are important factors in the development of type 2 diabetes. Insulin is known to stimulate cell proliferation and injection of insulin in rats promoted carcinogen-induced colon cancer.[23,35,36] Some large prospective studies in humans have enrolled cohorts of men and women, gathered anthropometric data and serum at baseline, and followed them periodically for many years to identify factors that may influence future cancer development. One such study, the Women's Health Initiative Observational Study (WHI-OS),

was conducted in 40 clinical centers across the United States. The study reported that women with endogenous insulin levels in the highest quartile of the normal range and those with insulin resistance had a higher risk of developing postmenopausal breast cancer compared to those with lower insulin levels and without insulin resistance.[37] Another smaller study examined insulin levels in women with early stage breast cancer and reported that those with insulin levels in the highest quartile had a risk of recurrence and death that was two to three times that of women with insulin levels in the lowest quartile.[38] The Physicians Health Study and Nurses Health Study both measured C-peptide (as a reflection of insulin secretion) and found that increased levels were strongly associated with an increased risk of colorectal cancer in men and weakly associated in women.[39,40] In Finnish men, who were a subset of the Alpha-Tocopherol, Beta-Carotene Cancer Prevention Study cohort, fasting insulin concentrations were found to be higher, as was insulin resistance in men who subsequently developed prostate cancer.[41] Although most studies have reported a positive association between insulin levels and breast cancer, the Nurse's Health Study II, which included predominantly premenopausal women, did not find an association between insulin and breast cancer. The discrepant associations between insulin and breast cancer in pre- and postmenopausal women may be due to differences in tumor hormone receptor status and the significance of insulin's indirect contribution to circulating estrogen levels in pre- and postmenopausal women. Additionally, premenopausal women may have a shorter duration of exposure to hyperinsulinemia and have other risk factors for breast cancer.[42] Overall, the majority of human epidemiological studies suggest that elevated insulin levels promote the development of certain cancers. Human tissue and animal *in vitro*, studies provide evidence that insulin may have both direct and indirect actions that promote cancer progression.

As noted previously, insulin resistance and hyperinsulinemia occur prior to the onset of hyperglycemia in the setting of type 2 diabetes. Hyperinsulinemia may have direct effects on tumor growth through its action on the insulin receptor (IR) and/or IGF-1 receptor (IGF-1R).[43] Additionally, hyperinsulinemia leads to increased hepatic IGF-1 production indirectly by increasing hepatic growth hormone receptor (GHR) levels, through which GH stimulates IGF-1 expression.[44] Higher circulating IGF-1 levels, even when within the normal range, were associated with an increased risk of cancer mortality in men over the age of 50 years in the Rancho Bernardo Study, and meta-analyses of other epidemiological studies have reported an increased risk of colorectal cancer, premenopausal breast cancer, and prostate cancer with increased IGF-1 levels.[45–49] Animal studies have demonstrated that low circulating IGF-1 levels, induced by either caloric restriction or genetic manipulation that resulted in liver IGF-1 deficiency, protected against cancer development, while administration of IGF-1 reversed this protective effect.[50,51] Therefore, in the setting of type 2 diabetes, insulin and IGF-1 may be involved in tumor development.

Insulin directly signals in cells by binding to the IR and/or IGF-IR, resulting in autophosphorylation of the beta subunit of the receptor and activation of downstream signaling pathways. Many tumors are known to express the IR, and studies of human breast cancer tissue demonstrate an increase in IR content in the tumors compared to normal breast tissue.[52–54] Similarly, human prostate and hepatocellular cancers have been shown to have greater IR content than benign prostate and normal hepatic tissue, respectively.[55,56] A subset of chronic lymphocytic leukemia (CLL) lymphocytes was recently shown to have significantly increased IR expression, compared to normal B lymphocytes. The increased IR expression occurred in the CLL subset that carried a mutation in the long arm of chromosome 11 (11q) and is associated with a more aggressive course.[57] In the same study, having higher IR expression was associated with shorter time to first therapy and overall survival than in those patients with CLL lymphocytes with lower IR content.[57] In breast cancer tissue from patients, the presence of detectable IR by immunohistochemistry was associated with a better prognosis than having no detectable IR. But there is contradictory data regarding how higher IR content affects prognosis, with one study reporting that higher IR content was associated with greater disease-free survival and another reporting that very high IR content is linked to decreased disease-free survival.[53,54] Differences in methodologies and arbitrary cutoffs for high versus low IR content most likely account for the conflicting results, and thus it remains to be determined

how IR content is linked to prognosis in human breast cancer. *In vitro* studies demonstrate that the IR has a significant role in cell transformation and tumor progression. One such study reported that knocking out the IGF-IR in mouse embryonal fibroblasts (MEFs) increased the sensitivity of the IR to insulin and promoted downstream signaling by concentrations of insulin that were close to physiological levels.[58] Other studies have demonstrated that signaling through the IR can compensate for a nonfunctioning IGF-IR and enhance tumor progression.[58–61] In T2DM, metabolic tissues demonstrate insulin resistance; in contrast, in one study of women with insulin resistance and breast cancer, the IR content of the tumors was not decreased compared to patients without insulin resistance.[54] In a nonobese mouse model, insulin-resistant, hyperinsulinemic mice developed greater breast cancer growth than control mice. The tumors of the hyperinsulinemic mice were found to have increased activation of the IR/IGF-IR signaling pathway and the mammary epithelial cells had increased expression of the IR isoform A, the more mitogenic isoform of the IR.[43] Therefore, the IR may play a role in tumor growth and proliferation, and in the setting of hyperinsulinemia, tumor cells do not develop insulin resistance. Therefore, in individuals with hyperinsulinemia, signaling downstream of the IR/IGF-IR may be increased.

Insulin binding to the IR leads to autophosphorylation of the IR beta subunit tyrosine kinase, which results in recruitment and tyrosine phosphorylation of the insulin receptor substrates (IRS) and then activation of downstream signaling pathways, including the phosphatidylinositol 3-kinase (PI3K)/Akt/mammalian target of rapamycin (mTOR) pathway and the mitogen-activated protein kinase (MAPK) pathway. Hyperinsulinemia has been shown to cause increased Akt phosphorylation in breast cancer xenografts in animal models[43] and is associated with increased tumor growth and, *ex vivo*, with CLL lymphocytes from humans that overexpress the IR.[57] Akt phosphorylation leads to the phosphorylation of mTOR. mTOR complex 1 (mTORC1), formed by the complex of mTOR, GbL, Raptor, and PRAS40, functions as a nutrient/energy sensor. mTOR is inhibited by the complex formed by tuberous sclerosis protein 1 (TSC1) and tuberous sclerosis protein 2 (TSC2) through the inhibition of the small GTPase Rheb.

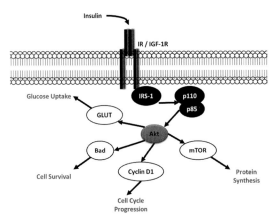

Figure 1. Pathways activated by Akt phosphorylation that increase tumor growth. This simplified schematic shows insulin binding to the insulin receptor (IR) and IGF-1R (insulin-like growth factor receptor), leading to phosphorylation of insulin-receptor substrate-1 (IRS-1), the phosphatidylinositol 3-kinase (p110 and p85), and activation of Akt. Akt then activates multiple pathways, as shown.

Activated Akt phosphorylates TSC2, which releases the inhibition of the TSC1/TSC2 complex on Rheb, allowing for the activation of mTORC1.[62] Akt also suppresses PRAS40, which leads to binding of 14-3-3 regulatory proteins and activation of mTORC1.[63] mTORC1 stimulates protein synthesis by activating S6 kinase and 4E-BP1/eukaryotic translation factor 4E (eIF4E).

Akt also activates many other signaling pathways (Fig. 1). It inhibits cell apoptosis by phosphorylating and thereby inhibiting the pro-apoptotic protein Bad, and by phosphorylating the forkhead transcription factors (FOXO), sequestering Bad and FOXO in the cytoplasm, rendering them unable to initiate the expression of apoptotic genes, such as FasL, TRAIL, and Bcl-XL. FOXO1 is phosphorylated by Akt in cancer cells lacking phosphatase and tensin homolog (PTEN), while FOXO3 and FOXO4 currently appear to be phosphorylated by Akt-independent pathways; however a detailed understanding of the FOXO proteins and their regulators remains to be determined.[64] In addition, Akt phosphorylation promotes the progression of cells from G1 to S phase of the cell cycle, when DNA replication occurs,[65] by phosphorylating p21 and increasing cyclin D translation, which drives the cell through the G1/S transition.[66] Activation of Akt also promotes glucose uptake into cells by promoting translocation of the glucose transporters (GLUT)

to the cell membrane. Therefore, insulin signaling and activation of Akt potentially activates multiple pathways involved in tumor growth.

Hyperglycemia

Glucose is a crucial nutrient for proliferating cells.[67] In the 1920s, Otto Warburg proposed that cancer cells develop an increased ability to produce energy from aerobic glycolysis and fermentation of pyruvate to lactate, even in the presence of abundant oxygen.[68] This observation, known as the "Warburg hypothesis," has become recognized as a common feature of many tumors. Producing energy from glucose in this manner contrasts the metabolism of glucose in normal, differentiated adult cells that have low rates of cell proliferation. Normal, nondividing adult cells derive most of their energy in the form of adenosine triphosphate (ATP) in two phases: first by the glycolysis of glucose to pyruvate, and second, by the oxidation of pyruvic acid to carbon dioxide and water. Although this method of glucose metabolism is the most efficient for producing ATP in nondividing cells, cancer cells are proliferating, and so are thought to rely on aerobic glycolysis as a mechanism of generating glycolytic intermediates that can then be used for protein synthesis and cell division.[31] By using this means of energy production, tumor cells have a greater uptake of glucose than do normal cells, a phenomenon that can be clinically exploited to diagnose cancers by visualization of fluorodeoxyglucose (FDG) uptake with positron emission tomography (PET).[68,69] Because tumor cells display such avid uptake of glucose, it is worth examining whether hyperglycemia in the setting of T2DM can feed tumor growth.

In epidemiological studies of individuals with diabetes, hyperglycemia and elevated hemoglobin A1c (A1c) have not been consistently associated with greater cancer incidence and mortality. A recent meta-analysis of prospective diabetes studies (VADT, ACCORD, UKPDS33, and UKPDS34) compared complications in patients with intensive glucose controls (A1c 6.9%, 6.4%, 7%, and 7.9%, respectively) compared to standard diabetes controls (A1c 8.4%, 7.5%, 7.9%, and 8.5%, respectively) and determined there was no difference in cancer incidence between standard and intensive glucose control groups.[70] Notably, cancer incidence was not the primary outcome of these studies, and the results may be confounded by higher rates of sulfonylurea and insulin usage, in addition to higher doses of insulin in the intensively treated group with lower A1c levels, which some studies have suggested may increase tumor incidence.[26,28] In contrast, a prospective study on over 60,000 individuals in the Vasterbotten Intervention Project in Sweden, and the Hong Kong diabetes registry study both reported an association between hyperglycemia and increased cancer risk. However, in these two studies, insulin resistance and other factors that could lead to increased tumor growth in the setting of hyperglycemia, such as chronic inflammation, were not analyzed.[71,72] Thus, human studies assessing the effect of hyperglycemia on tumor growth are inconclusive due to confounding effects of comorbidities and medications.

In vitro studies and animal models have been used to study the effects of hyperglycemia in the absence of these other factors. In cell lines, for example, including MCF-7 breast cancer and BxPC-3 and MIA PACA-2 pancreatic cell lines, increasing concentrations of glucose stimulate proliferation.[73,74] In a hyperglycemic mouse model, after tumor induction by carcinogens, the fatless diabetic (A-ZIP/F-1) mouse developed more aggressive skin and mammary tumors than the nondiabetic mouse.[75] The tumor tissues from the A-ZIP/F-1 mouse were found to have increased activation of PI3K/Akt/mTOR

and MAPK signaling pathways. These mice, however, also have elevated circulating insulin levels and inflammation cytokines, so it is not possible to conclude that the hyperglycemia alone is driving the accelerated tumor growth.[75] In rats, inducing insulin-deficient hyperglycemia using alloxan did not increase carcinogen-induced mammary tumor growth.[76] Therefore, despite the increased uptake of glucose in tumor cells, if glucose supplies are adequate to keep up with the demand of the tumor, studies do not conclusively demonstrate that hyperglycemia will further stimulate the growth of tumor cells.

The avid uptake of glucose and aerobic glycolysis seen in tumors can occur due to loss of tumor suppressor genes, oncogenic mutations, and the increased activation of the IR signaling pathway (Fig. 2).[68,77,78] GLUT1, GLUT3, and GLUT4, are known to be upregulated in certain tumors. GLUT1 is expressed in many cancers (gynecological, thyroid, gastrointestinal, lung, renal, brain, and skin[79–84]), whereas GLUT 4 is expressed less commonly but is found in some breast, gastric, and lung cancers, osteosarcomas, and rhabdomyosarcomas.[85–89] The expression of these transporters and their translocation to the cell membrane are regulated in different cells by the tumor suppressor gene p53, the oncogene c-Myc, and by insulin

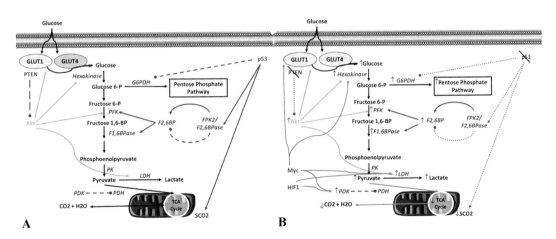

Figure 2. Aerobic glycolysis and its regulating enzymes and genes. This simplified schematic highlights important elements of the glycolytic pathway and oxidative phosphorylation that are regulated by tumor suppressor genes and the insulin-signaling pathway (Akt). Arrows indicate activation of one component by another, and circles indicate a component inhibiting another. Panel (A) indicates the elements that are regulating glycolysis and oxidative phosphorylation in normal cells. Panel (B) shows elements that are upregulated in tumor cells with loss of the tumor suppressor genes p53 and PTEN, the oncogene Myc, HIF, and increased Akt phosphorylation. Grayed out lines are pathways that are lost in tumor cells. Red arrows indicate components that are increased ($\uparrow$) or decreased ($\downarrow$).

signaling.[31,32,86,89–91] The tumor suppressor genes p53 and PTEN and the oncogenes Myc and RAS, as well as Akt signaling, also regulate many points in the glycolytic pathway (Fig. 2). Normally, p53 induces the transcription of TP53-induced glycolysis and apoptosis regulator (TIGAR), which lowers cellular levels of fructose 2,6 bisphosphate (a stimulator of glycolysis) and inhibits glucose-6-phosphate dehydrogenase, the rate-limiting enzyme in the pentose phosphate pathway.[92] In addition, p53 enhances the transcription of the gene for cytochrome c oxidase 1 (SCO2), which is a component of the mitochondrial oxidative phosphorylation complexes (Fig. 2A).[93] Loss of p53 therefore results in decreased SCO2, which prevents oxidative phosphorylation, promotes glycolysis by increasing fructose 2,6 bisphosphate, and activates the anabolic pentose phosphate pathway by activating glucose-6-phosphate dehydrogenase (Fig. 2B).[31,94] p53 also regulates the transcription of PTEN, TSC2, and the beta subunit of the AMP-activated protein kinase (AMPK), which are negative regulators of Akt and mTOR.[31] The PTEN gene encodes for the protein phosphatidylinositol-3,4,5-triphosphate 3-phosphatase, which dephosphorylates phosphatidylinositol 3,4,5-triphosphate (PIP_3) and results in the inhibition of Akt signaling. Loss of PTEN commonly occurs in many cancers and leads to phosphorylation and activation of Akt (Fig. 2B). Phosphorylation of Akt activates many pathways, as described earlier. In addition, the oncogene Myc and hypoxia-inducible factor-1 (HIF1) independently increase GLUT1 expression increasing glucose uptake by tumors. They activate hexokinase and pyruvate dehydrogenase kinase1 (PDK1), and increase lactate dehydrogenase A (LDH-A), which leads to conversion of pyruvate to lactate.[31,95–98] PDK phosphorylates and inactivates pyruvate dehydrogenase, which prevents pyruvate from entering Kreb's cycle and instead allows its conversion to lactate by LDH-A.[31] Higher tumor lactate levels have been demonstrated in cervical tumors with metastatic spread and are associated with decreased survival.[96] In the estrogen receptor (ER) positive MCF-7 breast cancer cell line, lactate increased in the expression of transcription factors, known to be associated with stem cells, which may contribute to tumor metastases.[99] The mechanisms through which lactate promote tumor spread are incompletely understood. Proposed mechanisms include

the conversion of lactate to acetyl-CoA, which can then be used to acetylate proteins, including histones, and thereby increase gene expression that leads to tumor metastasis. Alternatively, lactate may be converted to acetyl-CoA which then undergoes oxidative mitochondrial metabolism to yield ATP that can increase tumor growth and spreading.[99] In summary, insulin signaling, the loss of tumor suppressor genes, and overexpression of oncogenes lead to increased uptake of glucose into tumor cells where it undergoes aerobic glycolysis. This is an inefficient method for producing ATP, but results in the production of metabolic intermediates that can be used for cell growth and synthesis, and lactate production which creates an environment that promotes metastatic tumor spread. Aerobic glycolysis increases the tumor's demand for glucose and is enabled by the activation of transcription factors, which may occur due to mutations of the tumor suppressor genes or activation of components of the insulin signaling pathway, such as mTOR.

The interaction of glucose and insulin with estrogens and androgens

Hyperinsulinemia and hyperglycemia may indirectly affect estrogen and androgen signaling in tumor cells by increasing the circulating bioavailability of these hormones, particularly in the setting of obesity. By expressing aromatase, adipose tissue is capable of forming estrogens from androgenic precursors. In fact, adipose tissue is the main source of estrogens in men and postmenopausal women. Obese postmenopausal women are known to have circulating levels of estrogens 50–100% higher than their lean counterparts.[100] In addition, hyperglycemia and hyperinsulinemia reduce the hepatic production of sex hormone binding globulin (SHBG), which normally binds to circulating estrogens and androgens.[101] The increased production of estrogens and decreased SHBG leads to increased bioavailable estrogen and may contribute to the increased risk of hormone responsive cancers in women with T2DM and obesity. Additionally, in vitro studies of cell lines including breast cancer cell lines, have demonstrated that there is significant cross talk between ER, insulin receptor, and IGF-IR signaling, with IR and IGF-IR signaling enhancing ER signaling pathways.[102,103] Therefore, insulin resistance, hyperglycemia, hormonal alterations, and obesity all potentially interact in individuals with T2DM to increase the risk of hormone responsive cancers.

Considering the potential biological links between T2DM and cancer, is it possible that metformin inhibits tumor growth? Although human epidemiological data are limited, the ADA/ACS consensus statement reported that there is some support for the protective role of metformin in certain cancers. While further studies are needed to determine whether metformin truly improves cancer outcomes in humans, there are numerous proposed mechanisms through which metformin may work to reduce tumor growth and metastases.[19] Our present knowledge of the actions of metformin is incomplete and many of its effects are only now being elucidated. Therefore, we will discuss the current understanding of how metformin affects cancer growth.

Calorie restriction and cancer

In cancer cells, metformin mimics many of the effects of calorie restriction. Although diabetes, obesity, and insulin resistance are associated with increased cancer risk,[5,23,104,105] caloric restriction has been demonstrated for many years to reduce tumor growth.[51,106] The effect was first demonstrated in rodent models and later in the rhesus monkey.[107] Caloric restriction can potentially reduce tumor growth by multiple mechanisms. Insulin sensitivity increases with calorie restriction, therefore a decrease in circulating insulin and IGF-1 levels occurs. Calorie restriction also reduces PI3K/Akt/mTOR signaling, which decreases protein synthesis and cell proliferation.[108] Decreased caloric intake is associated with lower glucose levels and a decrease in ATP levels. As intracellular ATP levels decrease, the intracellular ratio of AMP:ATP increases, leading to activation of AMPK. AMPK phosphorylates TSC2 and raptor, leading to inhibition of mTORC1. Calorie restriction has many other effects on adipokines and inflammatory cytokines that may protect against cancer and are reviewed elsewhere.[109]

Metformin

In the past few years, some epidemiological studies have suggested that metformin is associated with a reduced cancer risk.[29,30,110–114] These studies report that both new and long-term users of metformin appear to be at lower risk of developing cancer.[29,30,110] Individuals who take metformin alone or in addition to sulfonylureas are also at lower risk compared to those taking either sulfonylureas or insulin alone, according to one cohort study from the Netherlands.[115] In one case-control study of insulin-treated patients with T2DM, taking metformin in addition to insulin appeared to protect against cancer development.[116] Furthermore, diabetic patients with breast cancer who take metformin along with neoadjuvant chemotherapy have been reported to have higher rates of pathological complete response than those not taking metformin.[117] Finally, cancer mortality appears to be decreased in diabetic metformin users.[115,118,119] Most of these epidemiological data are retrospective, and there are as yet no published randomized controlled trials designed to ascertain if metformin truly lowers cancer incidence and mortality, or improves the response to chemotherapy in those with cancer. There are ongoing metformin studies that are examining the clinical outcomes; those that are currently registered as "active" or "recruiting" (at http://clinicaltrials.gov/) are outlined in Table 2. There are *in vitro* and *in vivo* data from cell lines and animal models that support the hypothesis that metformin is protective against cancer. Some human studies are also beginning to examine the effects of metformin treatment on the molecular pathways in cancer cells.[120]

A recent randomized, unblinded study of women with stage I or II primary breast cancer without diabetes examined the effect of two weeks of metformin treatment on tumor proliferation and gene expression. Subjects had core biopsies of tumors taken before starting metformin and two weeks later. In the metformin treated group they found a decrease in cell proliferation and alterations in the gene expression for pathways involved in cell proliferation and phosphodiesterase 3B, a regulator of cyclic AMP and activator of AMPK,[120] which inhibits protein synthesis and cell cycle progression. Metformin does not appear to activate AMPK directly, but inhibits mitochondrial complex I of the respiratory chain, leading to an increase in the AMP:ATP ratio and thus activation of AMPK.[121] In MCF7 breast cancer cells, metformin was found to inhibit cell cycle progression by downregulating cyclin D1 and inhibiting the cell cycle G1/S phase transition of cells. This effect was lost by inhibiting AMPK.[122,123] A similar effect has also been described in ovarian cancer cells.[124] However, it has been reported that metformin in prostate cancer cells can inhibit

Table 2. Clinical trials examining the effects of metformin on cancer outcome or tumor signaling

Trial number	Type of trial	Phase	Tumor type	Stage	Primary outcome
NCT01266486	Single arm, open label	Phase II	Breast cancer	Early stage	pS6K, p4E-BP-1, pAMPK
NCT01302002	NonRandomized, open label	Phase 0	Breast cancer	Operable stage I and II	Proliferation and apoptosis
NCT00897884	Single arm, nonrandomized	–	Breast cancer	Operable T1–4 (T1 ≥ 1cm), Nx	Proliferation
NCT00984490	Single arm, open label	–	Breast cancer	Stage I and II	Proliferation
NCT01310231	Randomized, double-blind, placebo controlled	Phase II	Breast cancer	Metastatic	Progression-free survival
NCT01101438	Randomized, double blind, placebo controlled	Phase III	Breast cancer	Early stage	Invasive disease-free survival
NCT00930579	Nonrandomized, open label	Phase II	Breast cancer	DCIS or operable invasive breast cancer	AMPK/TOR signaling
NCT01205672	Single arm, open label	–	Endometrial cancer	All candidates for surgical staging	Insulin/glucose metabolism and mTOR signaling
NCT01333852	Randomized, double blind, placebo controlled	–	Head & neck cancer	Metastatic or recurrent	Disease control at 12 weeks
NCT01210911	Randomized, placebo controlled	Phase II	Pancreatic cancer	Locally advanced or metastatic	Six-month survival
NCT01167738	Randomized, open label	Phase II	Pancreatic cancer	Metastatic	Progression-free survival at six months
NCT01215032	Single arm, open label	–	Prostate cancer	Castration resistant	PSA response
NCT01243385	Single arm, open label	Phase II	Prostate cancer	Locally advanced or metastatic	Progression-free survival at 12 weeks

Active and recruiting clinical trials examining tumor outcomes of cancer tissue signaling from the http://ClinicalTrials.gov registry (last accessed July 18, 2011).

cell cycle progression in an AMPK-independent manner, with one study suggesting that this occurs through the activation of the HIF target gene REDD1 (RTP801/Dig2/DDIT4), which leads to mTOR inhibition and cell cycle arrest.[125,126] Further evidence that metformin has AMPK-independent effects comes not from tumors but from AMPK-deficient hepatocytes and mice with a liver deficiency of AMPK. These mice had no difference in hepatic glucose output, or gluconeogenic gene transcription.[127] Metformin suppresses glucose-6-phosphatase expression in the liver by inhibiting mitochondrial complex I, an affect that also appears to be independent of AMPK.[128] Although the effects of metformin in normal metabolic tissue and tumor cells may differ, these data suggest metformin may potentially affect AMPK-dependent and -independent pathways in cancers.

Metformin treats diabetes by inhibiting hepatic glucose output, and therefore reduces glucose levels.[129] It also improves insulin sensitivity by lowering circulating insulin levels.[130,131]

Metformin decreases Akt phosphorylation, in contrast to other inhibitors of mTOR, such as rapamycin, which actually increases Akt phosphorylation. In MCF7 cells, AMPK phosphorylates IRS-1 at serine 789 and has been reported by some to dampen signal transduction through IRS-1.[132] Metformin was also seen to reduce IGF-IR and IRS-1 levels in MCF7 cells.[132] As insulin signals through the IR and IGF-IR, it is possible that metformin may reduce insulin signaling by decreasing the level of the IGF-IR. In an animal model of colon cancer metformin reduced the accelerated growth of tumors induced by a high fat diet. Tumors from these animals treated with metformin were found to have decreased Akt phosphorylation and decreased expression of fatty acid synthase, along with activated AMPK. Akt stimulates GLUT1- and GLUT4-mediated glucose uptake, and therefore inhibition of Akt will reduce glucose uptake in cells. Along with the decreased circulating level of glucose due to decreased hepatic gluconeogenesis, metformin will reduce the supply of glucose to the tumor cells by preventing its uptake (Fig. 3). As mentioned, in tumors p53 mutations result in activation of the pentose phosphate pathway and production of precursors for the synthesis of fatty acids, amino acids, and nucleic acids.[94] Therefore, a decreased supply of

glucose will result in decreased ATP production by tumor cells and less metabolic intermediates, such as glucose 6-phosphate to enter the pentose phosphate pathway. Metformin also appears to inhibit cross talk between IR/IGF-IR and G protein-coupled receptor (GPCR) signaling pathways in pancreatic cancer by activating AMPK and thus inhibiting mTOR-mediated stimulation of GPCR signaling.[133] Additionally, AMPK activation by metformin has been shown to inhibit aromatase expression by inhibiting the activity of its promoter in human breast adipose tissue.[134] The inhibition of aromatase could also explain the reduced tumor incidence in diabetic patients taking metformin.

In summary, metformin may (1) decrease insulin signaling in tumor cells by decreasing circulating insulin levels; (2) inhibit the insulin signaling pathway in tumor cells by activating AMPK, which reduces glucose uptake; (3) prevent cell cycle progression through AMPK-dependent and -independent mechanisms; and (4) inhibit cross talk between receptors and decrease local estrogen production by breast adipose tissue by inhibiting aromatase expression (Fig. 3).

Metformin has also recently been shown to suppress breast cancer stem cells, which are thought to exist within tumors. These stem cells

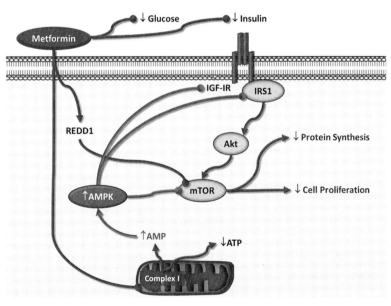

Figure 3. Effect of metformin on glucose and insulin signaling. This schematic represents some of the potential AMPK-dependent and -independent effects of metformin in tumors. Arrows indicate activation of one component by another; circles show one component that inhibits another.

have the ability to self-renew and give rise to differentiated cells and to form new tumors. After treatment with traditional chemotherapy, tumor size will decrease but the proportion of cancer stem cells will increase. Metformin has been shown to decrease the number of breast cancer stem cells and impair their ability to self-renew and proliferate.[135–138] Many of the pathways through which metformin is active in tumor cells and metabolic tissues are still being determined, therefore many studies are being performed to determine the clinical efficacy of metformin in human cancers and to uncover the details of its mechanism of action.

Conclusions

In conclusion, diabetes is associated with an increased risk of developing cancers at a variety of sites and is associated with worse outcomes, whereas calorie restriction in animal studies reduces tumor incidence. Elevated circulating insulin levels in animals and humans are associated with increased tumor growth, while hyperglycemia alone has proven difficult to assess due to confounding factors. Intracellular insulin signaling and the aerobic glycolysis of glucose promote the production of metabolic intermediates that can be used to form amino acids and nucleic acids needed for cell proliferation. Metformin reduces tumor proliferation by multiple mechanisms that involve the circulating levels of insulin and glucose, the expression of aromatase in surrounding tissues, and the intracellular regulation of insulin signaling and glucose metabolism. Randomized trials are anticipated to determine whether the potential of metformin to prevent tumor development, metastasis, and recurrence is real. Further studies are ongoing to expand our understanding of the pathways linking diabetes and cancer.

Conflicts of interest

The authors declare no conflicts of interest.

References

1. Maynard, G. 1910. A statistical study in cancer death-rates. *Biometrika* **7:** 276–304.
2. Pearson, K., A. Lee & E.M. Elderton. 1910. On the correlation of death-rates. *J. R. Stat. Soc.* **73:** 534–539.
3. Srokowski, T.P., S. Fang, G.N. Hortobagyi & S.H. Giordano. 2009. Impact of diabetes mellitus on complications and outcomes of adjuvant chemotherapy in older patients with breast cancer. *J. Clin. Oncol.* **27:** 2170–2176.
4. Barone, B.B., H.C. Yeh, C.F. Snyder, *et al.* 2008. Long-term all-cause mortality in cancer patients with preexisting diabetes mellitus: a systematic review and meta-analysis. *JAMA* **300:** 2754–2764.
5. Coughlin, S.S., E.E. Calle, L.R. Teras, *et al.* 2004. Diabetes mellitus as a predictor of cancer mortality in a large cohort of US adults. *Am. J. Epidemiol.* **159:** 1160–1167.
6. Everhart, J. & D. Wright. 1995. Diabetes mellitus as a risk factor for pancreatic cancer. A meta-analysis. *JAMA* **273:** 1605–1609.
7. Huxley, R., A. Ansary-Moghaddam, A. Berrington de Gonzalez, *et al.* 2005. Type-II diabetes and pancreatic cancer: a meta-analysis of 36 studies. *Br. J. Cancer* **92:** 2076–2083.
8. Friberg, E., N. Orsini, C.S. Mantzoros & A. Wolk. 2007. Diabetes mellitus and risk of endometrial cancer: a meta-analysis. *Diabetologia* **50:** 1365–1374.
9. El-Serag, H.B., H. Hampel & F. Javadi. 2006. The association between diabetes and hepatocellular carcinoma: a systematic review of epidemiologic evidence. *Clin. Gastroenterol. Hepatol.* **4:** 369–380.
10. Larsson, S.C., N. Orsini, K. Brismar & A. Wolk. 2006. Diabetes mellitus and risk of bladder cancer: a meta-analysis. *Diabetologia* **49:** 2819–2823.
11. MacKenzie, T., M.S. Zens, A. Ferrara, *et al.* 2010. Diabetes and risk of bladder cancer: evidence from a case-control study in New England. *Cancer* **117:** 1552–1556.
12. Larsson, S.C. & A. Wolk. 2011. Diabetes mellitus and incidence of kidney cancer: a meta-analysis of cohort studies. *Diabetologia* **54:** 1013–1018.
13. Larsson, S.C., N. Orsini & A. Wolk. 2005. Diabetes mellitus and risk of colorectal cancer: a meta-analysis. *J. Natl. Cancer Inst.* **97:** 1679–1687.
14. Larsson, S.C., C.S. Mantzoros & A. Wolk. 2007. Diabetes mellitus and risk of breast cancer: a meta-analysis. *Int. J. Cancer* **121:** 856–862.
15. Peairs, K.S., B.B. Barone, C.F. Snyder, *et al.* 2011. Diabetes mellitus and breast cancer outcomes: a systematic review and meta-analysis. *J. Clin. Oncol.* **29:** 40–46.
16. Kasper, J.S. & E. Giovannucci. 2006. A meta-analysis of diabetes mellitus and the risk of prostate cancer. *Cancer Epidemiol. Biomarkers Prev.* **15:** 2056–2062.
17. Bonovas, S., K. Filioussi & A. Tsantes. 2004. Diabetes mellitus and risk of prostate cancer: a meta-analysis. *Diabetologia* **47:** 1071–1078.
18. National diabetes fact sheet: national estimates and general information on diabetes and prediabetes in the United States, 2011. Centers for Disease Control and Prevention; 2011.
19. Giovannucci, E., D.M. Harlan, M.C. Archer, *et al.* 2010. Diabetes and cancer: a consensus report. *Diabetes Care* **33:** 1674–1685.
20. Martin, B.C., J.H. Warram, A.S. Krolewski, *et al.* 1992. Role of glucose and insulin resistance in development of type 2 diabetes mellitus: results of a 25-year follow-up study. *Lancet* **340:** 925–929.
21. American Diabetes Association. 2011. Standards of medical care in diabetes—2011. *Diabetes Care* **34**(Suppl 1): S11–S61.
22. West, K.M. & J.M. Kalbfleisch. 1971. Influence of nutritional factors on prevalence of diabetes. *Diabetes* **20:** 99–108.

23. Calle E.E., C. Rodriguez, K. Walker-Thurmond & M.J. Thun. 2003. Overweight, obesity, and mortality from cancer in a prospectively studied cohort of U.S. adults. *N. Engl. J. Med.* **348:** 1625–1638.

24. Poretsky, L. 2010. Chapter 36 in *Principles of Diabetes*. 2nd ed. Springer. New York

25. LeRoith, D. 2011. Chapter 3 in *Insulin-like Growth Factors and Cancer: From Basic Biology to Therapeutics*. Springer. New York.

26. Bowker, S.L., S.R. Majumdar, P. Veugelers & J.A. Johnson. 2006. Increased cancer-related mortality for patients with type 2 diabetes who use sulfonylureas or insulin. *Diabetes Care* **29:** 254–258.

27. Colhoun, H.M. 2009. Use of insulin glargine and cancer incidence in Scotland: a study from the Scottish Diabetes Research Network Epidemiology Group. *Diabetologia* **52:** 1755–1765.

28. Currie, C.J., C.D. Poole & E.A. Gale. 2009. The influence of glucose-lowering therapies on cancer risk in type 2 diabetes. *Diabetologia* **52:** 1766–1777.

29. Libby, G., L.A. Donnelly, P.T. Donnan, *et al.* 2009. New users of metformin are at low risk of incident cancer: a cohort study among people with type 2 diabetes. *Diabetes Care* **32:** 1620–1625.

30. Bodmer, M., C. Meier, S. Krahenbuhl, *et al.* 2010. Long-term metformin use is associated with decreased risk of breast cancer. *Diabetes Care* **33:** 1304–1308.

31. Levine, A.J. & A.M. Puzio-Kuter. 2010. The control of the metabolic switch in cancers by oncogenes and tumor suppressor genes. *Science* **330:** 1340–1344.

32. Peterson, C.W. & D.E. Ayer. 2011. An extended Myc network contributes to glucose homeostasis in cancer and diabetes. *Front. Biosci.* **17:** 2206–2223.

33. Paz-Filho, G., E.L. Lim, M.L. Wong & J. Licinio. 2011. Associations between adipokines and obesity-related cancer. *Front. Biosci.* **16:** 1634–1650.

34. DeBerardinis, R.J. & T. Cheng. 2010. Q's next: the diverse functions of glutamine in metabolism, cell biology and cancer. *Oncogene* **29:** 313–324.

35. Tran, T.T., A. Medline & W.R. Bruce. 1996. Insulin promotion of colon tumors in rats. *Cancer Epidemiol. Biomarkers Prev.* **5:** 1013–1015.

36. Tran, T.T., D. Naigamwalla, A.I. Oprescu, *et al.* 2006. Hyperinsulinemia, but not other factors associated with insulin resistance, acutely enhances colorectal epithelial proliferation in vivo. *Endocrinology* **147:** 1830–1837.

37. Gunter, M.J., D.R. Hoover, H. Yu, *et al.* 2009. Insulin, insulin-like growth factor-I, and risk of breast cancer in postmenopausal women. *J. Natl. Cancer Inst.* **101:** 48–60.

38. Goodwin, P.J., M. Ennis, K.I. Pritchard, *et al.* 2002. Fasting insulin and outcome in early-stage breast cancer: results of a prospective cohort study. *J. Clin. Oncol.* **20:** 42–51.

39. Ma, J., E. Giovannucci, M. Pollak, *et al.* 2004. A prospective study of plasma C-peptide and colorectal cancer risk in men. *J. Natl. Cancer Inst.* **96:** 546–553.

40. Wei, E.K., J. Ma, M.N. Pollak, *et al.* 2005. A prospective study of C-peptide, insulin-like growth factor-I, insulin-like growth factor binding protein-1, and the risk of colorectal cancer in women. *Cancer Epidemiol. Biomarkers Prev.* **14:** 850–855.

41. Albanes, D., S.J. Weinstein, M.E. Wright, *et al.* 2009. Serum insulin, glucose, indices of insulin resistance, and risk of prostate cancer. *J. Natl. Cancer Inst.* **101:** 1272–1279.

42. Eliassen, A.H., S.S. Tworoger, C.S. Mantzoros, *et al.* 2007. Circulating insulin and c-peptide levels and risk of breast cancer among predominately premenopausal women. *Cancer Epidemiol. Biomarkers Prev.* **16:** 161–164.

43. Novosyadlyy, R., D.E. Lann, A. Vijayakumar, *et al.* 2010. Insulin-mediated acceleration of breast cancer development and progression in a nonobese model of type 2 diabetes. *Cancer Res.* **70:** 741–751.

44. Baxter, R.C., A.S. Brown & J.R. Turtle. 1980. Association between serum insulin, serum somatomedin and liver receptors for human growth hormone in streptozotocin diabetes. *Horm. Metab. Res.* **12:** 377–381.

45. Major, J.M., G.A. Laughlin, D. Kritz-Silverstein, *et al.* 2010. Insulin-like growth factor-I and cancer mortality in older men. *J. Clin. Endocrinol. Metab.* **95:** 1054–1059.

46. Chen, W., S. Wang, T. Tian, *et al.* 2009. Phenotypes and genotypes of insulin-like growth factor 1, IGF-binding protein-3 and cancer risk: evidence from 96 studies. *Eur. J. Hum. Genet.* **17:** 1668–1675.

47. Rinaldi, S., R. Cleveland, T. Norat, *et al.* 2010. Serum levels of IGF-I, IGFBP-3 and colorectal cancer risk: results from the EPIC cohort, plus a meta-analysis of prospective studies. *Int. J. Cancer* **126:** 1702–1715.

48. Roddam, A.W., N.E Allen, P. Appleby, *et al.* 2008. Insulin-like growth factors, their binding proteins, and prostate cancer risk: analysis of individual patient data from 12 prospective studies. *Ann. Intern. Med.* **149:** 461–471, W83–W88.

49. Renehan, A.G., M. Zwahlen, C. Minder, *et al.* 2004. Insulin-like growth factor (IGF)-I, IGF binding protein-3, and cancer risk: systematic review and meta-regression analysis. *Lancet* **363:** 1346–1353.

50. Wu, Y., S. Yakar, L. Zhao, *et al.* 2002. Circulating insulin-like growth factor-I levels regulate colon cancer growth and metastasis. *Cancer Res.* **62:** 1030–1035.

51. Dunn, S.E., F.W. Kari, J. French, *et al.* 1997. Dietary restriction reduces insulin-like growth factor I levels, which modulates apoptosis, cell proliferation, and tumor progression in p53-deficient mice. *Cancer Res.* **57:** 4667–4672.

52. Papa, V., V. Pezzino, A. Costantino, *et al.* 1990. Elevated insulin receptor content in human breast cancer. *J. Clin. Invest.* **86:** 1503–1510.

53. Mathieu, M.C., G.M. Clark , D.C. Allred, *et al.* 1997. Insulin receptor expression and clinical outcome in node-negative breast cancer. *Proc. Assoc. Am. Physicians* **109:** 565–571.

54. Mulligan, A.M., F.P. O'Malley, M. Ennis, *et al.* 2007. Insulin receptor is an independent predictor of a favorable outcome in early stage breast cancer. *Breast Cancer Res. Treat.* **106:** 39–47.

55. Spector, S.A., E.T. Olson, A.A. Gumbs, *et al.* 1999. Human insulin receptor and insulin signaling proteins in hepatic disease. *J. Surg. Res.* **83:** 32–35.

56. Cox, M.E., M.E. Gleave, M. Zakikhani, *et al.* 2009. Insulin receptor expression by human prostate cancers. *Prostate* **69:** 33–40.

57. Saiya-Cork, K., R. Collins, B. Parkin, *et al.* 2011. A pathobiological role of the insulin receptor in chronic lymphocytic leukemia. *Clin. Cancer Res.* **17:** 2679–2692.

58. Dinchuk, J.E., C. Cao, F. Huang, *et al.* 2010. Insulin receptor (IR) pathway hyperactivity in IGF-IR null cells and suppression of downstream growth signaling using the dual IGF-IR/IR inhibitor, BMS-754807. *Endocrinology* **151:** 4123–4132.

59. Ulanet, D.B., D.L. Ludwig, C.R. Kahn & D. Hanahan. 2010. Insulin receptor functionally enhances multistage tumor progression and conveys intrinsic resistance to IGF-1R targeted therapy. *Proc. Natl. Acad. Sci. USA* **107:** 10791–10798.

60. Zhang, H., A.M. Pelzer, D.T. Kiang & D. Yee. 2007. Down-regulation of type I insulin-like growth factor receptor increases sensitivity of breast cancer cells to insulin. *Cancer Res.* **67:** 391–397.

61. Buck, E., P.C. Gokhale, S. Koujak, *et al.* 2010. Compensatory insulin receptor (IR) activation on inhibition of insulin-like growth factor-1 receptor (IGF-1R): rationale for cotargeting IGF-1R and IR in cancer. *Mol. Cancer Ther.* **9:** 2652–2664.

62. Levine, A.J., Z. Feng, T.W. Mak, *et al.* 2006. Coordination and communication between the p53 and IGF-1-AKT-TOR signal transduction pathways. *Genes Dev.* **20:** 267–275.

63. Gwinn, D.M., D.B. Shackelford, D.F. Egan, *et al.* 2008. AMPK phosphorylation of raptor mediates a metabolic checkpoint. *Mol. Cell* **30:** 214–226.

64. Fu, Z. & D.J. Tindall. 2008. FOXOs, cancer and regulation of apoptosis. *Oncogene* **27:** 2312–2319.

65. Smolewski, P. 2006. Recent developments in targeting the mammalian target of rapamycin (mTOR) kinase pathway. *Anticancer Drugs* **17:** 487–494.

66. Sen, P., S. Mukherjee, D. Ray & S. Raha. 2003. Involvement of the Akt/PKB signaling pathway with disease processes. *Mol. Cell Biochem.* **253:** 241–246.

67. Laporte, D., A. Lebaudy, A. Sahin, *et al.* 2011. Metabolic status rather than cell cycle signals control quiescence entry and exit. *J. Cell Biol.* **192:** 949–957.

68. Warburg, O. 1956. On the origin of cancer cells. *Science* **123:** 309–314.

69. Hsu, P.P. & D.M. Sabatini. 2008. Cancer cell metabolism: Warburg and beyond. *Cell* **134:** 703–707.

70. Johnson, J.A. & S.L. Bowker. 2011. Intensive glycaemic control and cancer risk in type 2 diabetes: a meta-analysis of major trials. *Diabetologia* **54:** 25–31.

71. Stattin, P., O. Bjor, P. Ferrari, *et al.* 2007. Prospective study of hyperglycemia and cancer risk. *Diabetes Care* **30:** 561–567.

72. Yang, X., G.T. Ko, W.Y. So, *et al.* 2010. Associations of hyperglycemia and insulin usage with the risk of cancer in type 2 diabetes: the Hong Kong diabetes registry. *Diabetes* **59:** 1254–1260.

73. Okumura, M., M. Yamamoto, H. Sakuma, *et al.* 2002. Leptin and high glucose stimulate cell proliferation in MCF-7 human breast cancer cells: reciprocal involvement of PKC-

74. alpha and PPAR expression. *Biochim. Biophys. Acta* **1592:** 107–1016.

75. Liu, H., Q. Ma & J. Li. 2011. High glucose promotes cell proliferation and enhances GDNF and RET expression in pancreatic cancer cells. *Mol. Cell Biochem.* **347:** 95–101.

76. Nunez, N.P., W.J. Oh, J. Rozenberg, *et al.* 2006. Accelerated tumor formation in a fatless mouse with type 2 diabetes and inflammation. *Cancer Res.* **66:** 5469–5476.

77. Heuson, J.C. & N. Legros. 1972. Influence of insulin deprivation on growth of the 7,12-dimethylbenz(a)anthracene-induced mammary carcinoma in rats subjected to alloxan diabetes and food restriction. *Cancer Res.* **32:** 226–232.

78. Frezza, C. & E. Gottlieb. 2009. Mitochondria in cancer: not just innocent bystanders. *Semin. Cancer Biol.* **19:** 4–11.

79. Macheda, M.L., S. Rogers & J.D. Best. 2005. Molecular and cellular regulation of glucose transporter (GLUT) proteins in cancer. *J. Cell Physiol.* **202:** 654–662.

80. Haber, R.S., K.R. Weiser, A. Pritsker, *et al.* 1997. GLUT1 glucose transporter expression in benign and malignant thyroid nodules. *Thyroid* **7:** 363–367.

81. Kurata, T., T. Oguri, T. Isobe, *et al.* 1999. Differential expression of facilitative glucose transporter (GLUT) genes in primary lung cancers and their liver metastases. *Jpn. J. Cancer Res.* **90:** 1238–1243.

82. Yamamoto, T., Y. Seino, H. Fukumoto, *et al.* 1990. Overexpression of facilitative glucose transporter genes in human cancer. *Biochem. Biophys. Res. Commun.* **170:** 223–230.

83. Younes, M., R.W. Brown, D.R. Mody, *et al.* 1995. GLUT1 expression in human breast carcinoma: correlation with known prognostic markers. *Anticancer Res.* **15:** 2895–2898.

84. Baer, S.C., L. Casaubon, M. Younes. 1997. Expression of the human erythrocyte glucose transporter Glut1 in cutaneous neoplasia. *J. Am. Acad. Dermatol.* **37:** 575–577.

85. Nagase, Y., K. Takata, N. Moriyama, *et al.* 1995. Immunohistochemical localization of glucose transporters in human renal cell carcinoma. *J. Urol.* **153:** 798–801.

86. Nagamatsu, S., H. Sawa, A. Wakizaka & T. Hoshino. 1993. Expression of facilitative glucose transporter isoforms in human brain tumors. *J. Neurochem.* **61:** 2048–2053.

87. Noguchi, Y., S. Sato, D. Marat, *et al.* 1999. Glucose uptake in the human gastric cancer cell line, MKN28, is increased by insulin stimulation. *Cancer Lett.* **140:** 69–74.

88. Armoni, M., M.J. Quon, G. Maor, *et al.* 2002. PAX3/forkhead homolog in rhabdomyosarcoma oncoprotein activates glucose transporter 4 gene expression in vivo and in vitro. *J. Clin. Endocrinol. Metab.* **87:** 5312–5324.

89. Ito, T., Y. Noguchi, S. Satoh, *et al.* 1998. Expression of facilitative glucose transporter isoforms in lung carcinomas: its relation to histologic type, differentiation grade, and tumor stage. *Mod. Pathol.* **11:** 437–443.

90. Schwartzenberg-Bar-Yoseph, F., M. Armoni & E. Karnieli. 2004. The tumor suppressor p53 down-regulates glucose transporters GLUT1 and GLUT4 gene expression. *Cancer Res.* **64:** 2627–2633.

91. Cifuentes, M., M.A. Garcia, P.M. Arrabal, *et al.* 2011. Insulin regulates GLUT1-mediated glucose transport in MG-63 human osteosarcoma cells. *J. Cell Physiol.* **226:** 1425–1432.

92. Ding, X.Z., D.M. Fehsenfeld, L.O. Murphy, *et al.* 2000. Physiological concentrations of insulin augment pancreatic

cancer cell proliferation and glucose utilization by activating MAP kinase, PI3 kinase and enhancing GLUT-1 expression. *Pancreas* **21:** 310–320.

92. Bensaad, K., A. Tsuruta, M.A. Selak, *et al.* 2006. TIGAR, a p53-inducible regulator of glycolysis and apoptosis. *Cell* **126:** 107–120.

93. Kawauchi, K., K. Araki, K. Tobiume & N. Tanaka. 2008. p53 regulates glucose metabolism through an IKK-NF-kappaB pathway and inhibits cell transformation. *Nat. Cell Biol.* **10:** 611–618.

94. Jiang, P., W. Du, X. Wang, *et al.* 2011. p53 regulates biosynthesis through direct inactivation of glucose-6-phosphate dehydrogenase. *Nat. Cell Biol.* **13:** 310–316.

95. Sun, Q., X. Chen, J. Ma, *et al.* 2011. Mammalian target of rapamycin up-regulation of pyruvate kinase isoenzyme type M2 is critical for aerobic glycolysis and tumor growth. *Proc. Natl. Acad. Sci. USA* **108:** 4129–4134.

96. Walenta, S., M. Wetterling, M. Lehrke, *et al.* 2000. High lactate levels predict likelihood of metastases, tumor recurrence, and restricted patient survival in human cervical cancers. *Cancer Res.* **60:** 916–921.

97. Shim, H., C. Dolde, B.C. Lewis, *et al.* 1997. c-Myc transactivation of LDH-A: implications for tumor metabolism and growth. *Proc. Natl. Acad. Sci. USA* **94:** 6658–6663.

98. Dang, C.V., J.W. Kim, P. Gao & J. Yustein. 2008. The interplay between MYC and HIF in cancer. *Nat. Rev. Cancer* **8:** 51–56.

99. Martinez-Outschoorn, U.E., M. Prisco, A. Ertel, *et al.* 2011. Ketones and lactate increase cancer cell "stemness," driving recurrence, metastasis and poor clinical outcome in breast cancer: achieving personalized medicine via Metabolo-Genomics. *Cell Cycle* **10:** 1271–1286.

100. Huang, Z., S.E. Hankinson, G.A. Colditz, *et al.* 1997. Dual effects of weight and weight gain on breast cancer risk. *JAMA* **278:** 1407–1411.

101. Pugeat, M, N. Nader, K. Hogeveen, *et al.* 2010. Sex hormone-binding globulin gene expression in the liver: drugs and the metabolic syndrome. *Mol. Cell Endocrinol.* **316:** 53–59.

102. Eertmans, F, W. Dhooge, O. De Wever, *et al.* 2007. Estrogen receptor alpha (ERalpha) and insulin-like growth factor I receptor (IGF-IR) cross-talk in the gonadotropic alphaT3–1 cell line. *J. Cell Physiol.* **212:** 583–590.

103. Richardson, A.E., N. Hamilton, W. Davis, *et al.* 2011. Insulin-like growth factor-2 (IGF-2) activates estrogen receptor-alpha and -beta via the IGF-1 and the insulin receptors in breast cancer cells. *Growth Factors* **29:** 82–93.

104. Rosato, V., C. Bosetti, R. Bosetti, *et al.* 2011. Metabolic syndrome and the risk of breast cancer in postmenopausal women. *Ann. Oncol.* [Epub ahead of Print]. doi:10.1093/annonc/mdr025.

105. Rosato, V., A. Zucchetto, C. Bosetti, *et al.* 2011. Metabolic syndrome and endometrial cancer risk. *Ann. Oncol.* **22:** 884–889.

106. Tannenbaum, A. & H. Silverstone. 1949. The influence of the degree of caloric restriction on the formation of skin tumors and hepatomas in mice. *Cancer Res.* **9:** 724–727.

107. Colman, R.J., R.M. Anderson, S.C. Johnson, *et al.* 2009. Caloric restriction delays disease onset and mortality in rhesus monkeys. *Science* **325:** 201–204.

108. Moore, T., S. Carbajal, L. Beltran, *et al.* 2008. Reduced susceptibility to two-stage skin carcinogenesis in mice with low circulating insulin-like growth factor I levels. *Cancer Res.* **68:** 3680–3688.

109. Hursting, S.D., S.M. Smith, L.M. Lashinger, *et al.* 2010. Calories and carcinogenesis: lessons learned from 30 years of calorie restriction research. *Carcinogenesis* **31:** 83–89.

110. Yang, X., W.Y. So, R.C. Ma, *et al.* 2011. Low HDL cholesterol, metformin use, and cancer risk in type 2 diabetes: the Hong Kong Diabetes Registry. *Diabetes Care* **34:** 375–380.

111. Donadon, V., M. Balbi, F. Valent & A. Avogaro. 2010. Glycated hemoglobin and antidiabetic strategies as risk factors for hepatocellular carcinoma. *World J. Gastroenterol.* **16:** 3025–3032.

112. Buchs, A.E. & B.G. Silverman. 2011. Incidence of malignancies in patients with diabetes mellitus and correlation with treatment modalities in a large Israeli health maintenance organization: a historical cohort study. *Metabolism.* **60:** 1379–1385.

113. Decensi, A., M. Puntoni, P. Goodwin, *et al.* 2010. Metformin and cancer risk in diabetic patients: a systematic review and meta-analysis. *Cancer Prev. Res. (Phila)* **3:** 1451–1461.

114. Evans, J.M., L.A. Donnelly, A.M. Emslie-Smith, *et al.* 2005. Metformin and reduced risk of cancer in diabetic patients. *BMJ* **330:** 1304–1305.

115. Landman, G.W., N. Kleefstra, K.J. van Hateren, *et al.* 2010. Metformin associated with lower cancer mortality in type 2 diabetes: ZODIAC-16. *Diabetes Care* **33:** 322–326.

116. Monami, M., C. Colombi, D. Balzi, *et al.* 2011. Metformin and cancer occurrence in insulin-treated type 2 diabetic patients. *Diabetes Care* **34:** 129–131.

117. Jiralerspong, S., S.L. Palla, S.H. Giordano, *et al.* 2009. Metformin and pathologic complete responses to neoadjuvant chemotherapy in diabetic patients with breast cancer. *J. Clin. Oncol.* **27:** 3297–3302.

118. He, X.X., S.M. Tu, M.H. Lee & S.C. Yeung. 2011. Thiazolidinediones and metformin associated with improved survival of diabetic prostate cancer patients. *Ann. Oncol.* [Epub ahead of Print]. doi:10.1093/annonc/mdr020.

119. Baur, D.M., J. Klotsche, O.P. Hamnvik, *et al.* 2010. Type 2 diabetes mellitus and medications for type 2 diabetes mellitus are associated with risk for and mortality from cancer in a German primary care cohort. *Metabolism.* **60:** 1363–1371.

120. Hadad, S., T. Iwamoto, L. Jordan, *et al.* 2011. Evidence for biological effects of metformin in operable breast cancer: a pre-operative, window-of-opportunity, randomized trial. *Breast Cancer Res. Treat.* **128:** 783–794.

121. El-Mir, M.Y., V. Nogueira, E. Fontaine, *et al.* 2000. Dimethylbiguanide inhibits cell respiration via an indirect effect targeted on the respiratory chain complex I. *J. Biol. Chem.* **275:** 223–228.

122. Zhuang, Y. & W.K. Miskimins. 2008. Cell cycle arrest in Metformin treated breast cancer cells involves activation of AMPK, downregulation of cyclin D1, and requires p27Kip1 or p21Cip1. *J. Mol. Signal.* **3:** 18-28.

123. Zakikhani, M., R. Dowling, I.G. Fantus, *et al.* 2006. Metformin is an AMP kinase-dependent growth inhibitor for breast cancer cells. *Cancer Res.* **66:** 10269–10273.

124. Gotlieb, W.H., J. Saumet, M.C. Beauchamp, *et al.* 2008. In vitro metformin anti-neoplastic activity in epithelial ovarian cancer. *Gynecol. Oncol.* **110:** 246–250.

125. Ben Sahra, I., C. Regazzetti, G. Robert, *et al.* 2011. Metformin, independent of AMPK, induces mTOR inhibition and cell-cycle arrest through REDD1. *Cancer Res.* **71:** 4366–4372.

126. Ben Sahra, I., K. Laurent, A. Loubat, *et al.* 2008. The antidiabetic drug metformin exerts an antitumoral effect in vitro and in vivo through a decrease of cyclin D1 level. *Oncogene* **27:** 3576–3586.

127. Foretz, M., S. Hebrard, J. Leclerc, *et al.* 2010. Metformin inhibits hepatic gluconeogenesis in mice independently of the LKB1/AMPK pathway via a decrease in hepatic energy state. *J. Clin. Invest.* **120:** 2355–2369.

128. Ota, S., K. Horigome, T. Ishii, *et al.* Metformin suppresses glucose-6-phosphatase expression by a complex I inhibition and AMPK activation-independent mechanism. *Biochem. Biophys. Res. Commun.* **388:** 311–316.

129. Caton, P.W., N.K. Nayuni, J. Kieswich, *et al.* 2010. Metformin suppresses hepatic gluconeogenesis through induction of SIRT1 and GCN5. *J. Endocrinol.* **205:** 97–106.

130. Algire, C., L. Amrein, M. Zakikhani, *et al.* 2010. Metformin blocks the stimulative effect of a high-energy diet on colon carcinoma growth in vivo and is associated with reduced expression of fatty acid synthase. *Endocr. Relat. Cancer* **17:** 351–360.

131. Goodwin, P.J., K.I. Pritchard, M. Ennis, *et al.* 2008. Insulin-lowering effects of metformin in women with early breast cancer. *Clin. Breast Cancer* **8:** 501–505.

132. Zakikhani, M., M.J. Blouin, E. Piura & M.N. Pollak. 2010. Metformin and rapamycin have distinct effects on the AKT pathway and proliferation in breast cancer cells. *Breast Cancer Res. Treat.* **123:** 271–279.

133. Kisfalvi, K., G. Eibl, J. Sinnett-Smith & E. Rozengurt. 2009. Metformin disrupts crosstalk between G protein-coupled receptor and insulin receptor signaling systems and inhibits pancreatic cancer growth. *Cancer Res.* **69:** 6539–6545.

134. Brown, K.A., N.I. Hunger, M. Docanto & E.R. Simpson. 2010. Metformin inhibits aromatase expression in human breast adipose stromal cells via stimulation of AMP-activated protein kinase. *Breast Cancer Res. Treat.* **123:** 591–596.

135. Hirsch, H.A., D. Iliopoulos, P.N. Tsichlis & K. Struhl. 2009. Metformin selectively targets cancer stem cells, and acts together with chemotherapy to block tumor growth and prolong remission. *Cancer Res.* **69:** 7507–7511.

136. Iliopoulos, D., H.A. Hirsch & K. Struhl. 2011. Metformin decreases the dose of chemotherapy for prolonging tumor remission in mouse xenografts involving multiple cancer cell types. *Cancer Res.* **71:** 3196–3201.

137. Vazquez-Martin, A., C. Oliveras-Ferraros, S. Cufi, *et al.* 2010. Metformin regulates breast cancer stem cell ontogeny by transcriptional regulation of the epithelial-mesenchymal transition (EMT) status. *Cell Cycle* **9:** 3807–3814.

138. Vazquez-Martin, A., C. Oliveras-Ferraros, S. Del Barco, *et al.* 2011. The anti-diabetic drug metformin suppresses self-renewal and proliferation of trastuzumab-resistant tumor-initiating breast cancer stem cells. *Breast Cancer Res. Treat.* **126:** 355–364.

Ann. N.Y. Acad. Sci. ISSN 0077-8923

ANNALS OF THE NEW YORK ACADEMY OF SCIENCES
Issue: *The Year in Diabetes and Obesity*

Prioritization of care in adults with diabetes and comorbidity

Neda Laiteerapong, Elbert S. Huang, and Marshall H. Chin

Section of General Internal Medicine, Department of Medicine, University of Chicago, Chicago, Illinois

Address for correspondence: Neda Laiteerapong, M.D., Department of Medicine, University of Chicago, 5841 S. Maryland Avenue, MC 2007, Chicago, IL 60637. nlaiteer@medicine.bsd.uchicago.edu

Approximately half of adults with diabetes have at least one comorbid condition. However, diabetes care guidelines focus on diabetes-specific care, and their recommendations may not be appropriate for many patients with diabetes and comorbidity. We describe Piette and Kerr's typology of comorbid conditions, which categorizes conditions based on if they are clinically dominant (eclipse diabetes management), symptomatic versus asymptomatic, and concordant (similar pathophysiologic processes as diabetes) versus discordant. We integrate this typology with clinical evidence and shared decision-making methods to create an algorithmic approach to prioritizing care in patients with diabetes and comorbidity. Initial steps are determining the patient's goals of care and preferences for treatment, whether there is a clinically dominant condition or inadequately treated symptomatic condition, and the risk of cardiovascular disease. With these data in hand, the clinician and patient prioritize diabetes treatments during a shared decision-making process. These steps should be repeated, especially when the patient's clinical status changes. This patient-centered process emphasizes overall quality of life and functioning rather than a narrow focus on diabetes.

Keywords: diabetes mellitus; comorbidity; multimorbidity; prioritization

Introduction

Approximately half of adults with diabetes and nearly 60% of elderly adults with diabetes have at least one comorbid chronic disease.[1–3] As many as 40% of elderly adults with diabetes have four or more comorbid diseases.[4] However, diabetes care guidelines typically focus on decreasing diabetes-related microvascular and cardiovascular complications[5–8] and may not apply to many patients with diabetes who are also burdened by other comorbid conditions.[1,9–11]

Comorbidity is defined by the presence of two or more medically diagnosed conditions in the same person.[12] Comorbidity includes conditions that are highly symptomatic with large effects on quality of life (e.g., depression)[13] and those that have no immediate effects on quality of life (e.g., hyperlipidemia).[14] When comorbidity is present, the status and treatment of one disease can improve,[15] worsen,[15–17] or have little effect on the other disease.

A comorbid chronic condition can influence the health outcomes of a patient with diabetes through multiple mechanisms. By their mere presence, some comorbid chronic conditions can directly worsen health-related quality of life (HRQL).[13,18] Comorbid chronic conditions, especially depression and chronic pain, can also impair the ability of patients to perform diabetes self-management and to adhere to treatments; these changes in self-care behavior can increase the probabilities of adverse health outcomes.[19–24] Having multiple chronic conditions or functional disabilities may also decrease the potential health benefits of intensive glucose control by increasing the risk of background mortality.[25,26]

The interactions of diabetes and comorbid conditions are becoming increasingly important due to the increasing prevalence of individuals with

doi: 10.1111/j.1749-6632.2011.06316.x

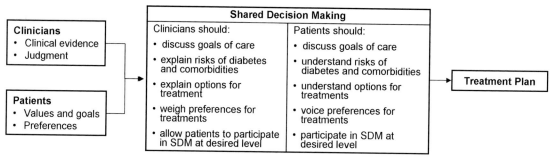

Figure 1. Shared decision-making framework for prioritization of care in adults with diabetes and comorbidity. SDM, shared decision making.

multiple chronic conditions. This trend can be partially attributed to progress in public health and medicine, which has increased life expectancy and led to an older population at greater risk for chronic diseases.[27] We have also become increasingly successful at decreasing the risk of mortality for specific chronic diseases such as diabetes, heart disease, and cerebrovascular disease, thus extending the life expectancy of those living with chronic disease.[28–30] At the same time, the recent obesity epidemic has increased the prevalence of diabetes.[31,32] The combined effect of these trends is that people are living longer with more chronic diseases, which increases the prevalence of patients with diabetes and comorbid conditions.

In light of the rising prevalence of diabetes and comorbidity, significant need exists for guidelines to address the interaction of diabetes with other conditions. The Veterans Affairs/Department of Defense (VA/DoD)[7] and the California Healthcare Foundation/American Geriatrics Society (CHF/AGS)[8] diabetes care guidelines include detailed discussions about specific comorbid conditions. The VA/DoD guideline recommends considering the patient's total health status when evaluating their diabetes management. As part of that consideration, the guideline identifies comorbid diseases that occur more frequently among patients with diabetes (e.g., coronary artery disease and hyperlipidemia), conditions that affect diabetes management (e.g., substance use disorder and depression), and diseases that may cause secondary diabetes (e.g., Cushing's disease). The CAF/AGS guidelines recommend screening patients for comorbid conditions, known as geriatric syndromes (depression, chronic pain, incontinence, and falls), which are highly prevalent in the elderly and are associated with lower HRQL.[13] Although

the previously mentioned guidelines are unusual because they discuss specific comorbid illnesses, many more guidelines do recommend considering life expectancy when setting glucose control targets.[5–8]

While these guidelines introduce some important considerations in patients with diabetes and comorbidity, numerous questions remain: How does one prioritize treatment decisions in adults with diabetes and comorbidity? Are there certain comorbid diseases that should be treated prior to others? And what key issues should be considered when caring for adults with diabetes and comorbidity?

In this review paper, we address these questions by suggesting an approach for prioritizing care decisions in patients with diabetes and comorbidity that integrates a typology for understanding comorbid conditions with the tenets of shared decision making. We describe the typology using three clinical conditions that highlight how comorbid conditions may guide diabetes treatment decisions (Table 1). We then outline a general approach to prioritizing care based on shared decision making—a marriage of the patient's preferences, population-based evidence, and the clinician's judgment (Fig. 1).[33]

Typology of comorbid chronic conditions

For patients with diabetes, Piette and Kerr published a typology of comorbid chronic conditions that serves as our starting point (Table 2).[34] They described three major types of comorbid diseases: clinically dominant comorbid conditions, symptomatic versus asymptomatic conditions, and concordant versus discordant conditions. Clinically dominant conditions are "conditions that are so complex or serious that they eclipse the management of other health problems." Examples include conditions that significantly shorten life expectancy, are

Table 1. Clinical evidence for relationships between diabetes and specific comorbid conditions

Author	Study design	Study population	Intervention	Measurements	Outcomes
Clinically dominant condition: end-stage diseases—limited life expectancy					
UKPDS 33 study[35]	Randomized controlled trial	3,867 U.K. adults with new-onset type 2 diabetes	Intensive (FPG <6 mmol/L) with sulfonylurea or insulin versus conventional glucose therapy (diet alone)	Any diabetes-related endpoint, diabetes-related death, all-cause mortality	Differences in diabetes-related death and all-cause mortality were not significant between groups. Compared to the conventional group, the intensive group had a 12% lower risk (CI: 1–21, $P = 0.03$) for any diabetes-related endpoint, especially due to a 25% risk reduction (CI: 7–40; $P = 0.01$) in microvascular endpoints. Kaplan–Meier plots for microvascular endpoints separated significantly only after nine years of follow-up. After 12 years of follow-up, results from most surrogate endpoints (ankle reflexes, cardiomegaly, and silent myocardial infarction) and end-stage complications (blindness and peripheral vascular disease) did not differ between groups.
Huang *et al.*[26]	Diabetes microsimulation model	Hypothetical population of adults 60–80 years old with type 2 diabetes and varied life expectancies estimated from a validated population-level mortality index	Intensive (A1C 7.0%) versus moderate glucose control (A1C 7.9%)	Lifetime difference in complications incidence and average quality-adjusted days	Expected benefits of intensive control declined as the mortality index increased (indicated by increasing levels of comorbid illness and functional impairment) for all age groups. For example, for adults 60–64 years old with new-onset diabetes, the benefits declined from 106 quality-adjusted days (CI: 95–117 days) at baseline good health to 44 days (CI: 38–50 days) with three additional mortality index points and eight days (CI: 5–10 days) with seven additional index points.

Continued

Table 1. *Continued*

Author	Study design	Study population	Intervention	Measurements	Outcomes
Greenfield et al.[25]	Five-year longitudinal observational study	3,074 patients with type 2 diabetes categorized into high- and low-to-moderate comorbidity based on responses to the TIBI questionnaire		Total mortality and five-year incident cardiovascular events. HR adjusted for age and sex.	A1C $\leq$6.5% at baseline was associated with lower cardiovascular events in the low-to-moderate comorbidity group (TIBI $\leq$12) (adjusted HR 0.60; CI: 0.42–0.85; $P = 0.005$). A1C <7.0% was associated with fewer cardiovascular events in the low-to-moderate comorbidity group (adjusted HR 0.61; CI: 0.44–0.83; $P = 0.001$). Neither A1C $\leq$6.5% nor A1C $\leq$7.0% was associated with lower cardiovascular events in the high comorbidity group (TIBI >12 points).
Symptomatic condition: chronic pain					
Laiteerapong et al.[13]	Cross-sectional survey	6,317 patients with diabetes receiving care through Kaiser Permanente Northern California		HRQL measured with a short survey based on the SF-8	Patients with chronic pain had lower physical HRQL scores (β-coefficient, –5.6; CI: –6.1 to –5.0; $P < 0.001$) to the same degree as participants who had myocardial infarction (β, –5.3; CI: –7.0 to –3.5; $P < 0.001$) stroke (β, –4.7; CI: –7.6 to –1.8; $P = 0.002$), or hypoglycemia (β, –4.7; CI: –8.2 to –1.3; $P < 0.001$).
Bair et al.[45]	Cross-sectional survey	11,689 participants with diabetes participating in a multisite prospective cohort study		HRQL measured by the SF-12	Patients with diabetes and chronic pain were more likely to report being depressed than patients without chronic pain (41.3% vs. 16.2%; $P < 0.001$). Patients who reported moderate pain were 1.3 times (OR, CI: 1.1–2.0) more likely to report depression, and those with extreme pain were 2.0 times (OR, CI: 1.6–2.5) more likely to report depression.

Continued

Table 1. *Continued*

Author	Study design	Study population	Intervention	Measurements	Outcomes
Krein *et al.*[21]	Cross-sectional survey	993 patients with diabetes receiving care through the Department of Veterans Affairs (VA)		Self-report of chronic pain, (pain present most of the time for $\geq$six months during past year) and diabetes self-management	Compared to patients who did not report chronic pain, patients with chronic pain ($n = 557$) had poorer overall diabetes self-management (β-coefficient, –5.0; CI: –7.8 to –2.2; $P = 0.002$) and greater difficulty following exercise (adjusted OR, 3.0; CI: 2.1–4.1) and eating plans (adjusted OR, 1.6; CI: 1.2–2.1). Patients who reported severe or very severe pain had significantly greater difficulty taking their diabetes medications (adjusted OR, 2.0; CI: 1.2–3.4) and exercising (adjusted OR, 2.5; CI: 1.3–5.0).
Krein *et al.*[46]	Prospective cohort study	1,169 patients with diabetes and a BP $\geq$140/90 prior to a PCP visit		For each visit, PCPs reported the top three issues discussed and whether hypertension medications were intensified or not intensified	A discussion of pain during visits significantly lowered the likelihood that blood pressure medications were intensified (35% vs. 46%; $P = 0.02$).
Concordant disease: cardiovascular disease					
ACCORD trial[54,55]	Randomized controlled trial	10,251 participants with type 2 diabetes aged $\geq$40 years with CVD or $\geq$55 years with a high risk of CVD	Intensive (A1C <6.0%) versus standard glucose therapy (A1C 7.0–7.9%	Nonfatal myocardial infarction, nonfatal stroke, or death from cardiovascular causes	After a mean follow-up of 3.5 years, the intensive therapy group had a higher risk of death (HR, 1.22; CI: 1.01–1.46) compared to the standard therapy group. At five-year follow-up, the intensive therapy group still had a higher risk of death (HR, 1.19; CI: 1.03–1.38) compared to the standard therapy group.

Continued

Table 1. *Continued*

Author	Study design	Study population	Intervention	Measurements	Outcomes
ADVANCE trial[56]	Randomized controlled trial	11,140 participants with type 2 diabetes ≥55 years with a history of major macrovascular or microvascular disease or at least one risk factor for vascular disease	Intensive (A1C <6.5%) versus standard glucose therapy based on local guidelines	Composite of macrovascular events and composite of microvascular events	After a mean follow-up of 5.6 years, the intensive therapy group had a 10% lower risk of the composite outcome of major macrovascular and microvascular events (HR, 0.90; CI: 0.82–0.98), due mostly to a reduction in nephropathy (HR, 0.79; CI: 0.66–0.93).
VADT[57]	Randomized controlled trial	1,791 military veterans with a suboptimal response to therapy for Type 2 diabetes	Intensive (A1C reduction of 1.5%) versus standard glucose therapy	Time to any CVE: death, CVE, and microvascular events	Intensive and standard glucose therapy groups did not differ in their time to CVE (HR, 0.88; CI: 0.74–1.05), mortality rates (HR, 1.07; CI: 0.81–1.42), CVE, or microvascular events
VADT sub-study[57]	Substudy of VADT	Subsample of 301 participants with type 2 diabetes in the VADT	Intensive (A1C reduction of 1.5%) versus standard therapy lowering	Baseline coronary artherosclerosis measured by CAC, CVE	Among participants randomized to intensive treatment, 11 of 62 individuals with a high CAC score (>100) had events, as compared to 1 of 52 individuals with low CAC scores (≤100). Participants with high CAC scores had a greater risk of CVE compared to those with low CAC scores (multivariable HR, 0.74; CI: 0.46–1.20; $P = 0.21$ vs. HR, 0.08; CI: 0.008–0.77; $P = 0.03$).

A1C, hemoglobin A1c; ACCORD, Action to Control Cardiovascular Risk in Diabetes Trial; ADVANCE, Action in Diabetes and Vascular Disease: Preterax and Diamicron MR Controlled Evaluation; CAC, coronary artery calcium; CI, 95% confidence interval; CVE, cardiovascular events; FBG, fasting blood glucose; HR, hazard ratio; HRQL, health-related quality of life; OR, odds ratio; PCP, primary care physician; RR, relative risk; TIBI, Total Illness Burden Inventory; UKPDS, United Kingdom Prospective Diabetes Study; VADT, Veterans Affairs Diabetes Trial.

severely symptomatic, or are recently diagnosed. Symptomatic conditions are conditions for which patients experience notable symptoms, as opposed to asymptomatic conditions, which are treated with the sole purpose of preventing future morbidity. Chronic pain is a classic symptomatic condition, whereas a typical asymptomatic condition is hyperlipidemia. Lastly, concordant conditions are conditions that are "parts of the same overall pathophysiologic risk profile," whereas discordant conditions have a less direct relationship to the condition of interest. In the case of diabetes, concordant conditions include hypertension and cardiovascular disease (CVD), whereas discordant conditions include cancer, chronic obstructive pulmonary disease, and anemia. This typology provides a simplified framework of the complex relationships between diabetes and comorbid conditions.

We use this typology to demonstrate how specific types of comorbid chronic conditions can guide the prioritization of care for diabetes treatments. For the clinically dominant condition, we describe end-stage diseases, since these diseases shorten life expectancy and thus may eclipse the potential benefit of intensive glucose control. We provide the example of chronic pain to show how a symptomatic condition can alter the priorities of diabetes care. Lastly, we describe the example of CVD, a key concordant condition that may increase mortality in patients who are treated with very intensive glucose targets. The clinical evidence for the relationships between diabetes and specific conditions are presented in Table 1.

Clinically dominant condition: end-stage diseases—limited life expectancy

For a patient with diabetes, clinically dominant conditions are those that determine prognosis and dictate everyday experiences. These include end-stage diseases, severely symptomatic conditions, and

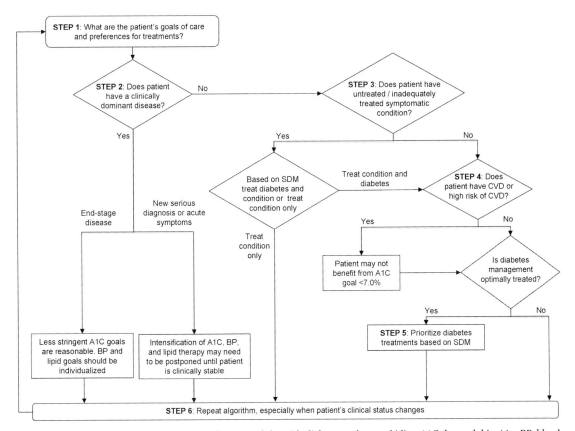

Figure 2. Algorithm for the prioritization of care in adults with diabetes and comorbidity. A1C, hemoglobin A1c; BP, blood pressure; SDM, shared decision making.

Table 2. Typology of comorbid chronic conditions[a]

Clinically dominant conditions
- Comorbid chronic conditions that are so complex or so serious that they eclipse the management of other health problems.
- Examples:
  - End-stage diseases: metastatic cancer, New York Heart Association Class 4 heart failure, advanced dementia, chronic obstructive pulmonary disease with severe hypoxia, severe decompensated liver disease, renal failure
  - Severe acute symptoms: chest pain, profound vomiting, unintentional weight loss (>5% body weight)
  - New serious diagnoses: cancer, pulmonary embolism, cerebrovascular accident

Symptomatic versus asymptomatic chronic conditions
- Treatment for symptomatic chronic conditions focuses on improving patients' symptom profiles, functioning and quality of life, and may also delay or prevent poor long-term outcomes.
  - Examples: chronic pain, depression, incontinence, falls/fear of falling, functional disability
- Treatment of asymptomatic chronic conditions focuses almost exclusively on preventing downstream adverse events and early mortality.
  - Examples: hyperlipidemia, mild hypertension

Concordant versus discordant chronic conditions
- Concordant conditions represent parts of the same overall pathophysiologic risk profile and are more likely to be the focus of the same disease and self-management plan.
  - Examples: cardiovascular disease, cerebrovascular disease
- Discordant treatments are not directly related in either their pathogenesis or management.
  - Examples: chronic obstructive pulmonary disease, cancer, anemia

---

[a]Adapted from Piette and Kerr.[34]

recently diagnosed diseases. Examples of end-stage diseases include metastatic cancer, New York Heart Association Class 4 heart failure, advanced dementia, chronic obstructive pulmonary disease with severe hypoxia, and severe decompensated liver disease (moderate ascites, bilirubin >3 mg/dL, albumin <2.8 g/dL, or elevated international normalized ratio >2.3). In these patients, end-stage diseases severely limit life expectancy to such an extent that the long-term benefits of optimally managed glycemic control would not be observed. In the United Kingdom Prospective Diabetes Study (UKPDS) intensive A1C treatment did not lower rates of diabetes-related mortality or CVD even after 10 years of follow-up. Intensive A1C control did significantly lower rates of microvascular disease (risk reduction, 25%; $P = 0.001$); however, the Kaplan–Meier plots only separated significantly after nine years of follow-up.[35] Even after 12 years of follow-up, results from most of the surrogate endpoints (ankle reflexes, cardiomegaly, and silent myocardial infarction) and end-stage complications (blindness and peripheral vascular disease) did not differ. Thus, if nearly a decade of intensive glucose control is needed prior to seeing improvements, then limited life expectancy may prevent patients from ever receiving the potential benefits of intensive glucose control.

Current evidence on the effects of life expectancy on glucose targets are based on microsimulation models and observational data. Microsimulation is a computer modeling technique that is used to predict outcomes for individuals.[36] Predictions for patient outcomes are calculated from transition probabilities that are generated from results of randomized controlled trials, epidemiologic studies (e.g., case-control and cohort), meta-analyses, and expert opinions. Microsimulation models often combine data from multiple sources to create a set of rules that can answer policy-relevant questions. Microsimulation models can be used to predict outcomes for populations that are not typically enrolled in clinical trials (e.g., the elderly and patients with multiple comorbid diseases). Additionally, some microsimulation models are flexible and allow researchers to alter individual patient characteristics (e.g., age, sex, and comorbidity). Several microsimulation models have been developed for diabetes, including the UKPDS Outcomes Model,[37] Centers for Disease Control and Prevention/Research Triangle Institute Diabetes Cost-Effectiveness Model,[38] Archimedes,[39] and the Michigan Model for Diabetes.[40]

Huang *et al.* used a diabetes microsimulation model to evaluate how life expectancy would affect the potential benefits of intensive glucose control (A1C level of 7.0%) compared to moderate control (A1C level of 7.9%).[26] This decision analytic study was performed on a hypothetical population of adults aged 60–80 years with type 2 diabetes and no history of diabetes-related complications. The population was based on the diabetes population aged >60 years old in the National Health and Nutrition Examination Surveys (NHANES) from 1999 to 2002. Huang *et al.* combined transition probabilities from the UKPDS[37] with a geriatric mortality prediction tool.[41] Transition probabilities from the UKPDS were based on a sample of 3,642 patients with new-onset type 2 diabetes who were randomized patients to intensive glucose control versus conventional therapy. The geriatric mortality prediction tool was developed from data based on community-dwelling U.S. adults older than 50 years who participated in the 1998 wave of the Health and Retirement Study (HRS). This tool accurately predicted four-year mortality in older adults. The mortality prediction tool used easy-to-collect clinical data (age, sex, comorbid conditions, and functional measures) to estimate a mortality index score, ranging from 1 to 26 points with higher values corresponding to greater risk of mortality.

Combining the diabetes model and the geriatric mortality tool, Huang *et al.* found that the expected benefits of intensive control were inversely related to the level of comorbid illness and functional impairment for all age groups.[26] For example, for adults aged 60–64 years with new-onset diabetes, the benefits declined from 106 quality-adjusted days (95% confidence interval (CI): 95–117 days) at baseline good health to 44 days (CI: 38–50 days) with three additional mortality index points and eight days (CI: 5–10 days) with seven additional index points. For patients with greater duration of diabetes, the expected benefits of intensive glucose control were

also negatively associated with life expectancy. For adults aged 60–64 years with diabetes for 10–15 years, the expected benefits of intensive glucose control decreased from 116 quality-adjusted days (CI: 103–129 days) to 36 days (CI: 29–43 days) with four additional index points and to eight days (CI: 6–11 days) with eight additional index points.

To verify whether the benefits of intensive A1C control were affected by comorbidity, Greenfield *et al.* conducted an observational study of 3,074 patients with type 2 diabetes who were characterized into high and low-to-moderate comorbidity groups at baseline and observed for five years.[25] The baseline comorbidity level was determined from patient responses on the Total Illness Burden Index (TIBI) questionnaire. The TIBI questionnaire assesses the presence and severity of eight comorbid conditions (atherosclerotic heart disease, lung disease, heart failure, arthritis, genitourinary disease, vision loss, gastrointestinal conditions, and foot disease). High comorbidity was defined by scores ≥ 12, whereas low-to-moderate comorbidity was defined by scores < 12. The TIBI has been validated as a predictor of 3.5-year mortality[42] and HRQL,[43] and a score of 12 points can discriminate greater and lesser risk for death.[42] Greenfield *et al.* found that patients in the low-to-moderate comorbidity group with baseline A1C levels $\leq 6.5\%$ had a lower five-year incidence of cardiovascular events (adjusted hazard ratio (HR), 0.60; CI: 0.42–0.85; $P = 0.005$). However, patients in the high comorbidity group experienced no significant benefit from A1C levels $\leq 6.5\%$. Similarly, only the low-to-moderate comorbidity group had fewer cardiovascular events after attaining an A1C level of 7.0% (adjusted HR, 0.61; CI: 0.44–0.83; $P = 0.001$). Together, these studies strongly suggest that moderate glucose targets may be reasonable in patients with diabetes and limited life expectancy.

Symptomatic condition: chronic pain
Symptomatic conditions cause patients to experience symptoms that negatively impact HRQL. Several symptomatic conditions are more prevalent among patients with diabetes compared to patients without diabetes, including chronic pain, depression, incontinence, falls/fear of falling, and functional disability.[8] To describe this typology, we highlight chronic pain as a classic example of a symptomatic condition.

Chronic pain is highly prevalent in patients with diabetes.[44] Chronic pain has been reported in over 40% of elderly adults with diabetes[13] and up to 60% of the VA population with diabetes.[22] In patients with diabetes, chronic pain may be caused by diabetes (e.g., peripheral neuropathy and peripheral vascular disease) or by common diseases (e.g., osteoarthritis and headache).

Chronic pain seriously impacts HRQL in patients with diabetes. It has been associated with similar declines in HRQL as cardiovascular and microvascular disease. In a study of 6,317 adults with diabetes, Laiteerapong *et al.* found that patients with chronic pain had lower physical HRQL scores (β-coefficient, -5.6; CI: -6.1 to -5.0; $P < 0.001$) to the same degree as participants who had myocardial infarction (β, -5.3; CI: -7.0 to -3.5; $P < 0.001$), stroke (β, -4.7; CI: -7.6 to -1.8; $P = 0.002$), or hypoglycemia (β, -4.7; CI: -8.2 to -1.3; $P < 0.001$).[13] Furthermore, a study by Bair *et al.* of 11,689 participants with diabetes found that patients with diabetes and chronic pain were more likely to report being depressed (41.3% vs. 16.2%; $P < 0.001$).[45] They also reported a dose-response relationship between chronic pain and depression with patients who report moderate pain being 1.3 times (odds ratio (OR), CI: 1.1–2.0) more likely to report depression and those with extreme pain being 2.0 times (OR, CI: 1.6–2.5) more likely to report depression.

The presence of chronic pain negatively impacts diabetes self-management. In a study by Krein *et al.*, 993 patients with diabetes were asked to report if they had chronic pain and if they had difficulty with diabetes self-management.[22] Diabetes self-management scores could range from 0 to 100, with higher scores indicating less difficulty with self-management. Even after adjustment for several factors including depressive symptoms and general health status, patients with chronic pain ($n = 557$) had poorer overall diabetes self-management (β-coefficient, -5.0; CI: -7.8 to -2.2; $P = 0.002$) compared to patients who did not report chronic pain. Patients with chronic pain also reported greater difficulty following exercise plans (adjusted OR, 3.0; CI: 2.1–4.1) and eating plans (adjusted OR, 1.6; CI: 1.2–2.1) compared to patients without chronic pain. Furthermore, compared to those with moderate pain, patients with diabetes who reported severe or very severe pain had significantly greater difficulty taking their diabetes medications (adjusted OR, 2.0; CI: 1.2–3.4) and exercising (adjusted OR, 2.5; CI: 1.3–5.0).

Because of the serious consequences of chronic pain to HRQL and diabetes self-management, deprioritizing chronic pain may impede both diabetes-specific and overall care. However, symptomatic conditions, like chronic pain, can be very challenging to treat. For example, Krein *et al.*[46] found that addressing pain significantly lowered the likelihood that blood pressure medications were intensified (35% vs. 46%, $P = 0.02$) during clinic visits. Their results may not be surprising since addressing any single clinical condition may take attention away from the care of any other clinical condition. This study is a reminder that it is important to consider managing diabetes while addressing symptomatic conditions. The severity of the patient's symptoms, degree of diabetes control, and patients' preferences should guide decisions to treat diabetes and symptomatic conditions simultaneously or sequentially.

Other examples of symptomatic conditions include depression, incontinence, falling/fear of falling, and functional disability. Compared to patients without diabetes, patients with diabetes have a two times greater odds of depression,[47] and symptomatic depression has been associated with a two times greater odds of poor adherence to diabetes medications among a cohort of 4,117 patients with diabetes.[19] Incontinence, falls, and functional disability are also especially prevalent in the elderly with diabetes and are associated with lower HRQL.[13,48–51] However, further evidence is needed to clarify whether these symptomatic conditions also negatively impact diabetes management.

Concordant condition: CVD

Concordant conditions have similar pathophysiological profiles as the disease of interest. As a result, the treatment of a concordant condition generally improves the status of both the concordant condition and the primary disease. Physicians may appropriately prioritize the treatment of concordant conditions over discordant conditions because a single treatment can improve the status of more than one condition.

Several studies have found that discordant conditions may be undertreated compared to concordant conditions. In a study of over one million elderly adults by Redelmeier *et al.*,[16] patients with diabetes were less likely to receive prescriptions for estrogen-replacement therapy (2.4% vs. 5.9%; $P < 0.001$; at a time when hormone replacement therapy was commonly prescribed in postmenopausal women). Another study by Turner *et al.* similarly reported that among 15,459 patients with uncontrolled hypertension, patients with more discordant conditions were less likely to have their blood pressure treatment intensified than patients with no discordant condition (one condition vs. none: adjusted OR, 0.85; CI: 0.80–0.90; ≥seven conditions vs. none: adjusted OR, 0.59; CI: 0.51–0.69).[17]

In patients with diabetes and CVD, both diseases have very similar treatment goals.[5,52,53] Increased physical activity and low cholesterol diets benefit both diabetes and CVD. Blood pressure (<130/80 mmHg) and cholesterol targets (low-density lipoprotein <100 mg/dL) are identical for patients with diabetes and patients with CVD. Aspirin therapy is very frequently recommended for patients with diabetes and almost universally recommended for patients with CVD. Thus, for the majority of patients, CVD management enhances the management of diabetes.

Although the benefits of cardiovascular management in diabetes patients with comorbid CVD are well accepted, the effects of glycemic management on CVD are far more uncertain. After the UKPDS trial showed improved outcomes in patients with new-onset diabetes from intensive glucose control,[35] several trials attempted to reproduce its results in patients with a history of diabetes, many of whom had CVD. Instead of confirming results, trial results were mixed and found either an increased mortality risk, a decreased risk of microvascular disease, or no benefit with intensive glucose therapy.

In the Action to Control Cardiovascular Risk in Diabetes (ACCORD) trial, 10,251 study participants with type 2 diabetes (mean duration, 10 years) were randomly assigned to intensive glucose therapy (A1C <6.0%) or standard therapy (A1C 7.0–7.9%).[54] In addition to having diabetes, participants were either ≥40 years old with CVD or ≥55 years old with a high risk of CVD. On average, the intensive therapy group achieved an A1C of 6.4% and the standard therapy group achieved an A1C of 7.5%. Unexpectedly, the trial ended early after a mean follow-up of 3.5 years because the intensive therapy group had a higher mortality rate than the standard therapy group (HR 1.22; 95% CI: 1.01–1.46). Recent five-year follow-up results from the ACCORD trial reconfirmed a greater mortality rate in the intensive glucose therapy group (HR, 1.19; CI: 1.03–1.38).[55]

Results from the Action in Diabetes and Vascular Disease: Preterax and Diamicron MR Controlled Evaluation (ADVANCE) trial differed from those of the ACCORD trial.[56] The ADVANCE trial included 11,140 participants with type 2 diabetes aged ≥55 years and randomized them to intensive glucose therapy (A1C <6.5%) or standard glucose therapy. Participants were required to have a history of major macrovascular or microvascular disease or at least one risk factor for vascular disease. Their median duration of diabetes was about eight years. The intensive therapy and standard therapy groups in ADVANCE achieved similar A1C levels as in the ACCORD trial (6.5% and 7.3%, respectively) at five years of follow-up. However, unlike the ACCORD trial, the intensive glucose therapy group had a 10% relative reduction in the combined outcome of major macrovascular and microvascular events (HR, 0.90; CI: 0.82–0.98), mostly due to a 21% relative reduction in nephropathy (HR, 0.79; CI: 0.66–0.93), and there were no significant effects on major macrovascular events or death.

The third study, the Veterans Affairs Diabetes Trial (VADT), randomized 1,791 veterans to intensive glucose therapy (an absolute reduction of 1.5% in A1C) versus standard therapy.[57] Patients had an average diabetes duration of 11.5 years, and 40% had a history of CVD. The A1C levels in both groups were higher in VADT compared to the ACCORD and ADVANCE trials. The intensive therapy group achieved a mean A1C of 6.9%, and the standard therapy group achieved a mean of 8.4%. However, unlike both the ACCORD and ADVANCE trials, there were no significant differences in major cardiovascular events, death, or microvascular events between the two groups after a median follow-up of 5.6 years. Additionally, a VADT substudy of 301 patients found that among patients in the intensive glucose therapy group, patients with higher baseline levels of coronary atherosclerosis experienced significantly more cardiovascular events than patients with lower levels of coronary atherosclerosis (multivariable HR, 0.08; CI: 0.008–0.77; $P = 0.03$ vs. HR, 0.74; CI: 0.46–1.20; $P = 0.21$).[58]

Because of these conflicting results, the optimal glucose target in patients with diabetes and CVD is still debated. Diabetes experts have recently

Table 3. Estimated prevalence of disease patterns in elderly adults with diabetes (*n*, %)[a]

	Men, aged 65 or older (Weighted $N = 2,592,800$)	Women, aged 65 or older (Weighted $N = 3,426,500$)
Diabetes only	703,120 (27)	585,280 (17)
One comorbid condition		
Arthritis	545,260 (21)	1,049,700 (31)
CHD	285,080 (11)	135,540 (4)
CLRT	110,890 (4)	97,480 (3)
CVA	82,780 (3)	–
Two comorbid conditions		
Arthritis and CHD	313,310 (12)	454,630 (13)
Arthritis and CLRT	83,450 (3)	369,870 (11)
Arthritis and CVA	79,260 (3)	98,590 (3)
Three comorbid conditions		
Arthritis, CHD, and CVA	79,420 (3)	123,310 (4)
Arthritis, CHD, and CLRT	–	192,380 (6)

CHD, coronary heart disease; CLRT, chronic lower respiratory tract disease; CVA, cerebrovascular disease.
[a]Prevalence estimates based on Weiss *et al.*[64] Only the chronic diseases of arthritis, CHD, CLRT, and CVA were included.

integrated diabetes trial results and have suggested that the A1C target should be 7.0% or greater in patients with CVD or a high risk of CVD.[59]

Although the presence of concordant conditions may appear to simplify diabetes treatment decisions, concordant conditions, like CVD, may not have simple relationships with diabetes. Achieving the treatment goals of CVD improves diabetes management, but intensive glucose therapy may increase mortality in patients with CVD. Thus, even with concordant conditions like CVD, treatment decisions for diabetes must be carefully considered.

Integrating comorbidities into diabetes care
The example clinical conditions (end-stage disease, chronic pain, and CVD) and the typology (clinically dominant, concordant vs. discordant, and symptomatic vs. asymptomatic) greatly simplify the complex interactions of comorbid diseases in patients with diabetes. For example, there can be significant overlap in the typology by conditions. End-stage diseases are often quite symptomatic (e.g., New York Heart Association Class IV heart failure). CVD is concordant and usually asymptomatic. Chronic pain is symptomatic but can be either concordant if the pain is due to diabetes complications, or discordant if the pain is due to other conditions.

Another reason this typology is frequently an oversimplification is because many adults with diabetes suffer from more than just one additional disease. Weiss *et al.* studied the prevalence of five major chronic diseases (arthritis, coronary heart disease, chronic lower respiratory tract disease, cerebrovascular accident, and diabetes) in older men and women from the NHANES 1999–2004 (Table 3).[60] Diabetes occurred with one comorbid disease in 39% of men and 37% of women, two comorbid conditions in 18% of men and 27% of women, and three comorbid conditions in 3% of men and 9% of women. Regarding specific combinations, in older men diabetes occurred most frequently alone (27%; 703,120 out of 2,592,800 older men with diabetes); in older women, diabetes occurred most frequently with arthritis (31%; 1,049,700 of 3,426,500 older women with diabetes). The second most common combination for diabetes was with arthritis in men (21%; 545,260) and alone in women (17%; 585,720). Among these five major chronic diseases, there were eight different combinations of diabetes and comorbidity.

The complex patterns of diabetes and comorbid chronic conditions likely preclude the development of a single rigid guideline. In situations where few guidelines exist and there is significant clinical uncertainty, shared decision making between patients and clinicians is a useful, and possibly necessary, tool for making individualized treatment decisions.[33] Components of shared decision making for clinicians and patients are noted in Figure 1. Key elements include discussions between clinicians and patients about the goals of care, risks of diabetes and comorbid conditions, options for treatments, and patient preferences for treatment. Additionally, patients should be allowed to participate in shared decision making at their desired level.

This strategy has been endorsed by the United States Preventive Services Task Force (USPSTF),[61] an independent panel that develops evidence-based recommendations on clinical preventive services. The USPSTF suggests a graded approach to shared decision making. For screening tests with strong evidence, lengthy and frequent discussion is likely unnecessary, but for screening tests with less certain evidence, engaging patients in shared decision making is necessary to assess the net benefit of the screening test. Thus, shared decision making is not necessary for hypertension screening, a recommendation with substantial net benefit. However, shared decision making should be used for mammography decisions in women <50 years because individual women may have a strong desire to be screened,[62] even though there may be only a small net benefit.[63]

Several critical reasons exist for using shared decision-making principles when caring for adults with diabetes and comorbidity. First, patients can vary greatly in their overall health priorities. A study of 81 elderly adults by Fried *et al.* found that nearly half ranked maintaining independence as their most important outcome;[64] however, 27% ranked staying alive, 21% ranked reducing/eliminating pain, and 10% ranked reducing/eliminating other symptoms as their most important outcome. Second, patients can be inconsistent in their overall health priorities. Fried *et al.* asked 189 elderly adults with advanced disease, if when faced with a fatal disease exacerbation, they would be willing to either undergo or forego high-burden therapy to possibly avoid death.[65] They found that 35% had an inconsistent preference trajectory (e.g., becoming more and then less willing over time and vice versa). Third, providers and patients often disagree on the relative importance of different comorbid conditions. In a study by Zulman *et al.*, 28% of providers did not agree with patients in the ranking of their most important health condition.[66] Providers were more likely to rank hypertension as the most important condition, and patients were more likely to prioritize symptomatic conditions like pain, depression, and breathing problems.

Fourth, patients with diabetes have been shown to vary greatly in their preferences for treatment (Table 4). In a study of 475 elderly adults with diabetes, Chin *et al.* found that patients varied greatly in their perceptions of diabetes complications and treatments.[67] Using utility values (range, 0 [death] to 1 [perfect health]), they found a large range in the utility values for blindness (0.39; standard deviation [SD]: 0.32), lower leg amputation (0.45; SD: 0.34), conventional glucose treatment (0.76; SD: 0.27), and intensive insulin treatment (0.64; SD: 0.32). In a separate study of elderly adults, Brown *et al.* evaluated whether patient perceptions of diabetes treatments differed according to patient vulnerability, as assessed by the Vulnerable Elders Scale.[68] In general, they found that vulnerable patients reported lower utilities than nonvulnerable patients for most treatments, including intensive glucose control (mean, 0.61 vs. 0.72, $P < 0.01$). However, within-group variation was large for both groups (SD >0.25). Similarly, Huang *et al.* studied a multi-ethnic sample of 701 elderly and nonelderly adults with diabetes and found large variation in patients' preferences for diabetes complications and treatments (e.g., intensive glucose control, mean 0.67; SD 0.34).[69] Last, there is limited evidence and, as a result, significant clinical uncertainty as to the net clinical benefit of diabetes treatments in most patients with diabetes and comorbid chronic conditions.

Because patients vary in their health priorities and diabetes treatment preferences, and because clinicians cannot predict their preferences, shared decision making is especially critical to guiding treatment decisions in patients with diabetes and comorbidity. Using the tenets of shared decision making and the typology of comorbidity presented earlier, we present an algorithm for prioritizing care in adults with diabetes and comorbid chronic conditions.

Algorithm for prioritization of care in patients with diabetes and comorbidity (Fig. 2)

1. Elicit patient's goals of care and preferences for treatment to develop a care plan using the tenets of shared decision making.

Table 4. Utility values for diabetes complications and treatments[a]

Study population	Chin et al.[67] 473 older adults with diabetes	Brown et al.[68] 332 vulnerable and nonvulnerable older adults with diabetes[b]		Huang et al.[69] 701 multi-ethnic adults with diabetes
		Vulnerable	Nonvulnerable	
Diabetes complications				
Neuropathy				0.66 ± 0.34
Amputation	0.45 ± 0.34			0.55 ± 0.36
Retinopathy				0.53 ± 0.36
Blindness	0.39 ± 0.32			0.38 ± 0.35
Nephropathy				0.64 ± 0.35
Kidney failure	0.36 ± 0.31			0.35 ± 0.33
Mild stroke				0.70 ± 0.31
Major stroke				0.31 ± 0.31
Angina				0.64 ± 0.31
Diabetes treatments				
Conventional glucose treatment	0.76 ± 0.27	0.71 ± 0.33	0.79 ± 0.28	0.76 ± 0.31
Intensive glucose therapy		0.61 ± 0.34	0.72 ± 0.32	0.67 ± 0.34
Intensive pill therapy	0.77 ± 0.27			
Intensive insulin therapy	0.64 ± 0.32			
Conventional blood pressure control		0.73 ± 0.32	0.80 ± 0.28	0.77 ± 0.30
Intensive blood pressure control		0.69 ± 0.33	0.76 ± 0.29	0.73 ± 0.32
Aspirin		0.79 ± 0.28	0.83 ± 0.28	0.80 ± 0.29
Cholesterol-lowering pill		0.72 ± 0.30	0.83 ± 0.26	0.78 ± 0.29
Diet		0.89 ± 0.23	0.90 ± 0.21	0.88 ± 0.24
Exercise		0.85 ± 0.26	0.91 ± 0.19	0.89 ± 0.23
Polypharmacy		0.58 ± 0.35	0.66 ± 0.32	
Comprehensive diabetes care				0.64 ± 0.34

[a]Utility values can range between 0 (death) and 1 (perfect health).
[b]Study population was categorized by vulnerability based on their score on the Vulnerable Elders Scale-13 (VES-13). Patients with scores ≥ 3 points were defined as vulnerable.

Patients should be asked what their goals of care are and to what degree they want to participate in shared decision making. Patients can vary greatly in their desire to actively engage in shared decision making. In a review of eight studies with different patient populations in different settings, interest in shared decision making ranged from 19% to 68%.[70] There can be a spectrum of participation in medical decision making, ranging from very little to full ownership. In the paternalistic decision-making model, the clinician implements what he/she believes is best for the patient after receiving their assent (not consent).

On the other end of the spectrum, patients who have complete autonomy in the decision-making process use clinicians for their clinical acumen, like technicians, and have complete control over their medical care.[71] Shared decision making contrasts with these extreme views because it stresses the partnership between the patients' values and preferences and the clinicians' knowledge of clinical evidence and judgment. Barriers such as the power differential between clinician and patient may impede shared decision making. Racial and ethnic minorities with diabetes may face additional barriers such as historical mistrust

despite wanting to engage in shared decision making,[72,73] and thus clinicians need to
be particularly sensitive in discussing patient
preferences.[74,75] If patients are interested
in participating in shared decision making, then clinicians should elicit the patients' overall health goals and specific treatment preferences. This conversation can
be framed by a discussion of the overall health priorities introduced by Fried
et al.[64] (e.g., maintaining independence, staying alive, reducing/eliminating pain, and re-
ducing/eliminating other symptoms) and by
discussion of diabetes treatment goals and
preferences (e.g., preventing diabetes complications, decreasing polypharmacy, avoiding
insulin therapy, avoiding hypoglycemia, and
improving quality of life).

2. Assess whether the patient with diabetes has
any clinically dominant conditions.
Clinically dominant conditions can include
end-stage diseases that limit life expectancy,
severe acute symptoms, and new serious diagnoses. Patients with diabetes and end-stage
diseases may not benefit from intensive glucose control. In this population, less stringent
glucose targets are reasonable. Blood glucose
levels at least <200 mg/dL are reasonable to
avoid symptoms of diabetes.[76] In patients with
diabetes, the benefits from tight blood pressure
control (144/82 mmHg) compared to standard
therapy (154/87 mmHg) were discernible in
Kaplan–Meier plots after one year of control.[77]
Similarly, in a large study by the Heart Protection Collaborative Group, participants with
diabetes randomized to cholesterol-lowering
medication (simvastatin) had a 22% lower risk
of vascular events ($P < 0.001$) compared to
those who received placebo therapy, and this
difference became apparent within one to two
years of follow-up.[78] Thus, patients with diabetes and end-stage diseases may still benefit
from blood pressure and lipid control, depending on their prognosis. Decisions about blood
pressure and cholesterol treatment should be
guided based on each patient's individual context, including their current levels, tolerance
of medications, interest in therapy, concern
about adverse effects, and overall prognosis.
For patients with severe acute symptoms or

new serious diagnoses, intensification of glucose, blood pressure, and lipid control may
need to be postponed until patients are clinically stable.

3. Screen the patient with diabetes for untreated
or inadequately treated symptomatic conditions and then treat.
All patients with diabetes should be screened
for untreated or inadequately treated symptomatic conditions, that is, chronic pain, depression, incontinence, falls/fear of falling, and
functional disability. Patients with diabetes
and these symptomatic conditions generally
have poor HRQL.[8,13] Additionally, patients
with chronic pain and depression often have
difficulty managing their diabetes.[22] Once diagnosed, symptomatic conditions should be
treated. Depending on the severity of symptoms and patients' preferences, diabetes treatments can also be managed alongside symptomatic conditions.

4. Determine whether the patient has CVD or a
high risk for CVD.
Though most CVD treatments are concordant
with the care of diabetes, much controversy
exists regarding the appropriate intensity of
glucose control in patients with CVD, or a high
risk of CVD, as previously described. For this
reason, A1C targets at or higher than 7.0%
should be considered in these patients.[59]

5. Decide which of the diabetes treatment goals
should be given priority.
The comparative benefit of three diabetes
treatments (blood glucose, blood pressure, and
lipid control) have been reviewed in studies by
Vijan and Hayward.[79,80] In one study, using
results from the UKPDS, Vijan and Hayward
found that the effectiveness of tight blood pressure control (achieved blood pressure, 144/82
[tight] vs. 154/87 [control]) was superior to intensive glucose control (A1C, 7.0% [intensive]
vs. 7.9% [usual]) for all major clinical endpoints.[79] To prevent one diabetes endpoint, 8.9
persons needed to be treated with tight blood
pressure control compared to 31.2 persons
with intensive glucose control. In a separate
review on the effectiveness of pharmacologic
lipid-lowering in patients with type 2 diabetes,
Vijan and Hayward found that the number
needed to treat to prevent one cardiovascular

outcome was 34.5 for primary prevention and 13.5 for secondary prevention.[80] Thus, on a population level, overall fewer people would need to be treated with tight blood pressure control than cholesterol-lowering therapy, or intensive glucose control, to benefit one person. For individual patients, however, the optimal strategy is still unknown for prioritizing these three treatment decisions. Will patients fare better if each of the three outcomes is addressed one at a time, or the outcome that is most out of range is addressed first, or if all three outcomes are addressed simultaneously? Because of this clinical uncertainty, the tenets of shared decision making should guide discussions about how to prioritize diabetes treatments along with the care of comorbidities. Also considerations should be made for the patients' cognitive status, financial situation, and social support. Clinicians and patients should discuss the treatment options to develop a care plan.

6. Prioritization is an iterative process and should be revisited, especially when the patient's clinical status changes significantly.

Patients' priorities may change and their priorities may not be predicated on past preferences. Additionally, clinical knowledge and patients' comorbidity, cognition, and resources may change. Clinicians should frequently revisit patients' priorities, potential constraints, and past care decisions to ensure patient-centered care.

Discussion

Despite the fact that about half of adults with diabetes have a comorbid chronic condition, diabetes care guidelines have concentrated their recommendations on patients who only have diabetes. This review paper summarizes the current understanding of the complex relationships between diabetes and comorbid diseases. Several comorbid conditions, such as end-stage diseases, chronic pain, and CVD, can help guide diabetes treatment decisions. For patients with diabetes and other comorbid conditions, we provide a general algorithm for prioritizing care, which integrates a typology of comorbid conditions with the framework of shared decision making.

Although our overall understanding of diabetes and comorbidity is still rudimentary, the relationships between diabetes and selected comorbid conditions have been well-studied. Further research on the relationship between diabetes and symptomatic conditions could enhance the care of patients with diabetes and comorbidity. Potential areas of research include determining whether symptomatic conditions should be managed prior to diabetes, or if both conditions can be addressed simultaneously. Additional research could clarify the relationships between diabetes and discordant conditions. For example, recent studies have suggested that patients with diabetes are at an increased risk for cancer and lung disease.[81–84] However, it is still unknown how the presence of these discordant conditions should factor into decisions about diabetes management.

Because of the complexity of caring for patients with diabetes and comorbidity, it may not be possible to create a diabetes care guideline that applies to all patients with diabetes. However, shared decision making allows for treatment decisions to be patient-centered, a key principle of the National Quality Strategy for health care.[85] Practical strategies for using shared decision making in patients with diabetes and comorbidity would benefit primary care clinicians who are already hampered by the number of guideline recommendations.[86] Some possible strategies include using computers to elicit goals and preferences, as well as the development of multicondition decision aids that can integrate treatment decisions for diabetes and several comorbid diseases.

Although the study of diabetes and comorbidities is still in its nascency, clinicians are already faced with the struggle of caring for these complex patients. Clinicians aim to improve their patients' overall HRQL and functioning; thus, explicitly addressing the role of comorbidities in diabetes care is essential. Future clinical research in diabetes should concentrate on the practical question of how to best care for patients with diabetes and common comorbid conditions.

Acknowledgments

N.L. is supported by Grant Number F32DK089973 from the National Institute of Diabetes and Digestive and Kidney Diseases (NIDDK). E.S.H. is supported by Grant Number R01-DK-081796 from the NIDDK. M.H.C. is supported by a NIDDK

Midcareer Investigator Award in Patient-Oriented Research (K24 DK071933). This project was also supported by the NIDDK Diabetes Research and Training Center (P60 DK20595) and NIDDK Chicago Center for Diabetes Translation Research (P30 DK092949). The content is solely the responsibility of the authors and does not necessarily represent the official views of the NIDDK or the National Institutes of Health.

Conflicts of interest

The authors declare no conflicts of interest.

References

1. Druss, B.G., S.C. Marcus, M. Olfson, *et al.* 2001. Comparing the national economic burden of five chronic conditions. *Health Aff. (Millwood)* **20:** 233–241.
2. Lee, P.G., C. Cigolle & C. Blaum. 2009. The co-occurrence of chronic diseases and geriatric syndromes: the health and retirement study. *J. Am. Geriatr. Soc.* **57:** 511–516.
3. Schneider, K.M., B.E. O'Donnell & D. Dean. 2009. Prevalence of multiple chronic conditions in the United States' Medicare population. *Health Qual. Life Outcomes* **7:** 82.
4. Wolff, J.L., B. Starfield & G. Anderson. 2002. Prevalence, expenditures, and complications of multiple chronic conditions in the elderly. *Arch. Intern. Med.* **162:** 2269–2276.
5. American Diabetes Association. 2011. Standards of medical care in diabetes—2011. *Diabetes Care* **34**(Suppl 1): S11–61.
6. Handelsman, Y., J.I. Mechanick, L. Blonde, et al. 2011. American Association of Clinical Endocrinologists Medical Guidelines for clinical practice for developing a diabetes mellitus comprehensive care plan. *Endocr. Pract.* **17**(Suppl 2): 1–53.
7. Management of Diabetes Mellitus Update Working Group. 2010. *VA/DoD Clinical Practice Guideline for the Management of Diabetes Mellitus. Version 4.0.* Veterans Health Administration and Department of Defense. Washington, DC.
8. Brown, A.F., C.M. Mangione, D. Saliba & C.A. Sarkisian. 2003. Guidelines for improving the care of the older person with diabetes mellitus. *J. Am. Geriatr. Soc.* **51:** S265–280.
9. Tinetti, M.E., S.T. Bogardus, Jr. & J.V. Agostini. 2004. Potential pitfalls of disease-specific guidelines for patients with multiple conditions. *N. Engl. J. Med.* **351:** 2870–2874.
10. Boyd, C.M., J. Darer, C. Boult, *et al.* 2005. Clinical practice guidelines and quality of care for older patients with multiple comorbid diseases: implications for pay for performance. *JAMA* **294:** 716–724.
11. Durso, S.C. 2006. Using clinical guidelines designed for older adults with diabetes mellitus and complex health status. *JAMA* **295:** 1935–1940.
12. Fried, L.P., L. Ferrucci, J. Darer, *et al.* 2004. Untangling the concepts of disability, frailty, and comorbidity: implications for improved targeting and care. *J. Gerontol. A. Biol. Sci. Med. Sci.* **59:** 255–263.
13. Laiteerapong, N., A.J. Karter, J.Y. Liu, *et al.* 2011. Correlates of quality of life in older adults with diabetes: the diabetes & aging study. *Diabetes Care* **34:** 1749–1753.
14. Wexler, D.J., R.W. Grant, E. Wittenberg, *et al.* 2006. Correlates of health-related quality of life in type 2 diabetes. *Diabetologia* **49:** 1489–1497.
15. Desai, M.M., R.A. Rosenheck, B.G. Druss & J.B. Perlin. 2002. Mental disorders and quality of diabetes care in the veterans health administration. *Am. J. Psychiatry* **159:** 1584–1590.
16. Redelmeier, D.A., S.H. Tan & G.L. Booth. 1998. The treatment of unrelated disorders in patients with chronic medical diseases. *N. Engl. J. Med.* **338:** 1516–1520.
17. Turner, B.J., C.S. Hollenbeak, M. Weiner, *et al.* 2008. Effect of unrelated comorbid conditions on hypertension management. *Ann. Intern. Med.* **148:** 578–586.
18. Chen, H.Y., D.J. Baumgardner & J.P. Rice. 2011. Health-related quality of life among adults with multiple chronic conditions in the United States, behavioral risk factor surveillance system, 2007. *Prev. Chronic Dis.* **8:** A09.
19. Katon, W., J. Russo, E.H. Lin, *et al.* 2009. Diabetes and poor disease control: is comorbid depression associated with poor medication adherence or lack of treatment intensification? *Psychosom. Med.* **71:** 965–972.
20. Ciechanowski, P.S., W.J. Katon & J.E. Russo. 2000. Depression and diabetes: impact of depressive symptoms on adherence, function, and costs. *Arch. Intern. Med.* **160:** 3278–3285.
21. Schoenberg, N.E. & S.C. Drungle. 2001. Barriers to non-insulin dependent diabetes mellitus (NIDDM) self-care practices among older women. *J. Aging Health* **13:** 443–466.
22. Krein, S.L., M. Heisler, J.D. Piette, *et al.* 2005. The effect of chronic pain on diabetes patients' self-management. *Diabetes Care* **28:** 65–70.
23. Krein, S.L., M. Heisler, J.D. Piette, *et al.* 2007. Overcoming the influence of chronic pain on older patients' difficulty with recommended self-management activities. *Gerontologist* **47:** 61–68.
24. Blaum, C., C.T. Cigolle, C. Boyd, *et al.* 2010. Clinical complexity in middle-aged and older adults with diabetes: the health and retirement study. *Med. Care* **48:** 327–334.
25. Greenfield, S., J. Billimek, F. Pellegrini, *et al.* 2009. Comorbidity affects the relationship between glycemic control and cardiovascular outcomes in diabetes: a cohort study. *Ann. Intern. Med.* **151:** 854–860.
26. Huang, E.S., Q. Zhang, N. Gandra, *et al.* 2008. The effect of comorbid illness and functional status on the expected benefits of intensive glucose control in older patients with type 2 diabetes: a decision analysis. *Ann. Intern. Med.* **149:** 11–19.
27. Vincent, G.K. & V.A. Velkoff. 2010. The next four decades, the older population in the United States: 2010 to 2050. U.S. Census Bureau. Washington, DC.
28. Preis, S.R., S.J. Hwang, S. Coady, *et al.* 2009. Trends in all-cause and cardiovascular disease mortality among women and men with and without diabetes mellitus in the Framingham Heart Study, 1950 to 2005. *Circulation* **119:** 1728–1735.
29. Xu, J., K.D. Kochanek, S.L. Murphy & B. Tejada-Vera. 2010. Deaths: Final Data for 2007. *National Vital Statistics Reports* **58, no. 19.** National Center for Health Statistics. Hyattsville, MD.
30. Tierney, E.F., B.L. Cadwell, M.M. Engelgau, *et al.* 2004. Declining mortality rate among people with diabetes in North Dakota, 1997–2002. *Diabetes Care* **27:** 2723–2725.

31. Flegal, K.M., M.D. Carroll, C.L. Ogden & L.R. Curtin. 2010. Prevalence and trends in obesity among US adults, 1999–2008. *JAMA* **303:** 235–241.

32. Huang, E.S., A. Basu, M. O'Grady & J.C. Capretta. 2009. Projecting the future diabetes population size and related costs for the U.S. *Diabetes Care* **32:** 2225–2229.

33. Woolf, S.H., E.C. Chan, R. Harris, *et al.* 2005. Promoting informed choice: transforming health care to dispense knowledge for decision making. *Ann. Intern. Med.* **143:** 293–300.

34. Piette, J.D. & E.A. Kerr. 2006. The impact of comorbid chronic conditions on diabetes care. *Diabetes Care* **29:** 725–731.

35. UK Prospective Diabetes Study (UKPDS) Group. 1998. Intensive blood-glucose control with sulphonylureas or insulin compared with conventional treatment and risk of complications in patients with type 2 diabetes (UKPDS 33). *Lancet* **352:** 837–853.

36. Rutter, C.M., A.M. Zaslavsky & E.J. Feuer. 2011. Dynamic microsimulation models for health outcomes: a review. *Med. Decis. Making* **31:** 10–18.

37. Clarke, P.M., A.M. Gray, A. Briggs, *et al.* 2004. A model to estimate the lifetime health outcomes of patients with type 2 diabetes: the United Kingdom Prospective Diabetes Study (UKPDS) Outcomes Model (UKPDS no. 68). *Diabetologia* **47:** 1747–1759.

38. CDC Diabetes Cost-effectiveness Group. 2002. Cost-effectiveness of intensive glycemic control, intensified hypertension control, and serum cholesterol level reduction for type 2 diabetes. *JAMA* **287:** 2542–2551.

39. Schlessinger, L. & D.M. Eddy. 2002. Archimedes: a new model for simulating health care systems—the mathematical formulation. *J. Biomed. Inform.* **35:** 37–50.

40. Zhou, H., D.J. Isaman, S. Messinger, *et al.* 2005. A computer simulation model of diabetes progression, quality of life, and cost. *Diabetes Care* **28:** 2856–2863.

41. Lee, S.J., K. Lindquist, M.R. Segal & K.E. Covinsky. 2006. Development and validation of a prognostic index for 4-year mortality in older adults. *JAMA* **295:** 801–808.

42. Litwin, M.S., S. Greenfield, E.P. Elkin, *et al.* 2007. Assessment of prognosis with the total illness burden index for prostate cancer: aiding clinicians in treatment choice. *Cancer* **109:** 1777–1783.

43. Greenfield, S., L. Sullivan, K.A. Dukes, *et al.* 1995. Development and testing of a new measure of case mix for use in office practice. *Med. Care* **33:** AS47–55.

44. Butchart, A., E.A. Kerr, M. Heisler, *et al.* 2009. Experience and management of chronic pain among patients with other complex chronic conditions. *Clin. J. Pain* **25:** 293–298.

45. Bair, M.J., E.J. Brizendine, R.T. Ackermann, *et al.* 2010. Prevalence of pain and association with quality of life, depression and glycaemic control in patients with diabetes. *Diabet. Med.* **27:** 578–584.

46. Krein, S.L., T.P. Hofer, R. Holleman, *et al.* 2009. More than a pain in the neck: how discussing chronic pain affects hypertension medication intensification. *J. Gen. Intern. Med.* **24:** 911–916.

47. Anderson, R.J., K.E. Freedland, R.E. Clouse & P.J. Lustman. 2001. The prevalence of comorbid depression in adults with diabetes: a meta-analysis. *Diabetes Care* **24:** 1069–1078.

48. Solomon, R., P. Kirwin, P.H. Van Ness, *et al.* 2010. Trajectories of quality of life in older persons with advanced illness. *J. Am. Geriatr. Soc.* **58:** 837–843.

49. Kanauchi, M., A. Kubo, K. Kanauchi & Y. Saito. 2008. Frailty, health-related quality of life and mental well-being in older adults with cardiometabolic risk factors. *Int. J. Clin. Pract.* **62:** 1447–1451.

50. Ozcan, A., H. Donat, N. Gelecek, *et al.* 2005. The relationship between risk factors for falling and the quality of life in older adults. *BMC Public Health* **5:** 90.

51. Salkeld, G., I.D. Cameron, R.G. Cumming, *et al.* 2000. Quality of life related to fear of falling and hip fracture in older women: a time trade off study. *BMJ* **320:** 341–346.

52. National Cholesterol Education Program (NCEP) Expert Panel on Detection, Evaluation, and Treatment of High Blood Pressure in Adults (Adult Treatment Panel III). 2002. Final report. *Circulation* **106:** 3143–3421.

53. Chobanian, A.V., G.L. Bakris, H.R. Black, *et al.* 2003. The Seventh Report of the Joint National Committee on Prevention, Detection, Evaluation, and Treatment of High Blood Pressure: the JNC 7 report. *JAMA* **289:** 2560–2572.

54. Gerstein, H.C., M.E. Miller, R.P. Byington, *et al.* 2008. Effects of intensive glucose lowering in type 2 diabetes. *N. Engl. J. Med.* **358:** 2545–2559.

55. Gerstein, H.C., M.E. Miller, S. Genuth, *et al.* 2011. Long-term effects of intensive glucose lowering on cardiovascular outcomes. *N. Engl. J. Med.* **364:** 818–828.

56. Patel, A., S. MacMahon, J. Chalmers, *et al.* 2008. Intensive blood glucose control and vascular outcomes in patients with type 2 diabetes. *N. Engl. J. Med.* **358:** 2560–2572.

57. Duckworth, W., C. Abraira, T. Moritz, *et al.* 2009. Glucose control and vascular complications in veterans with type 2 diabetes. *N. Engl. J. Med.* **360:** 129–139.

58. Reaven, P.D., T.E. Moritz, D.C. Schwenke, *et al.* 2009. Intensive glucose-lowering therapy reduces cardiovascular disease events in veterans affairs diabetes trial participants with lower calcified coronary atherosclerosis. *Diabetes* **58:** 2642–2648.

59. Ismail-Beigi, F., E. Moghissi, M. Tiktin, *et al.* 2011. Individualizing glycemic targets in type 2 diabetes mellitus: implications of recent clinical trials. *Ann. Intern. Med.* **154:** 554–559.

60. Weiss, C.O., C.M. Boyd, Q. Yu, *et al.* 2007. Patterns of prevalent major chronic disease among older adults in the United States. *JAMA* **298:** 1160–1162.

61. Sheridan, S.L., R.P. Harris & S.H. Woolf. 2004. Shared decision making about screening and chemoprevention: a suggested approach from the U.S. Preventive Services Task Force. *Am. J. Prev. Med.* **26:** 56–66.

62. Welch, H.G. 2010. Screening mammography—a long run for a short slide? *N. Engl. J. Med.* **363:** 1276–1278.

63. Mandelblatt, J.S., K.A. Cronin, S. Bailey, *et al.* 2009. Effects of mammography screening under different screening schedules: model estimates of potential benefits and harms. *Ann. Intern. Med.* **151:** 738–747.

64. Fried, T.R., M. Tinetti, J. Agostini, *et al.* 2011. Health outcome prioritization to elicit preferences of older persons with multiple health conditions. *Patient Educ. Couns.* **83:** 278–282.

65. Fried, T.R., J. O'Leary, P. Van Ness & L. Fraenkel. 2007. Inconsistency over time in the preferences of older persons with advanced illness for life-sustaining treatment. *J. Am. Geriatr. Soc.* **55:** 1007–1014.

66. Zulman, D.M., E.A. Kerr, T.P. Hofer, *et al.* 2010. Patient-provider concordance in the prioritization of health conditions among hypertensive diabetes patients. *J. Gen. Intern. Med.* **25:** 408–414.

67. Chin, M.H., M.L. Drum, L. Jin, *et al.* 2008. Variation in treatment preferences and care goals among older patients with diabetes and their physicians. *Med. Care* **46:** 275–286.

68. Brown, S.E., D.O. Meltzer, M.H. Chin & E.S. Huang. 2008. Perceptions of quality-of-life effects of treatments for diabetes mellitus in vulnerable and nonvulnerable older patients. *J. Am. Geriatr. Soc.* **56:** 1183–1190.

69. Huang, E.S., S.E. Brown, B.G. Ewigman, *et al.* 2007. Patient perceptions of quality of life with diabetes-related complications and treatments. *Diabetes Care* **30:** 2478–2483.

70. Frosch, D.L. & R.M. Kaplan. 1999. Shared decision making in clinical medicine: past research and future directions. *Am. J. Prev. Med.* **17:** 285–294.

71. Emanuel, E.J. & L.L. Emanuel. 1992. Four models of the physician-patient relationship. *JAMA* **267:** 2221–2226.

72. Peek, M.E., H. Tang, A. Cargill & M.H. Chin. 2011. Are there racial differences in patients' shared decision-making preferences and behaviors among patients with diabetes? *Med. Decis. Making* **31:** 422–431.

73. Peek, M.E., S.C. Wilson, R. Gorawara-Bhat, *et al.* 2009. Barriers and facilitators to shared decision-making among African-Americans with diabetes. *J. Gen. Intern. Med.* **24:** 1135–1139.

74. Peek, M.E., A. Odoms-Young, M.T. Quinn, *et al.* 2010. Race and shared decision-making: perspectives of African-Americans with diabetes. *Soc. Sci. Med.* **71:** 1–9.

75. Peek, M.E., A. Odoms-Young, M.T. Quinn, *et al.* 2010. Racism in healthcare: relationship to shared decision-making and health disparities. Response to Bradby's critique. *Soc. Sci. Med.* **71:** 13–17.

76. Kasper, D.L., E. Braunwald, A.S. Fauci, *et al.* 2005. *Harrison's Principles of Internal Medicine*, Vol. 2. McGraw-Hill.

77. UK Prospective Diabetes Study Group (UKPDS). 1998. Tight blood pressure control and risk of macrovascular and microvascular complications in type 2 diabetes: UKPDS 38. *BMJ* **317:** 703–713.

78. Collins, R., J. Armitage, S. Parish, *et al.* 2003. MRC/BHF Heart Protection Study of cholesterol-lowering with simvastatin in 5963 people with diabetes: a randomised placebo-controlled trial. *Lancet* **361:** 2005–2016.

79. Vijan, S. & R.A. Hayward. 2003. Treatment of hypertension in type 2 diabetes mellitus: blood pressure goals, choice of agents, and setting priorities in diabetes care. *Ann. Intern. Med.* **138:** 593–602.

80. Vijan, S. & R.A. Hayward. 2004. Pharmacologic lipid-lowering therapy in type 2 diabetes mellitus: background paper for the American College of Physicians. *Ann. Intern. Med.* **140:** 650–658.

81. Giovannucci, E., D.M. Harlan, M.C. Archer, *et al.* 2010. Diabetes and cancer: a consensus report. *CA Cancer J. Clin.* **60:** 207–221.

82. Larsson, S.C., S.O. Andersson, J.E. Johansson & A. Wolk. 2008. Diabetes mellitus, body size and bladder cancer risk in a prospective study of Swedish men. *Eur. J. Cancer* **44:** 2655–2660.

83. Barone, B.B., H.C. Yeh, C.F. Snyder, *et al.* 2008. Long-term all-cause mortality in cancer patients with preexisting diabetes mellitus: a systematic review and meta-analysis. *JAMA* **300:** 2754–2764.

84. Ehrlich, S.F., C.P. Quesenberry, Jr., S.K. Van Den Eeden, *et al.* 2010. Patients diagnosed with diabetes are at increased risk for asthma, chronic obstructive pulmonary disease, pulmonary fibrosis, and pneumonia but not lung cancer. *Diabetes Care* **33:** 55–60.

85. National Priorities Partnership. 2010. Input to the Secretary of Health and Human Services on Priorities for the 2011 National Quality Strategy. *National Quality Forum*. Washington, D.C.

86. Ostbye, T., K.S. Yarnall, K.M. Krause, *et al.* 2005. Is there time for management of patients with chronic diseases in primary care? *Ann. Fam. Med.* **3:** 209–214.

Ann. N.Y. Acad. Sci. ISSN 0077-8923

ANNALS OF THE NEW YORK ACADEMY OF SCIENCES
Issue: *The Year in Diabetes and Obesity*

Receptor for AGE (RAGE): signaling mechanisms in the pathogenesis of diabetes and its complications

Ravichandran Ramasamy, Shi Fang Yan, and Ann Marie Schmidt

Diabetes Research Program, Division of Endocrinology, Department of Medicine, New York University School of Medicine, New York, New York

Address for correspondence: Ann Marie Schmidt, M.D., Diabetes Research Program, Division of Endocrinology, Department of Medicine, New York University School of Medicine, 550 First Avenue, Smilow 901C, New York, NY 10016. annmarie.schmidt@nyumc.org

The receptor for advanced glycation endproducts (RAGE) was first described as a signal transduction receptor for advanced glycation endproducts (AGEs), the products of nonenzymatic glycation and oxidation of proteins and lipids that accumulate in diabetes and in inflammatory foci. The discovery that RAGE was a receptor for inflammatory S100/calgranulins and high mobility group box 1 (HMGB1) set the stage for linking RAGE to both the consequences and causes of types 1 and 2 diabetes. Recent discoveries regarding the structure of RAGE as well as novel intracellular binding partner interactions advance our understanding of the mechanisms by which RAGE evokes pathological consequences and underscore strategies by which antagonism of RAGE in the clinic may be realized. Finally, recent data tracking RAGE in the clinic suggest that levels of soluble RAGEs and polymorphisms in the gene encoding RAGE may hold promise for the identification of patients who are vulnerable to the complications of diabetes and/or are receptive to therapeutic interventions designed to prevent and reverse the damage inflicted by chronic hyperglycemia, irrespective of its etiology.

Keywords: diabetes; complications; RAGE; inflammation; signal transduction

Introduction

The problem of types 1 and 2 diabetes is a growing one. The incidence of type 1 diabetes, an autoimmune disorder whose pathogenesis is strongly rooted in genetic risk factors, is increasing worldwide at a rate not possibly explained solely by genetic factors.[1] Environmental influences such as diet and gut microbiota, pollution, practices of food preparation and preservation, and increased use of antibiotics, as examples, are being investigated as putative underlying mechanisms accounting for this recent acceleration.[2] Similarly, the global increase in obesity and greater physical inactivity has been suggested to underlie the alarming rise in the incidence of type 2 diabetes. In addition to the increased overall incidence of type 2 diabetes, it is apparent that an earlier age of onset, particularly in adolescents, is a contributing factor. According to the International Diabetes Federation, the number of adults with impaired glucose tolerance will rise from 344 million in 2010 to a projected 472 million by 2030.[3,4] The escalation of type 2 diabetes in the young has led to school-based initiatives to both identify the etiology and find solutions for the increase in type 2 diabetes in young people under 21 years of age to address the crisis.[5]

In this paper, we will discuss fundamental mechanisms triggered as a consequence of hyperglycemia underlying the pathogenesis of both macro- and microvascular complications in diabetes. In particular, we will focus on recent advances in the biology of the receptor for advanced glycation endproducts (RAGE), an immunoglobulin superfamily molecule whose multiple ligands have been shown to accumulate in diabetic tissues. RAGE was discovered as a receptor for advanced glycation endproducts (AGEs), such as carboxymethyl lysine (CML).[6] AGEs, the products of nonenzymatic glycation and oxidation of proteins, form to an accelerated degree in

doi: 10.1111/j.1749-6632.2011.06320.x

hyperglycemia. AGEs, largely via RAGE, activate signaling mechanisms that cause cell stress, contribute to cellular dysfunction, and damage target organs, leading to complications. The findings that RAGE interacts with non-AGE ligands, such as S100/calgranulins and high mobility group box 1 (HMGB1),[7,8] underscore the possibility that RAGE is involved not only in diabetes complications, but in the causes of types 1 and 2 diabetes as well.

RAGE and the cardiovascular complications of diabetes

The chief cause of morbidity and mortality in diabetes is cardiovascular disease, particularly heart attacks and strokes.[9] Hence, the mechanisms underlying accelerated atherosclerosis are essential to uncover in order that targeted therapeutic strategies might be developed. In type 1 diabetes, epidemiologic studies of the Diabetes Control and Complications Trials/Epidemiology of Diabetes Interventions and Complications (DCCT/EDIC) showed that intensive glycemic control was protective—even years after levels of glycosylated hemoglobin became indistinguishable from those of the control treated group—against cardiovascular events and death.[10] In type 2 diabetes, studies from the United Kingdom demonstrated that incremental rises in glycosylated hemoglobin level were associated with increased risk of cardiovascular disease.[11]

Prompted by the findings of these large-scale trials, three recent clinical trials addressed whether intensive control of glycemia would afford a beneficial impact in type 2 diabetes by reduction of cardiovascular risk. The outcomes of these three studies were somewhat surprising. The Action to Control Cardiovascular Risk in Diabetes (ACCORD) trial was interrupted prematurely because of more deaths in the intensive versus the standard treatment group. Further, all cause and cardiovascular mortality was not lower in the intensive treatment group versus the standard treatment group.[12] A recent follow-up study reported that even after glycosylated hemoglobin levels in the intensive treatment group rose to levels more similar to those in the control treatment groups (6.4–7.2%), five-year mortality was still higher in the previously intensively treated group.[13] In two other trials, the Action in Diabetes and Vascular Disease: Preterax and Diamicron Modified Release Evaluation (ADVANCE) and Glucose Control and Vascular Complications

in Veterans with Type 2 Diabetes (VADT), although premature deaths were not reported in the intensive treatment group, no benefits of such treatment on cardiovascular disease were observed.[14,15] Hence, one conclusion of these studies was that significant hypoglycemia may have been associated with adverse outcomes. Indeed, the investigators of ADVANCE recently published findings on examination of the associations between severe hypoglycemia and diabetic micro- and macrovascular complications. They concluded that severe hypoglycemia was associated with a range of adverse clinical outcomes and could contribute to cardiac ischemia.[16]

Taken together, these studies suggest that intensive treatment of hyperglycemia and the associated risk of severe hypoglycemia might have been detrimental and did not result in reduction in macrovascular complications, particularly in older subjects. Such findings strongly suggest that strategies directed at blocking the adverse effects of hyperglycemia are likely to be more effective and better tolerated. It is in this context that we propose that RAGE may be one such logical target.

RAGE in cardiovascular disease: studies in animal models

Atherosclerotic plaques retrieved from human subjects reveal that RAGE is expressed in these lesions, and to an enhanced degree in diabetes. RAGE expression colocalizes to smooth muscles (SMCs) and macrophages and to markers of oxidative stress.[17] Experiments in animal models of diabetes and accelerated atherosclerosis revealed that blockade of RAGE, using soluble RAGE (the extracellular ligand binding domain of the receptor) suppressed accelerated atherosclerosis in diabetic apolipoprotein E null mice.[18–20] Irrespective of the means by which diabetes was induced—chemical (e.g., streptozotocin) type 1 diabetes model or genetic (e.g., breeding into the *db/db* background) type 2 diabetes model—soluble RAGE prevented acceleration of diabetic atherosclerosis and suppressed the increased vascular inflammation associated with diabetes. Treatment with soluble RAGE had no effect on levels of glucose or lipids in the diabetic mice,[18–20] but it did suppress AGE levels in plasma and tissues,[18] suggesting that blocking RAGE attenuated inflammatory and oxidative stresses contributing to acceleration of vascular plaques and to perpetuation of ligand generation.

In other studies, genetically modified animals were used to test the hypothesis that RAGE contributed to acceleration of diabetic atherosclerosis. In apolipoprotein E null mice bred into the RAGE null background, induction of diabetes resulted in less atherosclerosis compared to RAGE-expressing apolipoprotein E null mice with diabetes, despite equal degrees of hyperglycemia and hyperlipidemia. Because we observed that AGEs and inflammatory ligands were present even in nondiabetic atherosclerosis, but to lesser degrees, we tested the effects of RAGE deletion in nondiabetic apolipoprotein E null mice and found that atherosclerosis lesion area and complexity were reduced by deletion of RAGE even in the absence of diabetes.[21,22] Consistent with key roles for endothelial RAGE signaling in the absence of diabetes on vascular inflammation, transgenic mice expressing cytoplasmic domain-deleted RAGE (dominant negative or DN RAGE) on the preproendothelin 1 promoter (PPET, largely expressed but not exclusively in endothelial cells), revealed less atherosclerosis in the apolipoprotein E null background versus control apolipoprotein E null mice. We retrieved endothelial cells from RAGE null mice, transgenic PPET DN RAGE mice, or littermate C57BL/6 mice, and found that stimulation with RAGE ligands and with AGE-containing oxidized low density lipoprotein (LDL) stimulated cytokine and adhesion molecule expression in a manner dependent on JNK signaling, and that these effects were significantly reduced in endothelial cells retrieved from RAGE null mice or transgenic PPET DN RAGE mice.[21] Of note, when RAGE null mice were bred into a distinct genetic model of hypercholesterolemia and atherosclerosis, the low density lipoprotein receptor (LDL receptor) null background, significantly less atherosclerosis was observed compared to LDL receptor null mice expressing RAGE.[23] These studies were performed in the absence of diabetes and solidified that, irrespective of the means by which hypercholesterolemia was induced, RAGE contributed to the acceleration of vascular inflammation and cellular stress leading to atherosclerosis.

To determine the mechanisms underlying the beneficial effects of RAGE deletion in apolipoprotein E null mice, we performed Affymetrix genomic arrays on aortas retrieved from diabetic and nondiabetic apolipoprotein E null mice expressing or devoid of RAGE. Experiments were performed at age nine weeks, after two weeks of established hyperglycemia, in order to determine the initiating factors linked to atherosclerosis and its RAGE- and diabetes-dependence. We found that a major pathway impacted both by diabetes and RAGE was the ROCK1 branch of the transforming growth factor-β (TGF-β) pathway and that smooth muscle cells principally expressed three molecules associated with this family: thrombospondin-1, ROCK1, and TGF-β.[24] Consistent with key roles for this pathway in mediating smooth muscle cell migration and proliferation, pretreatment of wild-type smooth muscle cells retrieved from mouse aorta with two different inhibitors of ROCK (fasudil and Y27632) resulted in decreased migration and proliferation stimulated by the RAGE ligand S100B.[24]

In other studies, generation of chimeric apolipoprotein E null mice (nondiabetic) after lethal irradiation and reconstitution with RAGE expressing or RAGE null bone marrow revealed that mice reconstituted with RAGE null bone marrow had decreased atherosclerosis and necrotic cores particularly at later stages, suggesting important roles for RAGE in atherosclerosis progression. Expression of key inflammatory molecules and the ligand HMGB1 in the lesions was also reduced by deletion of RAGE.[25]

In summary, these studies to date have suggested that RAGE expression in endothelial cells, macrophages, and smooth muscle cells contributes to the pathogenesis of atherosclerosis, and particularly its acceleration in diabetes. Certainly, pathogenic roles for RAGE expression in distinct cell types, such as lymphocytes, dendritic cells, stem, or progenitor cells, cannot be excluded at this time. Studies are in progress to rigorously test the signaling mechanisms impacted by RAGE in distinct cell types linked to atherosclerosis.

In addition to roles in macrovascular disease and atherosclerosis, RAGE also contributes to the pathogenesis of myocardial dysfunction, especially in diabetes. Work by Ramasamy *et al.* showed that hearts of diabetic mice subjected to ischemia/reperfusion in the isolated perfused mode displayed increased damage as assessed by release of higher levels of lactic dehydrogenase (LDH), reduced ATP levels in the heart, and higher left ventricular developed pressure (LVDP), the latter a marker of cardiac dysfunction, compared to nondiabetic mice, and that in the presence of soluble RAGE or by RAGE deletion, these parameters were greatly improved.[26] Studies *in vitro* in isolated primary adult ventricular cardiomyocytes revealed that cardiomyocytes devoid of RAGE were more resistant to apoptosis and oxidative stress compared to wild-type cardiomyocytes exposed to *in vitro* applied hypoxia.[27] Other studies have confirmed the importance of RAGE in cardiac ischemia.[28–31]

Studies in the isolated perfused heart or in isolated cardiomyocytes were complemented by experiments in which mice were subjected to transient ligation of the left anterior descending coronary artery, a model of myocardial infarction. Compared to wild-type mice, mice devoid of RAGE displayed highly significant reductions in infarct volume and increased cardiac function, as assessed by echocardiography, compared to wild-type control animals.[32,33]

Taken together, these findings support the potential benefits of RAGE antagonism in heart disease, especially in diabetes, and suggest that roles for RAGE blockade in cardioprotection are not limited to its potential impact on macrovascular disease and atherosclerosis, but to innate cardiac dysfunction as well.

RAGE and cardiovascular disease: studies in human subjects

In addition to the studies described above on expression of RAGE in human atherosclerotic plaques, the study of soluble levels of RAGE in cardiovascular disease has become a highly studied area of research. Two different forms of soluble RAGE may be detected in human plasma: "total" soluble RAGE (cell surface cleaved form) and endogenous secretory or esRAGE (derived from a splice variant of RAGE). Although mixed results have been reported suggesting either low[34] or high[35] levels of soluble RAGE as putative biomarkers of the presence or extent of cardiovascular disease, a very recent study examined total sRAGE and esRAGE levels at the prerandomization phase of a study testing atorvastatin in type 2 diabetic subjects. In this nested case–control study, the findings revealed that sRAGE and esRAGE were higher in those with low body mass index, higher adiponectin levels, lower estimated glomerular filtration rate, and white ethnicity. Independent of the treatment arm, sRAGE and esRAGE were associated with incident cardiovascular disease, but there was no association with stroke. Of note, treatment

with atorvastatin had no effect on sRAGE levels.[35] It is important to note that two other studies in diabetic and nondiabetic subjects showed that treatment with statins (atorvastatin) raised sRAGE levels.[36,37] Certainly, as recently reviewed by Wilson,[38] further analysis is needed to discern the predictive nature of sRAGE levels in cardiovascular disease. Indeed, in this context, it is critical to consider the status of renal function, as significantly impaired renal function has been linked to higher sRAGE levels.[39] Hence, interpretation of sRAGE levels must be made in the context of renal status, particularly in subjects with diabetes.

Lastly, in addition to effects of medications commonly used in cardiovascular or metabolic disease on plasma levels of soluble RAGE, these medications also may exert their benefit, at least in part, via suppression of cellular/tissue levels of RAGE. For example, treatment with simvastatin reduced atherosclerotic plaque expression of RAGE in human subjects,[40] treatment of streptozotocin-diabetic mice with the peroxisome proliferator activator receptor delta agonist L-165041 reduced RAGE expression in the kidneys,[41] treatment of mesangial cells with glucagon-like peptide 1 (GLP-1) inhibited RAGE expression,[42] and treatment of experimental animals with atorvastatin protects against middle cerebral artery occlusion, at least in part, via reduced expression of RAGE in the brain consequent to stroke.[43]

Taken together, evidence is mounting linking RAGE to mechanisms of atherosclerosis, especially in diabetes. Importantly, measurement of soluble RAGEs, under active investigation in cardiovascular disease, holds promise as a means of biomarking the state of diabetic macrovessels. In addition to macrovascular disease of diabetes, RAGE is also implicated in microvascular complications. In this review, we will discuss recent advances on the role of RAGE in one such complication, diabetic nephropathy.

RAGE and diabetic nephropathy

In the Western world, diabetes is the leading cause of end-stage renal disease, surpassing other etiologies, such as hypertension.[44,45] Likely support for the contribution of AGEs to the pathogenesis of diabetic kidney disease was obtained by studies in which pimagedine (aminoguanidine) was administered to types 1 and 2 diabetic subjects with nephropathy. Despite toxicity associated with the agent (glomerulonephritis), the use of pimagedine was associated with decreased 24-hour proteinuria in the treated subjects.[46] Notably, however, the outcome of estimated glomerular filtration rate was marginally but not statistically significantly improved in the treated group ($P = 0.05$).[46] Although pimagedine did not advance in clinical development for these reasons, its use nevertheless supported roles for AGEs in the pathogenesis of diabetic kidney disease.

It was in this context that we postulated roles for the chief AGE receptor RAGE in diabetic nephropathy. In human subjects, D'Agati *et al.* showed that AGEs and RAGE were both present and expressed in human diabetic kidneys to increased degrees compared to nondiabetic control subjects, particularly in the glomerulus and especially in glomerular epithelial cells (podocytes) and endothelial cells.[47] Based on these findings suggesting roles for AGE–RAGE in diabetic kidney disease, multiple pharmacological strategies were tested *in vivo* in animal models; examples of which include administration of soluble RAGE and antibodies to RAGE. In each case, targeting RAGE resulted in attenuation of functional and pathological endpoints of nephropathy in mouse models of types 1 and 2 diabetes.[48–50]

Studies in homozygous RAGE null mice confirmed important roles for RAGE in the pathogenesis of diabetic nephropathy.[48] Although earlier studies employed mice vulnerable to the earliest changes in the diabetic kidney but without frank loss of glomerular filtration rate (GFR), recent experiments in OVE26 mice, a mouse model of type 1 diabetes in the FVB genetic background, reveal significant loss of GFR as measured by inulin clearance. In OVE26/RAGE-null (OVE26 RKO) mice, significant protection from glomerular sclerosis, thickening of the glomerular basement membrane, podocyte effacement, and loss of GFR were noted compared to OVE26 littermates expressing RAGE.[51] Experiments performed on these animals revealed two key insights into the mechanisms by which RAGE deletion exerted beneficial effects in the diabetic kidney.

First, our data revealed the intriguing finding that despite equivalent degrees of hyperglycemia in OVE26 and OVE26 RKO mice, the levels of the AGE precursor methylglyoxal (MG) were lower in the kidneys of mice devoid of RAGE, and, indeed, in-

distinguishable from those in the kidneys of nondiabetic FVB mice. We reported that compared to OVE26 mice, kidneys from OVE26 RKO mice displayed higher levels of glyoxalase1 mRNA, protein and activity.[51] Hence, RAGE-dependent regulation of key pathways linked to AGE detoxification may explain these findings and add further support for the role of AGEs in the pathogenesis of nephropathy.

Second, in addition to RAGE-dependent regulation of glyoxalase1, additional studies using Affymetrix gene arrays were performed on isolated glomeruli from OVE26 and OVE26 RKO mice at two months of age. We reasoned that at such a time point, although microalbuminuria was evident, highly advanced glomerular lesions were not yet present. We identified significant changes in expression of Serpine1 (the gene for plasminogen activator inhibitor 1 or PAI 1) in the glomeruli. Serpine 1 levels were increased by 1.46-fold in OVE26 glomeruli versus wild-type FVB; this was verified by real-time PCR experiments. At seven months of age, kidney cortex from OVE26 mice revealed a 4.3-fold increase in levels of Serpine1 mRNA versus wild-type FVB mice. These levels were significantly lower in OVE26 RKO cortex. In parallel, levels of TGF-β, TGF-β–induced (active) and α I (IV) collagen were significantly higher in the cortex of OVE26 versus OVE26 RKO mice.[51] Lastly, ROCK1 activity, linked to TGF-β, was significantly higher in the kidney cortex of OVE26 versus OVE26 RKO mice (Fig. 1).[51] Interestingly, in renal tubular cells, others have shown that AGE-mediated induction of connective tissue growth factor (CTGF) occurs in a TGF-β–dependent manner via Smad3 signaling.[52]

Recent findings implicate RAGE in the angiotensin II (angII) axis. In cultured podocytes, angiotensin II induces RAGE expression in a manner dependent on the AT2 receptor. In mice devoid of AT2 receptor, angII treatment did not upregulate RAGE to the same degree as that observed in wild-type mice.[53] Such findings add further support to the concept that AT1 receptor blockade alone may not be sufficient for the treatment of diabetic nephropathy, and suggest that complementary strategies to block RAGE may impart benefit to the diabetic kidney.

Work from our laboratory and others has suggested that RAGE-dependent inflammation contributes to the pathogenesis of diabetic

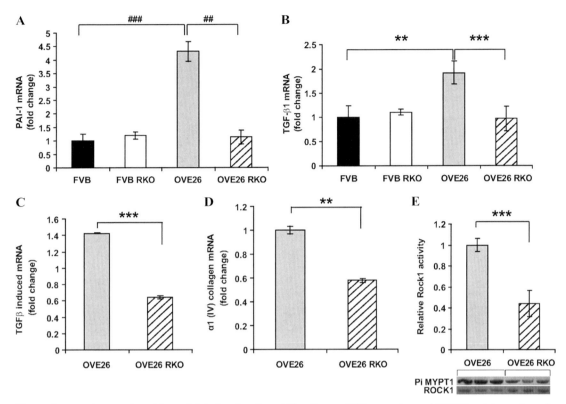

Figure 1. PAI-1 (Serpine1), Tgf-β1, Tgf-β–induced, and α1-(IV) collagen mRNA transcripts and ROCK1 activity are lower in OVE26 RKO kidney cortex than in OVE26 kidney cortex at age seven months. Real-time PCR for PAI-1 (A), Tgf-β1 (B), Tgf-β1–induced (C), and α1-(IV) collagen (D) gene products was performed, normalized to 18s transcript levels, and expressed as fold-change compared with the FVB or OVE26 group, as indicated in the figure (**$P < 0.01$, ***$P < 0.005$, ##$P < 0.0005$, ###$P < 0.0001$). $n = $ at least 6 per group. (E) ROCK1 activity was measured as the amount of phosphorylated MYPT1 compared with total ROCK1 (***$P = 0.005$). $n = $ at least 3 per group. Reprinted with permission from Ref. 51.

complications—both in the macro- and microvasculature. The discovery that RAGE bound S100/calgranulins and HMGB1 ligands suggested direct roles for RAGE in inflammation. In the section to follow, we discuss recent insights into the role of RAGE in propagation of inflammation.

RAGE and the inflammatory response: new twists

The earliest studies examining the effects of ligands on the *RAGE* gene promoter shed first light on the concept that RAGE upregulation and action is sustained in a ligand-enriched environment; contrary to other settings in which ligands downregulate expression of their receptors, RAGE ligands upregulate expression of RAGE.[54] In other studies, it has been shown that RAGE stimulation upregulates two key transcription factors implicated in inflammatory responses, NF-κB and early growth response-1

(Egr-1).[55,56] In diabetic tissues and in chronic inflammation, RAGE is implicated in the sustained activation of NF-κB that likely contributes to the chronicity and unrelenting nature of diabetic target cell stress and dysfunction.[57,58]

Given roles for RAGE in inflammatory mechanisms, experiments have been performed illustrating the effects of RAGE deletion or antagonism in a range of infectious settings, such as cecal ligation and puncture (sepsis), influenza A viral pneumonia, pneumococcal pneumonia, *Escherichia coli* pneumonia and sepsis, and *Listeria monocytogenes,* as examples.[59–63] In these settings, blocking RAGE action was beneficial and resulted in either improved survival and/or markedly reduced tissue damage.

In the particular context of periodontal disease, it is known that subjects with diabetes experience increased severity of periodontal disease; Lamster *et al.* showed that RAGE and AGEs were expressed in human diabetic gingival tissue retrieved at the time of surgery.[64] In murine models of accelerated alveolar bone loss and gingival inflammation in diabetes, administration of soluble RAGE suppressed exaggerated gingival inflammation, matrix metalloproteinase activity, and alveolar bone loss in mice treated by oral and anal gavage with the periodontal pathogen *Porphryomonas gingivalis (Pg)* strain 381.[65] Recently, Lalla *et al.* addressed the direct question, does RAGE play a role in the pathogenicity of *Pg*? Their intriguing findings linked RAGE directly to endothelial cell stress. Endothelial cells were retrieved from the aortas of wild-type or RAGE null mice and infected with *Pg* strain 381 or a fimbriae-deficient mutant strain known as DPG3. A number of findings emerged; first, in wild-type endothelial cells, *Pg* 381 resulted in increased expression of RAGE; second, levels of AGEs and monocyte chemoattractant peptide-1 (MCP-1) were increased by *Pg* 381 in wild-type but not in RAGE null endothelial cells, and not by DPG3 in wild-type endothelial cells; and third, treatment of human aortic endothelial cells with *Pg* 381 upregulated RAGE expression in a manner blocked by antioxidants or AGE blockade.[66]

Hence, these experiments suggested direct links of RAGE to endothelial stress induced by the pathogen *Pg* 381; the finding that DPG3 had no effect on AGE, RAGE, or MCP-1 production strongly suggested that invasion was required for the effects of RAGE in endothelial cells, and perhaps that RAGE influences this invasion process. Further experimentation is required to address this point. At this stage, however, such data provide further potential benefits to strategies aimed at pharmacological blockade of RAGE.

Taken together, these data reinforce roles for RAGE at multiple levels of the inflammatory response and support the concept of a RAGE-dependent gene regulatory network in inflammation. In mouse models, skin inflammation was shown to be mediated via key transcription factors regulated by RAGE, including Sp1, Tcfap2, E2f, myc, and Egr-1.[67] In human subjects, recent studies have shown direct correlations between RAGE polymorphism G82S and serum levels of C-reactive protein in the Chinese Han population.[68] From mouse to human, the role of RAGE as a key contributor to the inflammatory response is being confirmed.

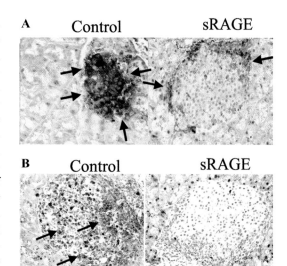

Figure 2. Treatment with sRAGE reduces the expression of IL-1β and TNF-α in islets in NOD/scid mice subjected to adoptive transfer of diabetogenic splenocytes from NOD mice. The islets of NOD/scid mice that received splenocytes from diabetic NOD mice were studied for expression of IL-1β (A) and TNF-α (B) by immunohistochemistry. The area of cells staining with the anticytokine antibodies is indicated with arrows and was determined for each treatment group (control versus soluble RAGE). Representative sections from three separate recipients in each category are shown. The expression levels of both IL-1β and TNF-α were reduced by treatment with sRAGE. Reprinted with permission from Ref. 69.

Therefore, although our work began in the context of complications of diabetes, it is not surprising that RAGE is linked to the pathogenesis of diabetes as well.

RAGE and the pathogenesis of diabetes

Previous studies demonstrated that administration of soluble RAGE to NOD/*scid* mice subjected to adoptive transfer of diabetogenic splenocytes from NOD mice delayed the time to diabetes compared to treatment with vehicle, murine serum albumin.[69] In parallel, levels of RAGE, S100/calgranulin, and T cells were significantly decreased in the islets of soluble RAGE treated mice.[69] Furthermore, levels of key cytokines implicated in inflammatory damage to the islets, TNF-α and IL-1β, were significantly reduced by treatment with sRAGE (Fig. 2).[69] On account of these findings, further studies were performed in a murine model of allogeneic, orthotopic heart transplantation in a mouse model, and revealed that administration of soluble RAGE significantly prolonged the time to allograft rejection.[70]

These findings led to the ultimate testing of RAGE in T cell responses and revealed that RAGE is inducibly upregulated during T cell activation. Clynes *et al.* showed that transfer of RAGE null OT II T cells (express T cell receptors recognizing ovalbumin) into OVA-immunized hosts resulted in reduced proliferative responses that were further diminished when RAGE null OT II T cells were transferred into RAGE null recipients. Although RAGE null dendritic cells displayed no overt abnormalities in antigen recognition responses, RAGE null T cells showed significantly impaired proliferative responses *in vitro* to nominal and alloantigens, in parallel with decreased production of interferon-γ and interleukin 2. Those findings indicated for the first time that RAGE expressed on T cells is required for efficient priming of T cells, and suggest that RAGE may play direct roles in the pathogenesis of autoimmune disorders such as type 1 diabetes.[71]

In the direct context of pancreatic islet β cell toxicity, two recent papers have suggested that RAGE may be implicated directly in this process, thereby further linking RAGE to the pathogenesis of diabetes. Lee *et al.* showed that RAGE was expressed on INS-1 cells (rat pancreatic β cell line) and on human islets. They showed that RAGE ligands S100B and HMGB1 induced apoptotic death of INS-1 cells and islets in a manner suppressed by an NADPH oxidase inhibitor.[72] In other studies, Zhu *et al.* showed that RAGE ligand-glycated serum induced upregulation of RAGE in INS-1 cells and induced apoptosis of these cells in parallel with Bcl-2 expression in a time- and dose-dependent manner. Both antibody to RAGE and RAGE knockdown blocked these adverse effects of glycated serum, thereby directly implicating RAGE in β cell death.[73] Those authors noted, however, that although glycated serum blocked glucose stimulated insulin secretion in rat islets, blockade of RAGE had no protective effects.[73] However, in further work, Shu *et al.* showed that AGEs decrease insulin secretion via repression of Pdx-1 protein expression and that antibodies to RAGE restored Pdx-1 expression and expression of insulin mRNA in INS-1 cells.[74] Taken together, these data suggest that RAGE ligand–RAGE interaction may play multiple roles in the steps causing and perpetuating islet dysfunction in types 1 and 2 diabetes. Given the varied effects of RAGE signaling in a range of disease-like settings, a question that arose was, how do the diverse ligands of RAGE all recognize this receptor?

RAGE structure and ligand identification: insights from structural biology

Prototypic of members of the immunoglobulin superfamily, RAGE is composed of immunoglobulin-like domains. Its extracellular region contains one V-type immunoglobulin domain followed by two distinct C-type immunoglobulin domains; this region of the molecule is followed by a single transmembrane domain, and then in the intracellular space, a short and highly charged cytoplasmic domain.[75]

We generated individual V, C1, and C2 domains and first showed that CML-AGEs bound selectively to the V-domain;[6] subsequent studies indicated that the S100/calgranulin, HMGB1, and amyloid-β peptide ligands all cross-competed with each other, suggesting that the V-domain was the key site of binding action.[76] Yet, despite these findings strongly suggesting a key characteristic of the V-domain, which yielded the multiligand nature of the receptor, the precise means by which these ligands might bind RAGE remained elusive.

In 2010, two papers appeared reporting the crystal structure of RAGE; remarkably, the findings were highly similar and laid the foundation for a much crisper understanding of RAGE and ligand binding.[77,78] In the first paper, Koch *et al.* studied the ligand S100B and RAGE. The X-ray crystal structure of the V-C1 domain of human RAGE was resolved at 1.85Å, and the V-C1 ligand-binding surface was mapped onto the structure from titrations with S100B monitored by heteronuclear NMR spectroscopy. A highly basic surface in the V-C1 domain was identified that accounted for the ligand-binding characteristics.[77] In the second work, Park *et al.* resolved the structure of RAGE to 1.5 Å; their work revealed that RAGE was a highly elongated molecule with a large basic patch and a large hydrophobic patch. They found that binding of RAGE to S100B was dependent on calcium and on residues in the C'D loop (residues 54–67) of the first domain. Interestingly, they showed that AGE binding was dependent on the recognition of negative charges on the AGE proteins. These authors also reported that RAGE binds to dsDNA and dsRNA.[78]

In recent work, Xue *et al.* reported on the mechanisms by which carboxyethyl lysine (CEL) ligands of RAGE interact with the receptor.[79] Their work showed that the CEL moiety fits inside a positively charged cavity of the V domain and that peptide backbone atoms make specific contacts with the V domain.[79] Importantly, they showed that the geometry of the bound CEL peptide was compatible with many CML- and CEL-modified sites within plasma proteins, thereby explaining how patterned ligands such as these specific AGEs may bind to RAGE.

Sarkany *et al.* recently reported on the structure of the soluble form of RAGE. These authors demonstrated that soluble RAGE displays concentration-dependent oligomerization behavior mediated by the presence of Ca^{2+} ions. They employed synchrotron small-angle X-ray scattering and determined the solution structure of human soluble RAGE in both the monomeric and dimeric forms. The model for the monomer is reported to display a J-like shape, and the dimer to be formed through the association of the two N-terminal domains with an elongated structure.[80]

Certainly, now that a crystal structure of RAGE is available, it is likely that such knowledge will accelerate the development of a range of chemical antagonists. In this context, exciting recent discoveries point to new targets for antagonizing RAGE in the intracellular space.

RAGE, signal transduction, and diaphanous-1

Ligand binding to RAGE in the extracellular space stimulates signal transduction mechanisms that ultimately are responsible for the diverse effects of RAGE on gene expression changes. It is well established that RAGE is expressed on multiple cell types and that ligand binding stimulates signal transduction cascades such as mitogen-activated protein kinases, phosphatidylinositol 3-kinase, Jak/STAT (signal transducers and activators of transcription), and the Rho GTPases Rac-1 and Cdc42.[6–8,81–84] To discern the precise mechanisms by which RAGE signals through the cytoplasmic domain, a yeast two hybrid assay in which the human RAGE cytoplasmic domain was used as bait to identify potential binding partners in a lung library; the lung was chosen since RAGE was initially identified from bovine lung extract.[85] From the yeast two hybrid assay, multiple clones of the FH1 domain of diaphanous-1 (mDia1) were identified as potential binding partners of the RAGE cytoplasmic domain.[86] The FH1 domain of

mDia1 is proline-rich and has been reported to interact with mediators of the actin cytoskeleton (profilin) and various signal transduction pathway molecules, such as c-Src.[87–88] To confirm the interaction, coimmunoprecipitation studies using his-tagged RAGE cytoplasmic domain and Myc-tagged mDia1 (as well as deletion mutants testing the roles of individual domains of mDia1) were performed and confirmed that the RAGE cytoplasmic domain bound the FH1 domain of mDia1.[86] Indeed, a recent publication confirmed this binding in cultured cells.[89] In other studies, C6 glioma cells expressing full-length or cytoplasmic domain-deleted or dominant negative (DN) RAGE showed that mDia1 was coimmunoprecipitated with RAGE but mDia1 did not coimmunoprecipitate with RAGE cytoplasmic domain-deleted DN RAGE–expressing C6 glioma cells.[86]

The key test of the mDia1 finding was whether mDia1 was implicated in RAGE-mediated cellular signaling and functional outcomes, such as cellular migration. In RAGE-expressing cells, but not DN RAGE-expressing cells, both Rac1 and Cdc42 were rapidly activated upon ligand stimulation. To test its role in RAGE ligand-stimulated cellular migration, use of siRNA knockdown mDia1 knockdown suppressed RAGE ligand-stimulated cellular migration but scramble siRNA controls had no inhibitory effects.[86] Interestingly, siRNA knockdown of mDia1 expression did not affect migration of cells in response to a non-RAGE ligand such as fetal bovine serum (10%). In parallel, siRNA knockdown of mDia1 blocked RAGE ligand-stimulated activation of rac1 and cd42, whereas scramble siRNAs had no effect.[86]

In addition to its actions as an effector of Rho GTPase signaling, mDia1 has also been shown to modulate serum response factors (SRFs),[90,91] key factors that bind to serum response elements (SRE) in the promoters of a number of genes, thereby regulating critical cellular functions, in a manner dependent on mDia1 effects on the actin cytoskeleton.[92] As Egr-1 is an SRF–SRE–dependent gene, we tested the role of mDia1. It is important to note that previous work had shown that in endothelial cells in hypoxia, RAGE upregulates Egr-1 in a manner dependent on rapid activation of protein kinase C-βII and JNK signaling.[56] Interestingly, when endothelial cells were placed in hypoxia, rapid (within 10 min) release of RAGE ligand AGE reactive

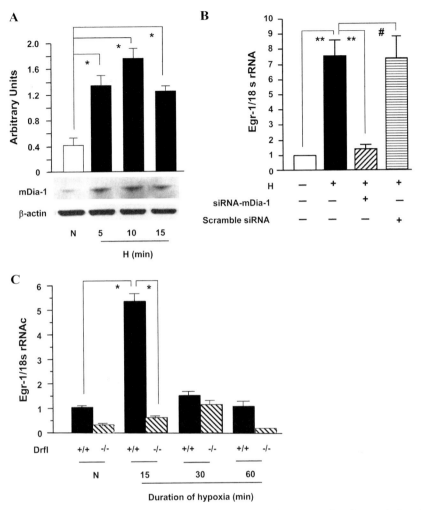

Figure 3. Hypoxia induces mDia-1 expression and mDia1 plays key roles in hypoxia-mediated upregulation of Egr-1. THP-1 cells and macrophages from mDia1 null mice were exposed to hypoxia (*H*; 0.5% of oxygen) or normoxia (*N*) for the indicated times. (A) Total protein was prepared from THP-1 cells, and immunoblotting with anti-mDia1 IgG was performed on 30 μg/lane of protein from THP-1 cells. Results of multiple experiments were quantified. (B and C) Total RNA was prepared from the indicated cells, and real-time PCR analysis of Egr-1 expression was performed. Data are represented as the relative expression of mRNA for Egr-1 normalized to 18 SirRNA. (B) RNA was prepared from THP-1 cells transfected with siRNA-mDia1 or scramble siRNA and then subjected to hypoxia for 15 min. (C) RNA was prepared from macrophages from wild-type or mDia1 (Drf1) null mice after exposure to hypoxia or normoxia for the indicated times. *$P < 0.0001$ and **$P < 0.001$ indicate statistical significance; #indicates no statistical significance. Note that Drf1 indicates mDia1. Adapted from Ref. 93.

epitopes into the cellular supernatants was observed. *In vivo*, pretreatment of mice with aminoguanidine, or *in vitro*, pretreatment of wild-type endothelial cells with anti-AGE IgG, blocked hypoxia-mediated upregulation of Egr-1.[56]

Hence, tests of human THP-1 cells showed that hypoxia increased expression of mDia1 versus control normoxia treatment of these cells. siRNA knockdown of mDia1 during hypoxia blocked hypoxia-stimulated upregulation of Egr-1 in THP-1 cells, whereas scrambled siRNA had no effect. Furthermore, thioglycollate-elicited murine macrophages retrieved from RAGE null or mDia1 null mice failed to upregulate Egr-1 in hypoxia compared to that observed in wild-type murine macrophages.[93] (Fig. 3) Taken together, these data demonstrated for the first time key roles for mDia1 in mediating RAGE ligand-stimulated activation of Rho GTPases, cellular migration, and hypoxia-stimulated upregulation of Egr-1.

Conclusions: what we have learned and where do we proceed from here?

As with any biological target, the chief goal is the translation of the findings to human subjects. In the case of RAGE, there appears to be multiple possible opportunities. From the standpoint of therapeutics, studies using pharmacological antagonists and RAGE null mice support that especially in the case of diabetic macro- and microvascular disease, blocking RAGE is beneficial. As discussed above, potent roles for RAGE in diabetic atherosclerosis, cardiac dysfunction, and nephropathy have been shown. In addition, but not covered in this review, from studies in human subjects suggesting links of *RAGE* gene polymorphisms and soluble RAGE levels to animal models of these disorders, evidence is mounting linking RAGE to diabetic retinopathy,[94–100] peripheral neuropathy,[101–104] and impaired wound healing.[105–108]

Despite this promise, key questions remain on the long-term safety and advisability of blocking RAGE. We and others have shown that even long-term (> 6 months) treatment with soluble RAGE is well tolerated by diabetic mice,[100] and that homozygous RAGE null mice display no overt abnormalities in viability or fertility. Rather, they appear to be protected against the chronic complications of diabetes, as discussed above.

These considerations prompt the question, what is the natural function of RAGE? We predict that the ligand families of RAGE, particularly certain members of the S100/calgranulin family and HMGB1, lead dual lives in cellular systems. We propose that in homeostatic systems, free of chronic inflammation, aging, hyperglycemia, or sustained oxidative stress, for example, release of these RAGE ligand families serves, together with the host of other such mediators, as key first lines of defense against infection, inflammation, or injury. However, in settings in which these molecules may accumulate in the microenvironments, both by failure of clearance or perpetuation of signals eliciting their release, the failure to quell these ligand responses tips the biological balance to favor the development of chronic disease.

Hence, it is in this context we speculate that our recent discovery that the RAGE cytoplasmic domain binds to the formin mDia1, and that mDia1 is required for RAGE ligand-stimulated activation of Rac1 and Cdc42 and cellular migration in transformed cells, and for hypoxia-stimulated upregulation of Egr-1 in macrophages, points to the RAGE cytoplasmic domain-mDia1 interaction as a focused target of RAGE signaling. Indeed, others have reported that the RAGE cytoplasmic domain may bind to ERK and to TIRAP (the latter an adaptor protein for toll like receptors 2/4).[89,109] In the latter two studies, however, the functional implications of this apparent binding relationship to *in vivo* pathobiology have yet to be shown. Is it possible that targeting RAGE cytoplasmic domain/mDia1 will antagonize the pathological impact of RAGE signaling, and that interactions of the RAGE cytoplasmic domain with distinct molecules affect adaptive functions of the molecule? The answers to these fundamental questions are under active investigation and are eagerly awaited.

Conflicts of interest

The authors declare no conflicts of interest.

References

1. Forlenza, G.P., N.M. Paradise Black, E.G. McNamara & S.E. Sullivan. 2010. Ankyloglossia, exclusive breastfeeding, and failure to thrive. *Pediatrics* **125:** e1500–e1504.
2. Peng, H. & W. Hagopian. 2006. Environmental factors in the development of Type 1 diabetes. *Rev. Endocr. Metab. Disord.* **7:** 149–162.
3. Hu, F.B. 2011. Globalization of diabetes: the role of diet, lifestyle, and genes. *Diabetes Care* **34:** 1249–1257.
4. International Diabetes Federation. IDF Diabetes Atlas. Epidemiology and Morbidity. In *International Diabetes Federation*. Available from: http://www.idf.org.
5. Sweat, V., J.M. Bruzzese, S. Albert, *et al.* 2011. The Banishing Obesity and Diabetes in Youth (BODY) Project: description and feasibility of a program to halt obesity-associated disease among urban high school students. *J. Community Health*. In press.
6. Kislinger, T., C. Fu, B. Huber, *et al.* 1999. N(epsilon)-(carboxymethyl)lysine adducts of proteins are ligands for receptor for advanced glycation end products that activate cell signaling pathways and modulate gene expression. *J. Biol. Chem.* **274:** 31740–31749.
7. Hofmann, M.A., S. Drury, C. Fu, *et al.* 1999. RAGE mediates a novel proinflammatory axis: a central cell surface receptor for S100/calgranulin polypeptides. *Cell* **97:** 889–901.
8. Taguchi, A., D.C. Blood, G. del Toro, *et al.* 2000. Blockade of RAGE-amphoterin signalling suppresses tumour growth and metastases. *Nature* **405:** 354–360.
9. Moss, S.E., R. Klein & B.E. Klein. 1991. Cause-specific mortality in a population-based study of diabetes. *Am. J. Public. Health* **81:** 1158–1162.

10. Nathan, D.M., P.A. Cleary, J.Y. Backlund, *et al.* & G. Diabetes Control and Complications Trial/Epidemiology of Diabetes Interventions and Complications Study Research. 2005. Intensive diabetes treatment and cardiovascular disease in patients with type 1 diabetes. *N. Engl. J. Med.* **353:** 2643–2653.

11. Khaw, K.T., N. Wareham, S. Bingham, *et al.* 2004. Association of hemoglobin A1c with cardiovascular disease and mortality in adults: the European prospective investigation into cancer in Norfolk. *Ann. Intern. Med.* **141:** 413–420.

12. Action to Control Cardiovascular Risk in Diabetes Study Group, H.C. Gerstein, M.E. Miller, R.P. Byington, *et al.* 2008. Effects of intensive glucose lowering in type 2 diabetes. *N. Engl. J. Med.* **358:** 2545–2559.

13. ACCORD Study Group, H.C. Gerstein, M.E. Miller, S. Genuth, *et al.* 2011. Long-term effects of intensive glucose lowering on cardiovascular outcomes. *N. Engl. J. Med.* **364:** 818–828.

14. ADVANCE Collaborative Group, A. Patel, S. MacMahon, J. Chalmers, *et al.* 2008. Intensive blood glucose control and vascular outcomes in patients with type 2 diabetes. *N. Engl. J. Med.* **358:** 2560–2572.

15. Duckworth, W., C. Abraira, T. Moritz, *et al.* 2009. Glucose control and vascular complications in veterans with type 2 diabetes. *N. Engl. J. Med.* **360:** 129–139.

16. Zoungas, S., A. Patel, J. Chalmers, *et al.* 2010. Severe hypoglycemia and risks of vascular events and death. *N. Engl. J. Med.* **363:** 1410–1418.

17. Cipollone, F., A. Iezzi, M. Fazia, *et al.* 2003. The receptor RAGE as a progression factor amplifying arachidonate-dependent inflammatory and proteolytic response in human atherosclerotic plaques: role of glycemic control. *Circulation* **108:** 1070–1077.

18. Park, L., K.G. Raman, K.J. Lee, *et al.* 1998. Suppression of accelerated diabetic atherosclerosis by the soluble receptor for advanced glycation endproducts. *Nat. Med.* **4:** 1025–1031.

19. Bucciarelli, L.G., T. Wendt, W. Qu, *et al.* 2002. RAGE blockade stabilizes established atherosclerosis in diabetic apolipoprotein E-null mice. *Circulation* **106:** 2827–2835.

20. Wendt, T., E. Harja, L. Bucciarelli, *et al.* 2006. RAGE modulates vascular inflammation and atherosclerosis in a murine model of type 2 diabetes. *Atherosclerosis* **185:** 70–77.

21. Harja, E., D.X. Bu, B.I. Hudson, *et al.* 2008. Vascular and inflammatory stresses mediate atherosclerosis via RAGE and its ligands in apoE-/- mice. *J. Clin. Invest.* **118:** 183–194.

22. Soro-Paavonen, A., A.M. Watson, J. Li, *et al.* 2008. Receptor for advanced glycation end products (RAGE) deficiency attenuates the development of atherosclerosis in diabetes. *Diabetes* **57:** 2461–2469.

23. Sun, L., T. Ishida, T. Yasuda, *et al.* 2009. RAGE mediates oxidized LDL-induced pro-inflammatory effects and atherosclerosis in nondiabetic LDL receptor-deficient mice. *Cardiovasc. Res.* **82:** 371–381.

24. Bu, D.X., V. Rai, X. Shen, *et al.* 2010. Activation of the ROCK1 branch of the transforming growth factor-beta pathway contributes to RAGE-dependent acceleration of atherosclerosis in diabetic ApoE-null mice. *Circ. Res.* **106:** 1040–1051.

25. Morris-Rosenfeld, S., E. Blessing, M.R. Preusch, *et al.* 2011. Deletion of bone marrow-derived receptor for advanced glycation end products inhibits atherosclerotic plaque progression. *Eur. J. Clin. Invest.* **41:** 1164–1171.

26. Bucciarelli, L.G., R. Ananthakrishnan, Y.C. Hwang, *et al.* 2008. RAGE and modulation of ischemic injury in the diabetic myocardium. *Diabetes* **57:** 1941–1951.

27. Shang, L., R. Ananthakrishnan, Q. Li, *et al.* 2010. RAGE modulates hypoxia/reoxygenation injury in adult murine cardiomyocytes via JNK and GSK-3beta signaling pathways. *PLoS One* **5:** e10092.

28. Wang, L.J., L. Lu, F.R. Zhang, *et al.* 2011. Increased serum high-mobility group box-1 and cleaved receptor for advanced glycation endproducts levels and decreased endogenous secretory receptor for advanced glycation endproducts levels in diabetic and nondiabetic patients with heart failure. *Eur. J. Heart Fail.* **13:** 440–449.

29. Ma, H., S.Y. Li, P. Xu, *et al.* 2009. Advanced glycation endproduct (AGE) accumulation and AGE receptor (RAGE) up-regulation contribute to the onset of diabetic cardiomyopathy. *J. Cell. Mol. Med.* **13:** 1751–1764.

30. Nielsen, J.M., S.B. Kristiansen, R. Nørregaard, *et al.* 2009. Blockage of receptor for advanced glycation end products prevents development of cardiac dysfunction in db/db type 2 diabetic mice. *Eur. J. Heart Fail.* **11:** 638–647.

31. Petrova, R., Y. Yamamoto, K. Muraki, *et al.* 2002. Advanced glycation endproduct-induced calcium handling impairment in mouse cardiac myocytes. *J. Mol. Cell. Cardiol.* **34:** 1425–1431.

32. Aleshin, A., R. Ananthakrishnan, Q. Li, *et al.* 2008. RAGE modulates myocardial injury consequent to LAD infarction via impact on JNK and STAT signaling in a murine model. *Am. J. Physiol. Heart Circ. Physiol.* **294:** H1823–H1832.

33. Andrassy, M., H.C. Volz, J.C. Igwe, *et al.* 2008. High-mobility group box-1 in ischemia-reperfusion injury of the heart. *Circulation* **117:** 3216–3226.

34. Falcone, C., E. Emanuele, A. D'Angelo, *et al.* 2005. Plasma levels of soluble receptor for advanced glycation end products and coronary artery disease in nondiabetic men. *Arterioscler. Thromb. Vasc. Biol.* **25:** 1032–1037.

35. Colhoun, H.M., D.J. Betteridge, P. Durrington, *et al.* 2011. Total soluble and endogenous secretory receptor for advanced glycation endproducts as predictive biomarkers of coronary heart disease risk in patients with type 2 diabetes: an analysis from the CARDS trial. *Diabetes* **60:** 2379–2385.

36. Tam, H.L., S.W. Shiu, Y. Wong, *et al.* 2010. Effects of atorvastatin on serum soluble receptors for advanced glycation end-products in type 2 diabetes. *Atherosclerosis* **209:** 173–177.

37. Santilli, F., L. Bucciarelli, D. Noto, *et al.* 2007. Decreased plasma soluble RAGE in patients with hypercholesterolemia: effects of statins. *Free Radic. Biol. Med.* **43:** 1255–1262.

38. Wilson, C. 2011. Cardiovascular endocrinology: RAGE-a biomarker for CHD in T2DM? *Nat. Rev. Endocrinol.* **7:** 561.

39. Kalousová, M., M. Hodková, M. Kazderová, *et al.* 2006. Soluble receptor for advanced glycation end products in patients with decreased renal function. *Am. J. Kidney Dis.* **47:** 406–411.

40. Cuccurullo, C., A. Iezzi, M.L. Fazia, *et al.* 2006. Suppression of RAGE as a basis of simvastatin-dependent plaque stabilization in type 2 diabetes. *Arterioscler. Thromb. Vasc. Biol.* **26:** 2716–2723.

41. Liang, Y.J., S.A. Chen & J.H. Jian. 2011. Peroxisome proliferator-activated receptor delta downregulates the expression of the receptor for advanced glycation end products and pro-inflammatory cytokines in the kidney of streptozotocin-induced diabetic mice. *Eur. J. Pharm. Sci.* **43:** 65–70.

42. Ishibashi, Y., Y. Nishino, T. Matsui, *et al.* 2011. Glucagon-like peptide-1 suppresses advanced glycation end product-induced monocyte chemoattractant protein-1 expression in mesangial cells by reducing advanced glycation end product receptor level. *Metabolism* **60:** 1271–1277.

43. Wang, L., X. Zhang, L. Liu, *et al.* 2010. Atorvastatin protects rat brains against permanent focal ischemia and down-regulates HMGB1, HMGB1 receptors (RAGE and TLR4), NF-kappaB expression. *Neurosci. Lett.* **471:** 152–156.

44. Ritz, E. & S.R. Orth. 1999. Nephropathy in patients with type 2 diabetes mellitus. *N. Engl. J. Med.* **341:** 1127–1133.

45. U.S. Renal Data System. 2004. *USRDS 2004 Annual Data Report: Atlas of End-Stage Renal Disease in the United States.* National Institutes of Health, National Institute of Diabetes an Digestive and Kidney Diseases, Bethesda, MD, USA.

46. Bolton, W.K., D.C. Cattran, M.E. Williams, *et al.* & ACTION I Investigator Group. 2004. Randomized trial of an inhibitor of formation of advanced glycation end products in diabetic nephropathy. *Am. J. Nephrol.* **24:** 32–40.

47. Tanji, N., G.S. Markowitz, C. Fu, *et al.* 2000. Expression of advanced glycation end products and their cellular receptor RAGE in diabetic nephropathy and nondiabetic renal disease. *J. Am. Soc. Nephrol.* **11:** 1656–1666.

48. Wendt, T.M., N. Tanji, J. Guo, *et al.* 2003. RAGE drives the development of glomerulosclerosis and implicates podocyte activation in the pathogenesis of diabetic nephropathy. *Am. J. Pathol.* **162:** 1123–1137.

49. Jensen, L.J., L. Denner, B.F. Schrijvers, *et al.* 2006. Renal effects of a neutralising RAGE-antibody in long-term streptozotocin-diabetic mice. *J. Endocrinol.* **188:** 493–501.

50. Flyvbjerg, A., L. Denner, B.F. Schrijvers, *et al.* 2004. Long-term renal effects of a neutralizing RAGE antibody in obese type 2 diabetic mice. *Diabetes* **53:** 166–172.

51. Reiniger, N., K. Lau, D. McCalla, *et al.* 2010. Deletion of the receptor for advanced glycation end products reduces glomerulosclerosis and preserves renal function in the diabetic OVE26 mouse. *Diabetes* **59:** 2043–2054.

52. Chung, A.C., H. Zhang, Y.Z. Kong, *et al.* 2010. Advanced glycation end-products induce tubular CTGF via TGF-beta-independent Smad3 signaling. *J. Am. Soc. Nephrol.* **21:** 249–260.

53. Rüster, C., S. Franke, U. Wenzel, *et al.* 2011. Podocytes of AT2 receptor knockout mice are protected from angiotensin II-mediated RAGE induction. *Am. J. Nephrol.* **34:** 309–317.

54. Li, J. & A.M. Schmidt. 1997. Characterization and functional analysis of the promoter of RAGE, the receptor for advanced glycation end products. *J. Biol. Chem.* **272:** 16498–16506.

55. Schmidt, A.M., O. Hori, J.X. Chen, *et al.* 1995. Advanced glycation endproducts interacting with their endothelial receptor induce expression of vascular cell adhesion molecule-1 (VCAM-1) in cultured human endothelial cells and in mice. A potential mechanism for the accelerated vasculopathy of diabetes. *J. Clin. Invest.* **96:** 1395–1403.

56. Chang, J.S., T. Wendt, W. Qu, *et al.* 2008. Oxygen deprivation triggers upregulation of early growth response-1 by the receptor for advanced glycation end products. *Circ. Res.* **102:** 905–913.

57. Bierhaus, A., S. Schiekofer, M. Schwaninger, *et al.* 2001. Diabetes-associated sustained activation of the transcription factor nuclear factor-kappaB. *Diabetes* **50:** 2792–2808.

58. Kislinger, T., N. Tanji, T. Wendt, *et al.* 2001. Receptor for advanced glycation end products mediates inflammation and enhanced expression of tissue factor in vasculature of diabetic apolipoprotein E-null mice. *Arterioscler. Thromb. Vasc. Biol.* **21:** 905–910.

59. Christaki, E., S.M. Opal, J.C. Keith, Jr., *et al.* 2011. A monoclonal antibody against RAGE alters gene expression and is protective in experimental models of sepsis and pneumococcal pneumonia. *Shock* **35:** 492–498.

60. van Zoelen, M.A., K.F. van der Sluijs, A. Achouiti, *et al.* 2009. Receptor for advanced glycation end products is detrimental during influenza A virus pneumonia. *Virology* **391:** 265–273.

61. van Zoelen, M.A., M. Schouten, A.F. de Vos, *et al.* 2009. The receptor for advanced glycation end products impairs host defense in pneumococcal pneumonia. *J. Immunol.* **182:** 4349–4356.

62. Ramsgaard, L., J.M. Englert, M.L. Manni, *et al.* 2011. Lack of the receptor for advanced glycation end-products attenuates E. coli pneumonia in mice. *PLoS One* **6:** e20132.

63. Lutterloh, E.C., S.M. Opal, D.D. Pittman, *et al.* 2007. Inhibition of the RAGE products increases survival in experimental models of severe sepsis and systemic infection. *Crit. Care* **11:** R122.

64. Schmidt, A.M., E. Weidman, E. Lalla, *et al.* 1996. Advanced glycation endproducts (AGEs) induce oxidant stress in the gingiva: a potential mechanism underlying accelerated periodontal disease associated with diabetes. *J. Periodont. Res.* **31:** 508–515.

65. Lalla, E., I.B. Lamster, M. Feit, *et al.* 2000. Blockade of RAGE suppresses periodontitis-associated bone loss in diabetic mice. *J. Clin. Invest.* **105:** 1117–1124.

66. Pollreisz, A., B.I. Hudson, J.S. Chang, *et al.* 2010. Receptor for advanced glycation endproducts mediates pro-atherogenic responses to periodontal infection in vascular endothelial cells. *Atherosclerosis* **212:** 451–456.

67. Riehl, A., T. Bauer, B. Brors, *et al.* 2010. Identification of the Rage-dependent gene regulatory network in a mouse model of skin inflammation. *BMC Genom.* **11:** 537.

68. Gao, J., Y. Shao, W. Lai, *et al.* 2010. Association of polymorphisms in the RAGE gene with serum CRP levels and

coronary artery disease in the Chinese Han population. *J. Hum. Genet.* **55:** 668–675.

69. Chen, Y., S.S. Yan, J. Colgan, *et al.* 2004. Blockade of late stages of autoimmune diabetes by inhibition of the receptor for advanced glycation end products. *J. Immunol.* **173:** 1399–1405.

70. Moser, B., M.J. Szabolcs, H.J. Ankersmit, *et al.* 2007. Blockade of RAGE suppresses alloimmune reactions in vitro and delays allograft rejection in murine heart transplantation. *Am. J. Transplant.* **7:** 293–302. *Erratum in Am. J. Transplant.* 2007 May; 2007(2005): 1318.

71. Moser, B., D.D. Desai, M.P. Downie, *et al.* 2007. Receptor for advanced glycation end products expression on T cells contributes to antigen-specific cellular expansion in vivo. *J. Immunol.* **179:** 8051–8058.

72. Lee, B.W., H.Y. Chae, S.J. Kwon, *et al.* 2010. RAGE ligands induce apoptotic cell death of pancreatic beta-cells via oxidative stress. *Int. J. Mol. Med.* **26:** 813–818.

73. Zhu, Y., T. Shu, Y. Lin, *et al.* 2011. Inhibition of the receptor for advanced glycation endproducts (RAGE) protects pancreatic beta-cells. *Biochem. Biophys. Res. Commun.* **404:** 159–165.

74. Shu, T., Y. Zhu, H. Wang, *et al.* 2011. AGEs decrease insulin synthesis in pancreatic beta-cell by repressing Pdx-1 protein expression at the post-translational level. *PLoS One* **6:** e18782.

75. Neeper, M., A.M. Schmidt, J. Brett, *et al.* 1992. Cloning and expression of a cell surface receptor for advanced glycosylation end products of proteins. *J. Biol. Chem.* **267:** 14998–15004.

76. Leclerc, E., G. Fritz, S.W. Vetter & C.W. Heizmann. 2009. Binding of S100 proteins to RAGE: an update. *Biochim. Biophys. Acta* **1793:** 993–1007.

77. Koch, M., S. Chitayat, B.M. Dattilo, *et al.* 2010. Structural basis for ligand recognition and activation of RAGE. *Structure* **18:** 1342–1352.

78. Park, H., F.G. Adsit & J.C. Boyington. 2010. The 1.5 Å crystal structure of human receptor for advanced glycation endproducts (RAGE) ectodomains reveals unique features determining ligand binding. *J. Biol. Chem.* **285:** 40762–40770.

79. Xue, J., V. Rai, D. Singer, *et al.* 2011. Advanced glycation end product recognition by the receptor for AGEs. *Structure* **19:** 722–732.

80. Sarkany, Z., T. Ikonen, F. Ferreira-da-Silva, *et al.* 2011. Solution structure of the soluble receptor for advanced glycation end-products (sRAGE). *J. Biol. Chem.* **286:** 37,525–37,534.

81. Huttunen, H.J., C. Fages & H. Rauvala. 1999. Receptor for advanced glycation end products (RAGE)-mediated neurite outgrowth and activation of NF-kappaB require the cytoplasmic domain of the receptor but different downstream signaling pathways. *J. Biol. Chem.* **274:** 19919–19924.

82. Lander, H.M., J.M. Tauras, J.S. Ogiste, *et al.* 1997. Activation of the receptor for advanced glycation end products triggers a p21(ras)-dependent mitogen-activated protein kinase pathway regulated by oxidant stress. *J. Biol. Chem.* **272:** 17810–17814.

83. Huang, J.S., J.Y. Guh, H.C. Chen, *et al.* 2001. Role of receptor for advanced glycation end-product (RAGE) and the JAK/STAT-signaling pathway in AGE-induced collagen production in NRK-49F cells. *J. Cell. Biochem.* **81:** 102–113.

84. Yeh, C.H., L. Sturgis, J. Haidacher, *et al.* 2001. Requirement for p38 and p44/p42 mitogen-activated protein kinases in RAGE-mediated nuclear factor-kappaB transcriptional activation and cytokine secretion. *Diabetes* **50:** 1495–1504.

85. Schmidt, A.M., M. Vianna, M. Gerlach, *et al.* 1992. Isolation and characterization of two binding proteins for advanced glycosylation end products from bovine lung which are present on the endothelial cell surface. *J. Biol. Chem.* **267:** 14987–14997.

86. Hudson, B.I., A.Z. Kalea, M. Del Mar Arriero, *et al.* 2008. Interaction of the RAGE cytoplasmic domain with diaphanous-1 is required for ligand-stimulated cellular migration through activation of Rac1 and Cdc42. *J. Biol. Chem.* **283:** 34457–34468.

87. Krebs, A., M. Rothkegel, M. Klar & B.M. Jockusch. 2001. Characterization of functional domains of mDia1, a link between the small GTPase Rho and the actin cytoskeleton. *J. Cell. Sci.* **114:** 3663–3672.

88. Tominaga, T., E. Sahai, P. Chardin, *et al.* 2000. Diaphanous-related formins bridge Rho GTPase and Src tyrosine kinase signaling. *Mol. Cell* **5:** 13–25.

89. Sakaguchi, M., H. Murata, K. Yamamoto, *et al.* 2011. TIRAP, an adaptor protein for TLR2/4, transduces a signal from RAGE phosphorylated upon ligand binding. *PLoS One* **6:** e23132.

90. Young, K.G. & J.W. Copeland. 2010. Formins in cell signaling. *Biochim. Biophys. Acta* **1803:** 183–190.

91. Geneste, O., J.W. Copeland & R. Treisman. 2002. LIM kinase and Diaphanous cooperate to regulate serum response factor and actin dynamics. *J. Cell Biol.* **157:** 831–838.

92. Copeland, J.W. & R. Treisman. 2002. The diaphanous-related formin mDia1 controls serum response factor activity through its effects on actin polymerization. *Mol. Biol. Cell.* **13:** 4088–4099.

93. Xu, Y., F. Toure, W. Qu, *et al.* 2010. Advanced glycation end product (AGE)-receptor for AGE (RAGE) signaling and up-regulation of Egr-1 in hypoxic macrophages. *J. Biol. Chem.* **285:** 23233–23240.

94. Balasubbu, S., P. Sundaresan, A. Rajendran, *et al.* 2010. Association analysis of nine candidate gene polymorphisms in Indian patients with type 2 diabetic retinopathy. *BMC Med. Genet.* **11:** 158.

95. Zong, H., M. Ward, A. Madden, *et al.* 2010. Hyperglycaemia-induced pro-inflammatory responses by retinal Muller glia are regulated by the receptor for advanced glycation end-products (RAGE). *Diabetologia* **53:** 2656–2666.

96. Zhang, H.M., L.L. Chen, L. Wang, *et al.* 2009. Association of 1704G/T and G82S polymorphisms in the receptor for advanced glycation end products gene with diabetic retinopathy in Chinese population. *J. Endocrinol. Invest.* **32:** 258–262.

97. Barile, G.R. & A.M. Schmidt. 2007. RAGE and its ligands in retinal disease. *Curr. Mol. Med.* **7:** 758–765.

98. Kaji, Y., T. Usui, S. Ishida, *et al.* 2007. Inhibition of diabetic leukostasis and blood-retinal barrier breakdown with

a soluble form of a receptor for advanced glycation end products. *Invest. Ophthalmol. Vis. Sci.* **48:** 858–865.

99. Pachydaki, S.I., S.R. Tari, S.E. Lee, *et al.* 2006. Upregulation of RAGE and its ligands in proliferative retinal disease. *Exp. Eye Res.* **82:** 807–815.

100. Barile, G.R., S.I. Pachydaki, S.R. Tari, *et al.* 2005. The RAGE axis in early diabetic retinopathy. *Invest. Ophthalmol. Vis. Sci.* **46:** 2916–2924.

101. Brussee, V., G. Guo, Y. Dong, *et al.* 2008. Distal degenerative sensory neuropathy in a long-term type 2 diabetes rat model. *Diabetes* **57:** 1664–1673.

102. Toth, C., L.L. Rong, C. Yang, *et al.* 2008. Receptor for advanced glycation end products (RAGEs) and experimental diabetic neuropathy. *Diabetes* **57:** 1002–1017.

103. Haslbeck, K.M., E. Schleicher, A. Bierhaus, *et al.* 2005. The AGE/RAGE/NF-(kappa)B pathway may contribute to the pathogenesis of polyneuropathy in impaired glucose tolerance (IGT). *Exp. Clin. Endocrinol. Diabetes* **113:** 288–291.

104. Bierhaus, A., K.M. Haslbeck, P.M. Humpert, *et al.* 2004. Loss of pain perception in diabetes is dependent on a receptor of the immunoglobulin superfamily. *J. Clin. Invest.* **114:** 1741–1751.

105. Berlanga, J., D. Cibrian, I. Guillen, *et al.* 2005. Methylglyoxal administration induces diabetes-like microvascular changes and perturbs the healing process of cutaneous wounds. *Clin. Sci.* **109:** 83–95.

106. Wear-Maggitti, K., J. Lee, A. Conejero, *et al.* 2004. Use of topical sRAGE in diabetic wounds increases neovascularization and granulation tissue formation. *Ann. Plast. Surg.* **52:** 519–521; Discussion 522.

107. Santana, R.B., L. Xu, H.B. Chase, *et al.* 2003. A role for advanced glycation end products in diminished bone healing in type 1 diabetes. *Diabetes* **52:** 1502–1510.

108. Goova, M.T., J. Li, T. Kislinger, *et al.* 2001. Blockade of receptor for advanced glycation end-products restores effective wound healing in diabetic mice. *Am. J. Pathol.* **159:** 513–525.

109. Ishihara, K., K. Tsutsumi, S. Kawane, *et al.* 2003. The receptor for advanced glycation end-products (RAGE) directly binds to ERK by a D-domain-like docking site. *FEBS Lett.* **550:** 107–113.

Ann. N.Y. Acad. Sci. ISSN 0077-8923

ANNALS OF THE NEW YORK ACADEMY OF SCIENCES

Issue: *The Year in Diabetes and Obesity*

Type 1 diabetes: role of intestinal microbiome in humans and mice

Brian P. Boerner[1] and Nora E. Sarvetnick[2,3]

[1]Department of Internal Medicine, [2]Department of Surgery, [3]Nebraska Regenerative Medicine Project, University of Nebraska Medical Center, Omaha, Nebraska

Address for correspondence: Nora Sarvetnick, Ph.D., Department of Surgery, University of Nebraska Medical Center, 985965 Nebraska Medical Center, Omaha, NE 68198-5965. noras@unmc.edu

Type 1 diabetes is a disease involving autoimmune destruction of pancreatic beta cells in genetically predisposed individuals. Identifying factors that trigger initiation and progression of autoimmunity may provide opportunities for directed prophylactic and therapeutic measures to prevent and/or treat type 1 diabetes. The human intestinal microbiome is a complex, symbiotic ecological community that influences human health and development, including the development and maintenance of the human immune system. The role of the intestinal microbiome in autoimmunity has garnered significant attention, and evidence suggests a particular role for intestinal microbiome alterations in autoimmune disease development, including type 1 diabetes. This review will examine the role of the intestinal microbiome in the development and function of the immune system and how this relates to the development of autoimmunity. Data from animal and human studies linking alterations in the intestinal microbiome and intestinal integrity with type 1 diabetes will be closely examined. Finally, we will examine the interactions between the intestinal microbiome and dietary exposures and how these interactions may further influence autoimmunity and type 1 diabetes development.

Keywords: type 1 diabetes; intestine, microbiome; gliadin

Introduction

Type 1 diabetes is an autoimmune disease resulting in the destruction of insulin-secreting beta cells of the pancreas. The resultant lack of insulin results in hyperglycemia that is secondarily associated with micro- and macrovascular complications. Lifelong exogenous insulin replacement remains the mainstay of therapy for the majority of patients with type 1 diabetes. Despite improvements in insulin therapy, glucose monitoring, and glycemic control, life expectancy is shorter, and quality of life is significantly compromised, compared to the general population.[1–3] The economic burden is also significant. Each year in the United States, type 1 diabetes accounts for 14.4 billion dollars in medical costs and lost income.[4] These factors have prompted substantial research efforts to define the pathophysiology of type 1 diabetes in order to develop more efficacious therapies or to prevent the disease all together. Recently, the intestinal microbiome, encompassing the entire bacterial community of the intestine, has garnered significant attention for its role in normal health and development and potential role in disease including type 1 diabetes. The following will review type 1 diabetes pathogenesis, the study of the intestinal microbiome, and the potential role that alterations in the microbiome and intestinal integrity may have in the development of type 1 diabetes.

Type 1 diabetes mellitus

Incidence

The incidence of type 1 diabetes has increased dramatically in developed countries over the past several decades. The majority of data collected regarding type 1 diabetes incidence comes from large registries, including a European registry, EURODIAB (Epidemiology and Prevention of Diabetes), and the DiaMond network, encompassing 57 countries, including the United States, China, and several European countries. The EURODIAB registries

doi: 10.1111/j.1749-6632.2011.06340.x

revealed a 3.9% annual increase in the incidence of type 1 diabetes from 1989 to 2003.[5] Similarly, DiaMond revealed a 2.4% annual increase in incidence between 1990 and 1994 and 3.4% between 1995 and 1999.[6] In the United States specifically, data previously revealed a steady or modestly increasing incidence of type 1 diabetes.[7] Recent data from the SEARCH for Diabetes in Youth study, however, suggest that the incidence of type 1 diabetes in the United States is higher than previously thought with 24.3 cases per 100,000 person-years, rivaling the incidence seen in other large, multinational registries.[8] The rapid increase in the incidence of type 1 diabetes in developed countries suggests that nongenetic factors contribute to the pathogenesis of the disease. Specifically, environmental factors including dietary changes, alterations in infectious disease exposures, and increased pharmaceutical use, especially antibiotics, may contribute to the development of the disease.

Pathophysiology

The pathophysiology of type 1 diabetes is complex and still not entirely understood. The clinical manifestations of type 1 diabetes represent the end stage of several distinct pathogenic processes. Genetic predisposition combined with environmental factors initiate the process of autoimmune destruction of the beta cells of the pancreas, a process that involves both the innate and adaptive immune systems. The beta cell destruction remains subclinical until approximately 80% of the beta cell mass is destroyed, at which time hyperglycemia ensues.[9] Eventually, near complete or complete loss of beta cells occurs resulting in significant insulin deficiency, worsening hyperglycemia, and the absolute necessity of exogenous insulin therapy.

Genetic susceptibility is a key factor in any individual's risk for developing type 1 diabetes. To date, several specific genetic risk factors for type 1 diabetes have been identified; and to further emphasize the role of genetics in the pathogenesis of type 1 diabetes, monozygotic twin siblings of individuals with type 1 diabetes have been shown to have a 50% risk of developing type 1 diabetes.[10] Specific polymorphisms in the major histocompatibility complex (MHC), immune molecules normally present on the surface of antigen presenting cells (APC), were the first genetic factors noted to be associated with an increased likelihood of type 1 diabetes. Specifically, the presence of HLA alleles DQ and DR significantly increases the likelihood of type 1 diabetes, though the amount of risk is in large part determined by environmental factors.[11,12] Underscoring the significance of HLA polymorphisms, greater than 90% of Caucasians with type 1 diabetes have a HLA DR3 or DR4 allele.[13]

Additional loci associated with, and thought to increase the risk for, type 1 diabetes have been identified and include a variable nucleotide terminal repeat (VNTR) of the insulin gene, polymorphisms of the lymphocyte-specific protein tyrosine phosphatase (*PTPN22*) gene, and cytotoxic T lymphocyte-associated protein 4 (CTLA-4).[14–16] The International Type 1 Diabetes Genetics Consortium (http://www.t1dgc.org), established in 2002, continues to expand the knowledge of the genetic factors that predispose to type 1 diabetes, for example knowledge obtained from genome-wide association studies to identify novel loci that increase risk for type 1 diabetes.[17,18] To date more than 40 loci associated with type 1 diabetes have been identified, including interferon-induced helicase (*IFIH1*), interleukin 2 receptor alpha (*ILR2A*), and three recently identified loci: LIM domain only 7 (*LMO7*), protein EFR3 homolog B (*EFR3B*), and an intergenic region on 6q27.[18–21]

The fact that the risk is not 100% for monozygotic twins of individuals with type 1 diabetes suggests an additional component in the pathogenesis. This prompted the hypothesis that environmental factors are required to trigger islet autoimmunity and initiate the process of islet destruction in genetically predisposed individuals. Specific triggers in human type 1 diabetes are relatively unknown but proposed factors include viral infections, such as coxsackievirus; certain dietary components including gliadin, cereal, and method of infant feeding (breastfeeding versus cow's milk); and improved sanitation and decreased childhood infections, the aptly named "hygiene hypothesis." The exact immunological events leading to insulitis (islet inflammation), beta cell loss, and subsequent diabetes are complex and not entirely understood. A full review of the current knowledge of these events is beyond the scope of this paper. In general, however, both the innate and adaptive immune systems are inappropriately activated and recruited to the pancreas by a triggering event, initiating an immune cascade that ultimately results in loss of self-tolerance and islet destruction.

Murine models have provided much of the background knowledge into the immunology of type 1 diabetes, though data in humans are growing. In studies of NOD mice, APC, such as macrophages and dendritic cells (DC), are the first to infiltrate the pancreas, presumably returning to pancreatic lymph nodes to present beta cell antigens to naive CD4[+] T cells, "priming" these CD4[+] T cells, and transforming them into a Th1 subtype.[22,23] Once triggered, autoreactive T cells converge on the pancreas and insulitis ensues. Damage to the islets produces additional self-antigens, which further amplifies T cell activation. B cells are also involved in the pathogenesis of diabetes in the NOD mouse via antigen presentation and production of proinflammatory cytokines as well as production of islet cell antibodies.[24,25] Furthermore, impaired production and action of Foxp3[+] regulatory T cells (T$_{reg}$ cells) results in abnormal Th1 and Th2 cell responses.[26,27] Th1 cells subsequently produce additional cytokines, attracting CD8[+] cytotoxic T cells that function to initiate cell death or apoptosis of beta cells, which leads to loss of insulin secretion and clinical manifestations of type 1 diabetes.[28]

Although studying type 1 diabetes immunology in humans has proven more difficult, many of the findings to date are similar to those in animal models. Specifically, autoreactive T cells clearly play a prominent role in human type 1 disease development. Studying cadaveric pancreases of individuals with new-onset type 1 diabetes, Wilcox et al. revealed that CD8[+] cells, along with macrophages, were the predominant cell types in islet infiltrates.[29] Ineffective function of T$_{reg}$ cells is also thought to contribute to disease development in humans.[30,31] Deciphering the triggering and propagating event(s) in the autoimmune cascade could potentially allow for targeted screening, prophylaxis, and therapy for type 1 diabetes.

The intestinal microbiome

Background

Humans are colonized and live in a symbiotic relationship with a vast number and variety of microorganisms, termed the "microbiome," that influence development and general health. The majority of these organisms are bacteria, and it is estimated that the average human microbiome contains 10^{14} bacte-

ria. While these organisms colonize many epithelial surfaces, including skin and upper airways, the intestinal tract, especially the large intestine, harbors the largest number of bacteria.

Early in the neonatal period the microbiome is established and continues to develop over several months to a year toward an adult microbiome. The route of delivery (vaginal vs. cesarean section) and method of nutrition (breastfeeding vs. formula) strongly influence an infant's core microbiota. Vaginal delivery exposes the neonate to the mother's vaginal and intestinal flora. The intestinal microbiome of infants born by cesarean section, however, is initially dominated by skin flora, namely *Staphylococcus*, with delayed acquisition of *Bacteroides*, *Bifidobacterium*, *Lactobacillus*, and *Escherichia coli*.[32–34] The alterations in flora between cesarean section and vaginal delivery persist well beyond infancy.[34] Of particular relevance to this paper, risk of type 1 diabetes onset in childhood is higher in children delivered by cesarean section.[35] Adult microbiota remain relatively stable over time, as reported by Manichanh et al., who showed over two years that an individuals microbiome will maintain phylotypes with 60% similarity.[36]

External factors influence the composition and function of the intestinal microbiome in humans. In particular, dietary exposures likely affect the functional diversity by altering the proportion of various members of the microbiome within the intestine. A poignant example of this phenomenon was presented in a study of twins that revealed obese individuals have reduced diversity of the intestinal microbiome compared to their lean, twin controls.[37] Specifically, the intestinal microbiome of obese individuals had a reduced abundance of Bacteroidetes and an enhanced abundance of Firmicutes and Actinobacteria associated with a reduced functional diversity compared to lean controls. Recently, Muegge et al. sampled fecal DNA from 33 mammalian species and 18 humans to understand the effects of diet on a wide range of species and dietary habits.[38] Differences in the structure and function of the intestinal microbiome were influenced by whether the host was an herbivore or carnivore. Interestingly, in the human subjects, who were asked to maintain meticulous food diaries, differences in the structure and function of the intestinal microbiome could be seen among these individuals based on their dietary intake. Taken together, these findings suggest that dietary exposures can directly influence the diversity and function of the intestinal microbiome that can further affect immune development.

The intestinal microbiome is vast and diverse and the bacterial 16S ribosomal RNA gene sequence (16S) provides a useful tool for analyzing the scope and diversity of the intestinal microbiome. The near ubiquitous expression of 16S in bacteria and the ease of use compared to DNA–DNA hybridization explain the widespread application of 16S gene sequencing in studies of bacterial communities. Utilizing 16S analysis, 395 phylotypes have been identified in the intestinal microbiome, and approximately 80% of these species were not able to be cultured with current methods.[39] Though many phyla are represented, the human intestinal microbiome comprises mainly four phyla: Firmicutes, Bacteroidetes, Actinobacteria, and Proteobacteria, with Firmicutes and Bacteroidetes being the two most prominent phyla.[40,41] Between individuals, however, significant variability exists in the bacterial composition of the intestinal microbiome.[37]

While 16S studies provide information on the number of known species in the microbiome, no information is provided on the function of these bacteria. Metagenomics has evolved as a powerful method to obtain and analyze the genetic diversity of the microbiome. Utilizing a "shotgun sequence" approach, massively parallel pyrosequencing, and complex computer software, metagenomics allows for evaluation of large samples of microbial genes including genes related directly to function. Initial studies utilizing metagenomic analysis of the human intestinal microbiome revealed multiple genes not normally found in the human genome.[42] Many of these gene products were involved in processes of amino acid, glycan, xenobiotic, and vitamin metabolism and biosynthesis. More recently, Qin et al. performed metagenomics on a larger cohort of 124 healthy Europeans, revealing the presence of approximately 1,150 bacterial species within the cohort.[43] Each individual's intestinal microbiome was estimated to comprise 160 bacterial species that contributed 150-fold more genes compared to the human gene set.

Despite the variability of microbiota between individuals, a recent metagenomics study of 22 individuals from four countries suggests the existence of "enterotypes," distinct groups of human microbiota that may respond differently to environmental stim-uli.[44] The ongoing Human Microbiome Project was developed to form a more concrete understanding of the composition of the human microbiome and the role the microbiome plays in normal physiology and development of disease.[45]

Though much knowledge is gained with metagenomics studies, the methods whereby intestinal bacterial samples are collected and analyzed must be emphasized and standardized, as variable methods can yield inconsistent results. Colonic bacteria samples collected from the same individual via a stool sample or intestinal biopsy may reveal different bacteria.[39] Methods used to extract samples may also influence the bacterial composition data.[46] Momozawa et al. recently confirmed the differences seen in bacterial yield between stool and biopsy samples, and that methods of stool sample recovery, either from colonoscopy or fresh stool sample, can identify different bacteria.[47] The authors contend that only biopsy specimens should be used for high-throughput analysis of human colonic bacteria.

Intestinal microbiome and autoimmunity

The intestinal microbiome is a complex system that acts in a symbiotic relationship with the host to influence development, nutrition, immunity, and disease. The intestinal mucosa is a common entry site for pathogens and harbors a significant proportion of the cells of the immune system. An intact mucosa provides the first line of defense against pathogens and other pathogenic antigens. Research in animal models and humans continues to define the vital role the intestinal flora plays in protecting the mucosa from invading pathogens and influencing the development and maintenance of both the systemic and innate immune systems.

Epidemiological data have revealed a disproportionate prevalence of autoimmune diseases in developed countries. This constitutes the original basis for the "hygiene hypothesis," the suggestion that decreased exposure to microorganisms, both pathogenic and symbiotic, in childhood alters natural development of the immune system predisposing to the loss of self-tolerance.[48] This hypothesis has fostered the concept that altered intestinal microbiota may be one of the predisposing factors for the development of autoimmunity. In addition to the knowledge that intestinal microbiota contribute significantly to the development and maintenance of the immune system, recent animal model and human studies of several different autoimmune diseases lend additional credence to the claim that altered intestinal flora may be at the forefront of the pathogenesis of these diseases.

Crohn's disease and ulcerative colitis, known broadly as inflammatory bowel disease (IBD), are autoimmune diseases of the intestinal tract that lead to mucosal inflammation and development of intestinal lesions. IBD is also associated with several extraintestinal manifestations. The exact etiology of IBD is unclear but likely involves environmental, genetic, and immune factors. The role of the microbiome in IBD development is becoming more established. Animal studies have revealed that the severity of experimentally-induced intestinal inflammation can be modulated via introduction of anaerobic bacteria.[49] Interestingly, germ-free animals appear to be protected from experimentally induced colitis but show rapid development of disease upon colonization with enteric bacteria.[50–52] Metagenomic evaluation of fecal samples from patients with Crohn's disease has revealed a reduced diversity of the Firmicutes phyla compared to healthy controls.[53] Similarly, Frank et al. characterized subsets of patients with Crohn's disease and ulcerative colitis who had reduced bacteria in the Firmicutes and Bacteroidetes phyla.[54] Willing et al. provided further evidence of an altered intestinal microbiome in Crohn's disease in their study of monozygotic twins.[55] Small intestine biopsies of twins concordant or discordant for ileal Crohn's disease revealed a preponderance of E. coli and a reduced abundance of Faecalibacterium prausnitzii, compared to individuals with colonic Crohn's or healthy controls.

Alterations in intestinal flora have been hypothesized to contribute to the pathogenesis of several other autoimmune diseases including celiac sprue, allergy, multiple sclerosis, rheumatoid arthritis, and ankylosing spondylitis.[56–60] Identifying specific intestinal microorganisms that alter risk of a disease will not only assist in defining pathogenesis but also provide a method of screening and the ability to tailor therapy specifically.

The intestinal microbiome: effects on immunity and risk of autoimmune diabetes

Much of the knowledge regarding the role that the intestinal microbiome may play in the development of autoimmune diabetes comes from animal studies using diabetes-prone and germ-free animals. These studies, combined with epidemiological data from humans, have begun to establish the many facets of the intestinal microbiome that directly affect the risk for, and development of, autoimmune diabetes. Additionally, early therapeutic studies have also been established directly targeting the intestinal microbiome. As illustrated in Figure 1, several environmental factors thought to be triggers of autoimmune diabetes may, at least in part, increase risk for diabetes due to their effects on the composition of the intestinal microbiome.

Animal studies

Animal models have provided a wealth of information regarding the influence of the intestinal flora on autoimmunity and autoimmune diabetes development.

Alterations in flora. Using mice raised in germ-free environments and subsequently exposed to microorganisms of choice (gnotobiology), much has been ascertained about the structural and functional effects of the intestinal flora on the immune system. Peyer's patches, splenic germinal centers, and mesenteric lymph nodes of germ-free mice are significantly smaller and fewer in number compared to mice raised in a normal environment.[61] Deficiencies in the development of mucosal-associated lymphoid tissue, specifically plasma cells and CD4+ T cells, are other consequences of a germ-free environment.[62,63] In germ-free animals, reintroduction of normal gut flora can normalize size and cellularity of lymphoid structures and increase antibody production.[64] In fact, colonization of germ-free mice with a single organism, segmented filamentous bacterium (SFB), is sufficient to stimulate production of IL-17–producing CD4+ T cells.[65] The intestinal microbiome affects several other components of immune development and function, as will be outlined throughout this section.

The sentinel studies suggesting a role for microorganism exposure in the pathogenesis of autoimmune diabetes employed diabetes-prone animals, NOD mice, and BioBreeding diabetes-prone (BB-DP) rats in particular, raised germ-free and/or exposed to a variety of infectious organisms or antigens.

Early studies revealed that in NOD mice, chronic viral infections were associated with a lower incidence of diabetes.[66,67] Active infection with mycobacteria and stimulus with bacterial antigens also

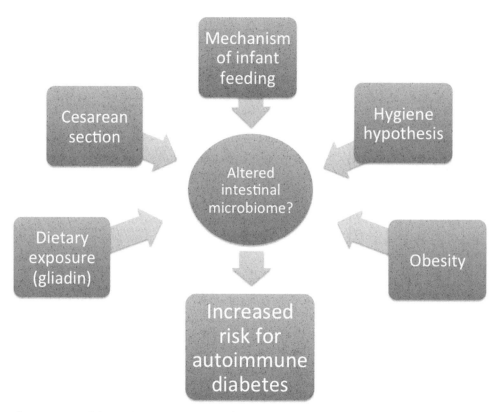

Figure 1. Environmental factors that may directly or indirectly alter the intestinal microbiome and therefore affect risk of autoimmune diabetes.

decreased the rate of development of autoimmune diabetes in NOD mice.[68–71] Extrapolation of these findings has led to the concept that a germ-free environment specifically increases the risk of diabetes development in NOD mice. However, we have shown that diabetes incidence in female NOD mice is not necessarily affected by germ-free conditions; rather, monoculture of these animals with *Bacillus cereus* delayed onset of diabetes, suggesting specific bacteria or bacterial products affect the risk of disease more so than a specific germ-free environment.[72] The protective effect of bacterial extracts may require functional natural killer cells (NKC) and involve increased production of TGF-β.[73] The ability to stimulate T_{reg} cell production, through induction of FoxP3 expression, may explain the protective effect of TGF-β.[74] Controversy exists over the protective role of NKC in autoimmune diabetes, however, as these cells have also been implicated in the pathogenesis.[75]

Identifying specific organisms associated with the development of autoimmune diabetes would allow for targeted screening and potential therapies. Initial attempts to identify specific intestinal flora alterations that increased risk for type 1 diabetes used diabetes-prone animal models. Performing fluorescent *in situ* hybridization to target 16S rRNA of *Bacteroides*, *Clostridium*, and *Lactobacillus* species in fecal samples of BB-DP rats, Brugman *et al.* revealed that *Bacteroides* sp. were more prominent in those rats that developed diabetes compared to rats that remained diabetes free.[76] More in-depth experiments revealed significantly higher proportion of *Lactobacillus* and *Bifidobacterium* genera in bio-breeding diabetes-resistant (BB-DR) rats compared to BB-DP rats, while BB-DP rats were found to have a higher abundance of *Bacteroides* genera.[77]

Innate immunity and intestinal integrity. The innate immune system relies on the microbiome for appropriate development of several cell types. Of particular interest is the intestinal epithelial cell (IEC). IECs contain tight junctions that normally function to regulate passage of nutrients and inhibit translocation of pathogenic organisms. IECs also express direct interaction with immune cells and produce and respond to a variety of cytokine stimuli. Many changes in IEC development and function are observed when alterations are made to the intestinal flora of animal models. For example, IECs of germ-free mice turn over at a slower rate than mice with normal intestinal microflora.[78] Additionally, mice depleted of their normal flora by antibiotics also show diminished IEC replication, significant alteration in IEC gene expression, and impaired production of antimicrobial factors including RegIIIγ, a Gram-positive specific antimicrobial peptide.[79] Reintroduction of colonic bacteria induces proliferation of IECs in germ-free mice via toll-like receptor (TLR) recognition of the microbes.[80]

IECs play a prominent role in the development and regulation of the immune system. An intact intestinal epithelium serves to regulate passage of antigens to DC and increased gut permeability due to a compromised epithelium results in exposure to antigens that is a potential trigger for an autoimmune response in predisposed individuals. IECs also function to uptake, process, and present antigen and can promote activation of CD8$^+$ T cells, as reviewed.[81] Additionally, IEC modulate function of DC via production of factors such as IL-10 that promote a tolerogenic DC response.[82] IEC may also play a role in T$_{reg}$ cell expansion.[83] Taken together, this evidence suggests that IEC are critical to the proper development of the innate immune system and dysregulation of IEC by an altered intestinal flora may result in the development of autoimmunity.

Evidence in the BB-DP rat model has suggested that *Lactobacillus johnsonii* N6.2 is a specific organism that may delay the onset of autoimmune diabetes via modulation of intestinal integrity.[84] In their study, Valladares *et al.* also noted a significant increase in the tight junction protein claudin-1 and decreased oxidative stress in the ileal mucosa of the *L. johnsonii* treated animals. These findings suggest that autoimmune diabetes may be the result of an inflammatory response initiated by a leaky gut epithelium, which is the result of an altered intestinal flora.

Further evidence from animal studies suggests that the integrity of the gut epithelium plays a prominent role in autoimmune diabetes development. BB-DP rats express less of the tight junction protein claudin and display increased intestinal permeability compared to control Wistar rats.[85] Translating further, increased gut permeability was associated with a higher rate of diabetes development in BB-DP rats on a regular diet.[86] Watts *et al.* additionally demonstrated that upregulation of zonulin—a protein that serves to regulate tight junctions—and, subsequently, increased intestinal permeability significantly increased the rate of diabetes development in BB-DP rats.[87]

More recently, Wen *et al.* sought to establish how the interaction between microorganisms and the intestinal epithelium could trigger autoimmunity and diabetes development.[88] The specific target of this study was myeloid differentiation factor 88 (MyD88), an adaptor molecule used by multiple TLR to regulate the innate immune response. Wildtype NOD mice developed diabetes quickly. NOD mice with a MyD88 knockout (KO), however, were protected from diabetes development while germ-free, MyD88-KO NOD mice developed diabetes in a rapid fashion. Furthermore, recolonization of the MyD88-KO mice decreased diabetes development, suggesting protection from diabetes is microorganism dependent. Knockdown of TLR2, TLR3, and TLR4 did not attenuate diabetes development, however, suggesting that while some microorganisms protect the host from developing diabetes, this protection is independent of the TLR system.

Adaptive immune system. The development and function of the adaptive immune system is also directly affected by the intestinal microbiota, a process that may influence risk of disease. T$_{reg}$ cells secrete anti-inflammatory cytokines IL-10 and TGF-β and function to temper the immune response through down-regulation of both the innate and adaptive immune systems.[89] Intestinal T$_{reg}$ cells in particular play a prominent role in tolerance of oral antigens and microbes.[90] Evidence from animal models suggests the presence of the intestinal microbiota is vital for the production of adequate numbers of functional T$_{reg}$ cells from the intestine. In germ-free mice, T$_{reg}$ cells are less prominent and less effective in suppressing T cell activity compared to T$_{reg}$ cells in conventional mice.[91] In an experimental model of colitis, IL-10 production from T$_{reg}$ cells of germ-free mice is also suppressed, as is the ability of these cells to modulate disease.[92] Conversion of CD4$^+$ T cells to T$_{reg}$ cells was stimulated by *B. fragilis* monocolonization of germ-free mice, a process dependent on the *B. fragilis*-produced polysachharide A (PSA).[93] IL-10 production and T cell suppressive activity of T_{reg} cells were also enhanced in a PSA-dependent fashion.

T helper 17 cells (Th17) are a proinflammatory subset of T cells that secrete interleukin 17 (IL-17), have antimicrobial activities, and have been implicated in many autoimmune diseases including multiple sclerosis, inflammatory bowel disease, and psoriasis.[94] The intestine harbors the largest number of Th17 cells, and the intestinal microbiota is likely required for the production and expansion of these cells.[95–97]

In a recent report, Lau *et al.* sought to understand the mechanisms by which *L. johnsonii* exposure can delay diabetes in BB-DP rats.[98] Interestingly, the study demonstrated enhanced Th17 differentiation in the mesenteric lymph nodes of animals fed *L. johnsonii*. The authors suggested that although Th17 cells are associated with insulitis the Th17 bias seen with *L. johnsonii* feeding limits the necessary conversion to the diabetogenic Th1 cell type, thereby inhibiting or delaying onset of diabetes. Others have suggested that a Th17 bias may reduce the risk of autoimmune diabetes via mucosal protection produced by IL-17 upregulation.[99] Other undefined mechanisms may also explain the effect seen with *L. johnsonii* exposure.

Other important regulatory cells of the immune system are directly influenced by the intestinal microbiome, including DC, which do not develop in appropriate numbers in germ-free mice, and B cells, which produce IgA at a reduced amount in germ-free mice, compared to wild-type mice.[100,101]

Dietary factors. The intestinal microbiota's influence on nutrition and the potential role of these factors in autoimmune diabetes pathogenesis has also been explored in animal models. The initial evidence suggesting a role for nutrition in autoimmune diabetes came from Hoorfar *et al.* in 1993.[102] Using NOD mice exposed to wheat-flour diet or hydrolyzed casein, this study revealed a significantly lower incidence of diabetes in mice receiving the hydrolyzed diet. Expanding further, Brugman *et al.* completely prevented diabetes by providing antibiotics and a hydrolyzed casein diet to BB-DP rats.[76]

Additional studies have expanded on the dietary hypothesis to more precisely pinpoint the components and associated mechanisms of diet that may increase risk for autoimmune diabetes. Gliadin, a glycoprotein implicated in the intestinal damage of celiac sprue, is the most extensively studied dietary component in the pathogenesis of type 1 diabetes. NOD mice that lack exposure to dietary gluten develop diabetes at a significantly lower rate than mice fed a standard diet.[103–105] BB-DP rats fed a cereal-based diet develop diabetes associated with a pancreatic Th1 cytokine pattern, compared to BB-DP rats on a protein-based diet who had less insulitis, a Th2 cytokine pattern, and overall lower incidence of diabetes.[106] Investigation into the mechanisms leading to development of insulitis and diabetes in animals on a gliadin diet suggests that these proteins increase small intestine inflammation and intestinal permeability.[86,107] Furthermore, BB-DP rats have a significantly higher proportion of Th1 cells in the mesenteric lymph nodes upon exposure to wheat proteins.[108] Pancreatic lymph node dendritic cells sample gut antigens and, upon recognizing protein products, stimulate production of activated T cells, a process that leads to increased beta cell apoptosis.[109] Finally, gliadin exposure also suppresses T_{reg} cell production in NOD mice, which is another potential mechanism by which dietary exposure may enhance genetic diabetes risk.[110]

The known association of alterations in diet and intestinal flora with diabetes development suggests that these two entities work in concert to affect disease risk. With this in mind, the interactions between intestinal bacteria and gliadin peptides are being closely examined. Hansen *et al.* examined the effect of a gluten-free versus standard diet on bacterial composition in NOD mice.[111] Diabetes developed in 47% of the standard-fed mice compared to only 5% in the mice fed a gluten-free diet. Examination of intestinal bacteria revealed a significantly lower prevalence of aerobic, microaerophilic, and anaerobic bacteria in the mice fed a gluten-free diet, compared to mice on a standard diet. Much of the difference in bacterial composition was directly attributable to Gram-positive bacteria.

In vitro studies have provided additional information regarding the interactions between gliadin and intestinal flora. As shown by Laparra *et al.*, intestinal epithelial cells (Caco-2) in culture exposed to gliadin-derived peptides produce inflammatory cytokines, a process that was downregulated when these cell preparations were inoculated with *Bifidiobacteria*, an intestinal bacteria that has been associated with lower incidence of diabetes in animal models.[112] The effect was most pronounced with *Bifidobacterium longum*. Gliadin peptide sequences were modified upon exposure to *B. longum*, suggesting a mechanism by which "protective" intestinal bacteria can indirectly maintain intestinal integrity. The same research group recently examined the proteome of Caco-2 cells after exposure to gliadin peptides in the presence or absence of *B. longum*.[113] Protein expression was altered in Caco-2 cells treated with gliadin peptides in the absence of *B. longum*; specifically, expression of proteins involved in cytoskeletion formation and apoptosis was altered. These effects were ameliorated when *B. longum* was added to the cell culture.

Whereas *B. longum* may protect the intestinal epithelium from gliadin-induced structural changes, other species of bacteria have been shown to act with gliadin to synergistically alter the integrity of the intestinal epithelium. Germ-free rats exposed to gliadin were found to have fewer goblet cells in the small intestine, a sign of early enteropathy, and this finding was more pronounced in animals inoculated with *Escherichia coli* CBL2 or *Shigella* CBL2.[114] *Shigella* CBL2 also augmented interferon-γ–induced impairment of tight junctions, allowing enhanced translocation of gliadin into the lamina propria.

The results from the above studies indicate that gliadin exposure increases the risk for diabetes through mechanisms involving both the integrity on the intestinal epithelium and the composition of the intestinal flora.

Probiotics. Expanding further on the concept of a protective intestinal flora, modification of the intestinal flora by probiotics has been investigated as a method to modulate the risk for diabetes. *Lactobacillus casei*-treated NOD mice were protected from diabetes onset and were found to have reduced numbers of splenic $CD8^+$ T cells and systemic inflammatory markers.[115] IL-2 levels were also higher in probiotic-treated mice, and the enhanced expression of this cytokine may serve to stabilize $FoxP3^+$ T_{reg} cells, as recently described by Chen *et al.*[116] NOD mice administered the probiotic compound VSL#3 showed a reduced severity of insulitis, reduced beta cell destruction, and lower rates of diabetes development compared to control.[117] In this study, IL-10 expression was significantly increased

in the Peyer's patches, spleen, and pancreas, suggesting an immunomodulatory effect of the probiotic. Another potential mechanism behind the protective effect of probiotics may include these organisms' ability to inhibit adherence of enteropathogenic bacteria by binding to intestinal epithelial cells and up-regulating mucin production.[118,119]

Human studies

Using discoveries in animal models, studies are beginning to emerge establishing the role of intestinal flora and integrity in the development of autoimmune diabetes in humans.

Alterations in flora. Attempts have been made to define an understanding of the underlying intestinal flora alterations underlying autoimmune diabetes development in humans. Using 16S RNA amplification techniques, Giongo *et al.* set out to define specific taxa that differed between children with type 1 diabetes and healthy controls.[120] Over time, the intestinal microbiota of children who developed type 1 diabetes consisted of a higher proportion of the Bacteroidetes phyla and a lower proportion of the Firmicutes phyla. Opposite findings were observed in control patients, in whom Bacteroidetes phyla sequences decreased over time while Firmicutes sequences increased. Additionally, within the Bacteroidetes phyla, the *Bacteroides ovatus* species represented 24% of the total increase in cases. Though this study was small, comprising eight case subjects and four controls, the findings represented some of the first evidence of specific changes in the composition of intestinal bacteria in humans with type 1 diabetes. Larger cohort studies such as The Environmental Determinants of Diabetes in the Young (TEDDY, currently in progress), are needed to further define alterations in the composition of the intestinal microbiome in humans and the underlying mechanisms that lead to autoimmunity and diabetes development.[121]

Intestinal integrity and immunity. Similar to animal models of autoimmune diabetes, several studies of intestinal integrity in human subjects with type 1 diabetes have revealed evidence of increased intestinal permeability.[122–124] Furthermore, the intestinal permeability seen in individuals with type 1 diabetes is detectable prior to clinical onset of disease, suggesting that the intestine is directly involved in the disease development.[125] A recent study by Brown *et al.* used metagenomics to determine the potential function of bacteria that differ between individuals with type 1 diabetes and healthy controls.[126] Findings from this study may begin to explain the contribution of the intestinal microbiome to maintenance of intestinal integrity. Bacteria from individuals with type 1 diabetes tended to have higher expression of genes related to motility and adhesion compared to controls. Additionally, evaluation of 16S demonstrated a higher proportion of butyrate-producing and mucin-degrading bacteria in controls compared to cases. Both butyrate and mucin are thought to be directly involved in maintaining intestinal epithelial integrity. The authors suggest a hypothesis whereby healthy individuals harbor a higher proportion of butyrate-producing bacteria that help to maintain intestinal integrity and prevent autoimmunity. These preliminary findings may help to advance the knowledge of the role of intestinal integrity in autoimmunity and type 1 diabetes development.

Inflammatory changes in the intestine of patients with type 1 diabetes lend further evidence for the involvement of the intestinal mucosa and altered intestinal immunity in the pathogenesis of type 1 diabetes. Though sometimes structurally normal, small intestine biopsies of patients with type 1 diabetes reveal increased expression of HLA-DR, HLA-DP, and intercellular adhesion molecule-1 (ICAM-1).[127] Frequently, microstructural intestinal changes are seen in patients with type 1 diabetes, including changes to the microvilli and tight junctions.[128] Higher densitites of IL-1α^+ and IL-4$^+$ cells in these biopsies also point toward a heightened intestinal inflammatory state in type 1 diabetes. Jejunal biopsies of patients with type 1 diabetes show evidence of mucosal inflammation and, upon *in vitro* exposure to gliadin, an exaggerated inflammatory response compared to control.[129] Finally, T_{reg} cell production in the intestinal mucosa is suppressed in patients with type 1 diabetes, as demonstrated by reduced numbers of FoxP3$^+$ cells in small intestine biopsies of children with type 1 diabetes.[130]

Dietary factors. As in animal models, human intestinal integrity appears to be compromised upon exposure to gliadin peptides. Human intestinal samples exposed to gliadin *ex vivo* display amplified release of zonulin and increased permeability.[129] Intestinal samples from patients with celiac disease

had more robust and sustained permeability compared to nonceliac disease controls, consistent with the theory of genetic predisposition enhancing risk in those with celiac disease. The role of gliadin in the pathogenesis of type 1 diabetes likely goes beyond affecting intestinal integrity. Small bowel biopsies of patients with type 1 diabetes exposed to gliadin reveal an exaggerated inflammatory response.[129] Production of cytokines TNF-α and IL-8—both involved in the pathogenesis of type 1 diabetes—by monocytes of susceptible humans is also stimulated by gliadin.[131] Finally, islet cell autoimmunity appears to be exaggerated in individuals who are exposed to gliadin-containing foods prior to six months of age.[132] Given the association of type 1 diabetes and celiac disease, and the role of gliadin in both, it is likely that these disease processes share specific risk factors and etiologies. Similar genetic susceptibility between the two diseases, as revealed by Smyth *et al.*, further enhances the concept of shared pathogenic mechanisms.[133]

Probiotics. Based on initial promising results in animal models, the use of probiotics to delay or prevent type 1 diabetes in humans has become an area of interest. Studies in healthy humans have demonstrated that exposure to *Lactobacillus plantarum* enhanced the expression of tight junction proteins,

Table 1. Organisms and other factors that may alter risk for autoimmune diabetes in diabetes-prone animal models and humans

May delay or prevent autoimmune diabetes	May promote autoimmune diabetes
Chronic viral infections[a]	*Bacteroides* sp.[a,b]
Mycobacterial infection[a]	*Bacteroides* genera[a,b]
Bacterial antigens[a]	Gliadin[a,b]
Monoculture with *B. cereus*[a]	Impaired intestinal epithelial integrity[a,b]
Lactobacillus genera[a,b]	Cow's milk[b]
Lactobacillus johnsonii N6.2[a]	Delivery by cesarean section[b]
Lactobacillus casei[a]	Hygiene hypothesis[b]
Probiotic VSL #3[a]	Acute viral infections[b] (coxsackievirus)
Bifidobacterium genera[a]	

[a]Animal models, [b]humans.

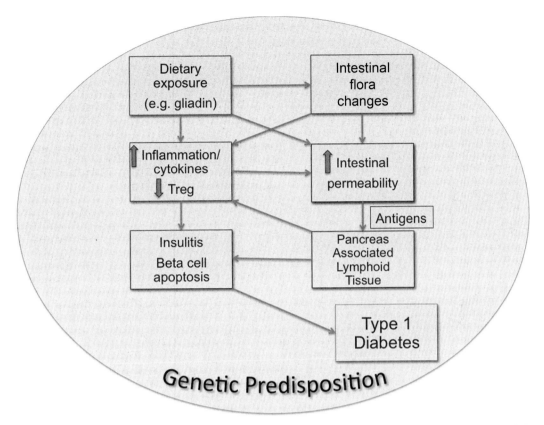

Figure 2. General schema outlining proposed relationships between intestinal flora/integrity and development of type 1 diabetes in genetically predisposed individuals.

suggesting the ability of these organisms to improve endothelial integrity.[134] The PRODIA study, currently ongoing in Finland, is investigating children with genetic susceptibility to type 1 diabetes and the ability of probiotics to decrease diabetes autoantibodies in this group.[135]

Conclusion

Type 1 diabetes is a complex series of events culminating in autoimmune destruction of pancreatic beta cells, hyperglycemia, and risk for subsequent vascular complications. In those with genetic predisposition, environmental factors affect disease risk and pathogenesis. Table 1 briefly summarizes some of the specific organisms and factors that have been identified to potentially alter risk of autoimmune diabetes development in diabetes-prone animal models and humans. Evidence to date strongly suggests that intestinal microbiota, through their impact on immune development and intestinal structure and function, are vital to the patho-

genesis of type 1 diabetes, though the exact mechanisms whereby intestinal bacteria are altered and how those alterations influence type 1 diabetes development are still unclear. Figure 2 presents a general view of the knowledge to date regarding potential mechanisms in the development of type 1 diabetes in genetically predisposed individuals and how the intestinal microbiome may play a direct role in this process. Continued exploration into the specific role of the intestinal microbiome in the development of type 1 diabetes will allow for targeted screening and development of novel therapies to treat and ideally prevent the disease.

Acknowledgment

This work was supported by a generous grant from the J.W. Kieckhefer Foundation.

Conflicts of interest

The authors declare no conflicts of interest.

References

1. Kalyva, E., E. Malakonaki, C. Eiser & D. Mamoulakis. 2011. Health-related quality of life (HRQoL) of children with type 1 diabetes mellitus (T1DM): self and parental perceptions. *Pediatr. Diabetes* **12:** 34–40.

2. Cameron, F.J., C. Clarke, K. Hesketh, *et al.* 2002. Regional and urban Victorian diabetic youth: clinical and quality-of-life outcomes. *J. Paediatr. Child. Health* **38:** 593–596.

3. Miller R.G., Secrest A.M., Sharma R.K., *et al.* 2011. Improvements in life expectancy of type 1 diabetes: The Pittsburgh Epidemiology of Diabetes Complications Study. 71st Scientific Sessions of the American Diabetes Association Abstract Number 0078-OR.

4. Tao, B., M. Pietropaolo, M. Atkinson, *et al.* 2010. Estimating the cost of type 1 diabetes in the U.S.: a propensity score matching method. *PLoS One* **5:** e11501–e11512.

5. Green, A. & C.C. Patterson. 2001. Trends in the incidence of childhood-onset diabetes in Europe 1989–1998. *Diabetologia* **44**(Suppl 3): B3–B8.

6. DIAMOND Project Group. 2006. Incidence and trends of childhood type 1 diabetes worldwide 1990–1999. *Diabet. Med.* **23:** 857–866.

7. Libman, I.M. & R.E. LaPorte. 2005. Changing trends in epidemiology of type 1 diabetes mellitus throughout the world: how far have we come and where do we go from here. *Pediatr. Diabetes* **6:** 119–121.

8. Dabelea, D., R.A. Bell, R.B. D'Agostino, Jr, *et al.* 2007. Incidence of diabetes in youth in the United States. *JAMA* **297:** 2716–2724.

9. Notkins, A.L. & A. Lernmark. 2001. Autoimmune type 1 diabetes: resolved and unresolved issues. *J. Clin. Invest.* **108:** 1247–1252.

10. Redondo, M.J., P.R. Fain & G.S. Eisenbarth. 2001. Genetics of type 1A diabetes. *Recent Prog. Horm. Res.* **56:** 69–89.

11. Altobelli, E., A. Blasetti, R. Petrocelli, *et al.* 2005. HLA DR/DQ alleles and risk of type I diabetes in childhood: a population-based case–control study. *Clin. Exp. Med.* **5:** 72–79.

12. Sanjeevi, C.B., S.K. Sedimbi, M. Landin-Olsson, *et al.* 2008. Risk conferred by HLA-DR and DQ for type 1 diabetes in 0- to 35-year age group in Sweden. *Ann. N.Y. Acad. Sci.* **1150:** 106–111.

13. Thomson, G., W.P. Robinson, M.K. Kuhner, *et al.* 1988. Genetic heterogeneity, modes of inheritance, and risk estimates for a joint study of Caucasians with insulin-dependent diabetes mellitus. *Am. J. Hum. Genet.* **43:** 799–816.

14. Bell, G.I., S. Horita & J.H. Karam. 1984. A polymorphic locus near the human insulin gene is associated with insulin-dependent diabetes mellitus. *Diabetes* **33:** 176–183.

15. Bottini, N., L. Musumeci, A. Alonso, *et al.* 2004. A functional variant of lymphoid tyrosine phosphatase is associated with type I diabetes. *Nat. Genet.* **36:** 337–338.

16. Ueda, H., J.M. Howson, L. Esposito, *et al.* 2003. Association of the T-cell regulatory gene CTLA4 with susceptibility to autoimmune disease. *Nature* **423:** 506–511.

17. Cooper, J.D., D.J. Smyth, A.M. Smiles, *et al.* 2008. Meta-analysis of genome-wide association study data identifies additional type 1 diabetes risk loci. *Nat. Genet.* **40:** 1399–1401.

18. Barrett, J.C., D.G. Clayton, P. Concannon, *et al.* 2009. Genome-wide association study and meta-analysis find that over 40 loci affect risk of type 1 diabetes. *Nat. Genet.* **41:** 703–707.

19. Smyth, D.J., J.D. Cooper, R. Bailey, *et al.* 2006. A genome-wide association study of nonsynonymous SNPs identifies a type 1 diabetes locus in the interferon-induced helicase (IFIH1) region. *Nat. Genet.* **38:** 617–619.

20. Lowe, C.E., J.D. Cooper, T. Brusko, *et al.* 2007. Large-scale genetic fine mapping and genotype-phenotype associations implicate polymorphism in the IL2RA region in type 1 diabetes. *Nat. Genet.* **39:** 1074–1082.

21. Bradfield, J.P., H.Q. Qu, K. Wang, *et al.* 2011. A genome-wide meta-analysis of six type 1 diabetes cohorts identifies multiple associated Loci. *PLoS Genet.* **7:** e1002293–e1002301.

22. Gagnerault, M.C., J.J. Luan, C. Lotton & F. Lepault. 2002. Pancreatic lymph nodes are required for priming of beta cell reactive T cells in NOD mice. *J. Exp. Med.* **196:** 369–377.

23. Turley, S., L. Poirot, M. Hattori, *et al.* 2003. Physiological beta cell death triggers priming of self-reactive T cells by dendritic cells in a type-1 diabetes model. *J. Exp. Med.* **198:** 1527–1537.

24. Wong, F.S., L. Wen, M. Tang, *et al.* 2004. Investigation of the role of B-cells in type 1 diabetes in the NOD mouse. *Diabetes* **53:** 2581–2587.

25. Serreze, D.V., S.A. Fleming, H.D. Chapman, *et al.* 1998. B lymphocytes are critical antigen-presenting cells for the initiation of T cell-mediated autoimmune diabetes in nonobese diabetic mice. *J. Immunol.* **161:** 3912–3918.

26. Sgouroudis, E. & C.A. Piccirillo. 2009. Control of type 1 diabetes by CD4+Foxp3 +regulatory T cells: lessons from mouse models and implications for human disease. *Diabetes Metab. Res. Rev.* **25:** 208–218.

27. Tang, Q., J.Y. Adams, C. Penaranda, *et al.* 2008. Central role of defective interleukin-2 production in the triggering of islet autoimmune destruction. *Immunity* **28:** 687–697.

28. Wang, B., A. Gonzalez, C. Benoist & D. Mathis. 1996. The role of CD8+ T cells in the initiation of insulin-dependent diabetes mellitus. *Eur. J. Immunol.* **26:** 1762–1769.

29. Willcox, A., S.J. Richardson, A.J. Bone, *et al.* 2009. Analysis of islet inflammation in human type 1 diabetes. *Clin. Exp. Immunol.* **155:** 173–181.

30. Lindley, S., C.M. Dayan, A. Bishop, *et al.* 2005. Defective suppressor function in CD4(+)CD25(+) T-cells from patients with type 1 diabetes. *Diabetes* **54:** 92–99.

31. Tree, T.I., B.O. Roep & M. Peakman. 2006. A mini meta-analysis of studies on CD4+CD25+ T cells in human type 1 diabetes: report of the Immunology of Diabetes Society T Cell Workshop. *Ann. N.Y. Acad. Sci.* **1079:** 9–18.

32. Dominguez-Bello, M.G., E.K. Costello, M. Contreras, *et al.* 2010. Delivery mode shapes the acquisition and structure of the initial microbiota across multiple body habitats in newborns. *Proc. Natl. Acad. Sci. USA* **107:** 11971–11975.

33. Gronlund, M.M., O.P. Lehtonen, E. Eerola & P. Kero. 1999. Fecal microflora in healthy infants born by different methods of delivery: permanent changes in intestinal flora

after cesarean delivery. *J. Pediatr. Gastroenterol. Nutr.* **28:** 19–25.

34. Salminen, S., G.R. Gibson, A.L. McCartney & E. Isolauri. 2004. Influence of mode of delivery on gut microbiota composition in seven year old children. *Gut* **53:** 1388–1389.

35. Cardwell, C.R., L.C. Stene, G. Joner, *et al.* 2008. Caesarean section is associated with an increased risk of childhood-onset type 1 diabetes mellitus: a meta-analysis of observational studies. *Diabetologia* **51:** 726–735.

36. Manichanh, C., E. Varela, C. Martinez, *et al.* 2008. The gut microbiota predispose to the pathophysiology of acute postradiotherapy diarrhea. *Am. J. Gastroenterol.* **103:** 1754–1761.

37. Turnbaugh, P.J., M. Hamady, T. Yatsunenko, *et al.* 2009. A core gut microbiome in obese and lean twins. *Nature* **457:** 480–484.

38. Muegge, B.D., J. Kuczynski, D. Knights, *et al.* 2011. Diet drives convergence in gut microbiome functions across mammalian phylogeny and within humans. *Science* **332:** 970–974.

39. Eckburg, P.B., E.M. Bik, C.N. Bernstein, *et al.* 2005. Diversity of the human intestinal microbial flora. *Science* **308:** 1635–1638.

40. Frank, D.N., A.L. St Amand, R.A. Feldman, *et al.* 2007. Molecular-phylogenetic characterization of microbial community imbalances in human inflammatory bowel diseases. *Proc. Natl. Acad. Sci. USA* **104:** 13780–13785.

41. Ley, R.E., C.A. Lozupone, M. Hamady, *et al.* 2008. Worlds within worlds: evolution of the vertebrate gut microbiota. Nature reviews. *Microbiology* **6:** 776–788.

42. Gill, S.R., M. Pop, R.T. Deboy, *et al.* 2006. Metagenomic analysis of the human distal gut microbiome. *Science* **312:** 1355–1359.

43. Qin, J., R. Li, J. Raes, *et al.* 2010. A human gut microbial gene catalogue established by metagenomic sequencing. *Nature* **464:** 59–65.

44. Arumugam, M., J. Raes, E. Pelletier, *et al.* 2011. Enterotypes of the human gut microbiome. *Nature* **473:** 174–180.

45. Turnbaugh, P.J., R.E. Ley, M. Hamady, *et al.* 2007. The human microbiome project. *Nature* **449:** 804–810.

46. Wu, G.D., J.D. Lewis, C. Hoffmann, *et al.* 2010. Sampling and pyrosequencing methods for characterizing bacterial communities in the human gut using 16S sequence tags. *BMC Microbiol.* **10:** 206–210.

47. Momozawa, Y., V. Deffontaine, E. Louis & J.F. Medrano. 2011. Characterization of bacteria in biopsies of colon and stools by high throughput sequencing of the V2 region of bacterial 16S rRNA gene in human. *PLoS One* **6:** e16952–e16962.

48. Okada, H., C. Kuhn, H. Feillet & J.F. Bach. 2010. The 'hygiene hypothesis' for autoimmune and allergic diseases: an update. *Clin. Exp. Immunol.* **160:** 1–9.

49. Verdu, E.F., P. Bercik, B. Cukrowska, *et al.* 2000. Oral administration of antigens from intestinal flora anaerobic bacteria reduces the severity of experimental acute colitis in BALB/c mice. *Clin. Exp. Immunol.* **120:** 46–50.

50. Dieleman, L.A., F. Hoentjen, B.F. Qian, *et al.* 2004. Reduced ratio of protective versus proinflammatory cytokine

responses to commensal bacteria in HLA-B27 transgenic rats. *Clin. Exp. Immunol.* **136:** 30–39.

51. Stepankova, R., F. Powrie, O. Kofronova, *et al.* 2007. Segmented filamentous bacteria in a defined bacterial cocktail induce intestinal inflammation in SCID mice reconstituted with CD45RBhigh CD4 +T cells. *Inflam. Bowl Dis.* **13:** 1202–1211.

52. Veltkamp, C., S.L. Tonkonogy, Y.P. De Jong, *et al.* 2001. Continuous stimulation by normal luminal bacteria is essential for the development and perpetuation of colitis in Tg(epsilon26) mice. *Gastroenterology* **120:** 900–913.

53. Manichanh, C., L. Rigottier-Gois, E. Bonnaud, *et al.* 2006. Reduced diversity of faecal microbiota in Crohn's disease revealed by a metagenomic approach. *Gut* **55:** 205–211.

54. Frank, D.N., A.L. St Amand, R.A. Feldman, *et al.* 2007. Molecular-phylogenetic characterization of microbial community imbalances in human inflammatory bowel diseases. *Proc. Natl. Acad. Sci. USA* **104:** 13780–13785.

55. Willing, B., J. Halfvarson, J. Dicksved, *et al.* 2009. Twin studies reveal specific imbalances in the mucosa-associated microbiota of patients with ileal Crohn's disease. *Inflam. Bowl Dis.* **15:** 653–660.

56. Ou, G., M. Hedberg, P. Horstedt, *et al.* 2009. Proximal small intestinal microbiota and identification of rod-shaped bacteria associated with childhood celiac disease. *Am. J. Gastroenterol.* **104:** 3058–3067.

57. Adlerberth, I., D.P. Strachan, P.M. Matricardi, *et al.* 2007. Gut microbiota and development of atopic eczema in 3 European birth cohorts. *J. Allergy Clin. Immunol.* **120:** 343–350.

58. Ochoa-Reparaz, J., D.W. Mielcarz, L.E. Ditrio, *et al.* 2009. Role of gut commensal microflora in the development of experimental autoimmune encephalomyelitis. *J. Immunol.* **183:** 6041–6050.

59. Toivanen, P. 2003. Normal intestinal microbiota in the aetiopathogenesis of rheumatoid arthritis. *Ann. Rheum. Dis.* **62:** 807–811.

60. Rehakova, Z., J. Capkova, R. Stepankova, *et al.* 2000. Germ-free mice do not develop ankylosing enthesopathy, a spontaneous joint disease. *Hum. Immunol.* **61:** 555–558.

61. Macpherson, A.J. & N.L. Harris. 2004. Interactions between commensal intestinal bacteria and the immune system. *Nat. Rev. Immunol.* **4:** 478–485.

62. Macpherson, A.J., L. Hunziker, K. McCoy & A. Lamarre. 2001. IgA responses in the intestinal mucosa against pathogenic and non-pathogenic microorganisms. *Microbes Infection/Institut Pasteur* **3:** 1021–1035.

63. Macpherson, A.J., M.M. Martinic & N. Harris. 2002. The functions of mucosal T cells in containing the indigenous commensal flora of the intestine. *Cell. Mol. Life Sci.* **59:** 2088–2096.

64. Pabst, O., H. Herbrand, M. Friedrichsen, *et al.* 2006. Adaptation of solitary intestinal lymphoid tissue in response to microbiota and chemokine receptor CCR7 signaling. *J. Immunol.* **177:** 6824–6832.

65. Ivanov, II, K. Atarashi, N. Manel, *et al.* 2009. Induction of intestinal Th17 cells by segmented filamentous bacteria. *Cell* **139:** 485–498.

66. Oldstone, M.B. 1988. Prevention of type I diabetes in nonobese diabetic mice by virus infection. *Science* **239:** 500–502.

67. Wilberz, S., H.J. Partke, F. Dagnaes-Hansen & L. Herberg. 1991. Persistent MHV (mouse hepatitis virus) infection reduces the incidence of diabetes mellitus in non-obese diabetic mice. *Diabetologia* **34:** 2–5.

68. Martins, T.C. & A.P. Aguas. 1996. Changes in B and T lymphocytes associated with mycobacteria-induced protection of NOD mice from diabetes. *J. Autoimmunity* **9:** 501–507.

69. Satoh, J., S. Shintani, K. Oya, et al. 1988. Treatment with streptococcal preparation (OK-432) suppresses anti-islet autoimmunity and prevents diabetes in BB rats. *Diabetes* **37:** 1188–1194.

70. Sai, P. & A.S. Rivereau. 1996. Prevention of diabetes in the nonobese diabetic mouse by oral immunological treatments. Comparative efficiency of human insulin and two bacterial antigens, lipopolysacharide from *Escherichia coli* and glycoprotein extract from *Klebsiella pneumoniae*. *Diabetes Metab.* **22:** 341–348.

71. Qin, H.Y. & B. Singh. 1997. BCG vaccination prevents insulin-dependent diabetes mellitus (IDDM) in NOD mice after disease acceleration with cyclophosphamide. *J. Autoimmun.* **10:** 271–278.

72. King, C. & N. Sarvetnick. 2011. The incidence of type-1 diabetes in NOD mice is modulated by restricted flora not germ-free conditions. *PLoS One* **6:** e17049–e17052.

73. Alyanakian, M.A., F. Grela, A. Aumeunier, et al. 2006. Transforming growth factor-beta and natural killer T-cells are involved in the protective effect of a bacterial extract on type 1 diabetes. *Diabetes* **55:** 179–185.

74. Fu, S., N. Zhang, A.C. Yopp, et al. 2004. TGF-beta induces Foxp3 + T-regulatory cells from CD4 + CD25—precursors. *Am. J. Transplant.* **4:** 1614–1627.

75. Shi, F.D., M. Flodstrom, B. Balasa, et al. 2001. Germ line deletion of the CD1 locus exacerbates diabetes in the NOD mouse. *Proc. Natl. Acad. Sci. USA* **98:** 6777–6782.

76. Brugman, S., F.A. Klatter, J.T. Visser, et al. 2006. Antibiotic treatment partially protects against type 1 diabetes in the Bio-Breeding diabetes-prone rat. Is the gut flora involved in the development of type 1 diabetes? *Diabetologia* **49:** 2105–2108.

77. Roesch, L.F., G.L. Lorca, G. Casella, et al. 2009. Culture-independent identification of gut bacteria correlated with the onset of diabetes in a rat model. *ISME J.* **3:** 536–548.

78. Pull, S.L., J.M. Doherty, J.C. Mills, et al. 2005. Activated macrophages are an adaptive element of the colonic epithelial progenitor niche necessary for regenerative responses to injury. *Proc. Natl. Acad. Sci. USA* **102:** 99–104.

79. Reikvam, D.H., A. Erofeev, A. Sandvik, et al. 2011. Depletion of murine intestinal microbiota: effects on gut mucosa and epithelial gene expression. *PLoS One* **6:** e17996–e18009.

80. Rakoff-Nahoum, S., J. Paglino, F. Eslami-Varzaneh, et al. 2004. Recognition of commensal microflora by toll-like receptors is required for intestinal homeostasis. *Cell* **118:** 229–241.

81. Campbell, N., X.Y. Yio, L.P. So, et al. 1999. The intestinal epithelial cell: processing and presentation of antigen to the mucosal immune system. *Immunol. Rev.* **172:** 315–324.

82. Jarry, A., C. Bossard, C. Bou-Hanna, et al. 2008. Mucosal IL-10 and TGF-beta play crucial roles in preventing LPS-driven, IFN-gamma-mediated epithelial damage in human colon explants. *J. Clin. Invest.* **118:** 1132–1142.

83. Westendorf, A.M., D. Fleissner, L. Groebe, et al. 2009. CD4+Foxp3+ regulatory T cell expansion induced by antigen-driven interaction with intestinal epithelial cells independent of local dendritic cells. *Gut* **58:** 211–219.

84. Valladares, R., D. Sankar, N. Li, et al. 2010. Lactobacillus johnsonii N6.2 mitigates the development of type 1 diabetes in BB-DP rats. *PLoS One* **5:** e10507–e10516.

85. Neu, J., C.M. Reverte, A.D. Mackey, et al. 2005. Changes in intestinal morphology and permeability in the biobreeding rat before the onset of type 1 diabetes. *J. Pediatr. Gastroenterol. Nutr.* **40:** 589–595.

86. Meddings, J.B., J. Jarand, S.J. Urbanski, et al. 1999. Increased gastrointestinal permeability is an early lesion in the spontaneously diabetic BB rat. *Am. J. Physiol.* **276:** G951–G957.

87. Watts, T., I. Berti, A. Sapone, et al. 2005. Role of the intestinal tight junction modulator zonulin in the pathogenesis of type I diabetes in BB diabetic-prone rats. *Proc. Natl. Acad. Sci. USA* **102:** 2916–2921.

88. Wen, L., R.E. Ley, P.Y. Volchkov, et al. 2008. Innate immunity and intestinal microbiota in the development of Type 1 diabetes. *Nature* **455:** 1109–1113.

89. Campbell, D.J. & M.A. Koch. 2011. Phenotypical and functional specialization of FOXP3 +regulatory T cells. Nature reviews. *Immunology* **11:** 119–130.

90. Dubois, B., G. Joubert, M. Gomez de Aguero, et al. 2009. Sequential role of plasmacytoid dendritic cells and regulatory T cells in oral tolerance. *Gastroenterology* **137:** 1019–1028.

91. Ostman, S., C. Rask, A.E. Wold, et al. 2006. Impaired regulatory T cell function in germ-free mice. *Eur. J. Immunol.* **36:** 2336–2346.

92. Strauch, U.G., F. Obermeier, N. Grunwald, et al. 2005. Influence of intestinal bacteria on induction of regulatory T cells: lessons from a transfer model of colitis. *Gut* **54:** 1546–1552.

93. Round, J.L. & S.K. Mazmanian. 2010. Inducible Foxp3+ regulatory T-cell development by a commensal bacterium of the intestinal microbiota. *Proc. Natl. Acad. Sci. USA* **107:** 12204–12209.

94. Hu, Y., F. Shen, N.K. Crellin & W. Ouyang. 2011. The IL-17 pathway as a major therapeutic target in autoimmune diseases. *Ann. N.Y. Acad. Sci.* **1217:** 60–76.

95. Ivanov, II, L. Frutos Rde, N. Manel, et al. 2008. Specific microbiota direct the differentiation of IL-17-producing T-helper cells in the mucosa of the small intestine. *Cell Host Microbe* **4:** 337–349.

96. Zaph, C., Y. Du, S.A. Saenz, et al. 2008. Commensal-dependent expression of IL-25 regulates the IL-23-IL-17 axis in the intestine. *J. Exp. Med.* **205:** 2191–2198.

97. Gaboriau-Routhiau, V., S. Rakotobe, E. Lecuyer, et al. 2009. The key role of segmented filamentous bacteria in the coordinated maturation of gut helper T cell responses. *Immunity* **31:** 677–689.

98. Lau, K., P. Benitez, A. Ardissone, *et al.* 2011. Inhibition of type 1 diabetes correlated to a Lactobacillus johnsonii N6.2-mediated Th17 bias. *J. Immunol.* **186:** 3538–3546.

99. Vaarala, O. 2011. The gut as a regulator of early inflammation in type 1 diabetes. *Curr. Opin. Endocrinol. Diabetes Obes.* **18:** 241–247.

100. Williams, A.M., C.S. Probert, R. Stepankova, *et al.* 2006. Effects of microflora on the neonatal development of gut mucosal T cells and myeloid cells in the mouse. *Immunology* **119:** 470–478.

101. Hapfelmeier, S., M.A. Lawson, E. Slack, *et al.* 2010. Reversible microbial colonization of germ-free mice reveals the dynamics of IgA immune responses. *Science* **328:** 1705–1709.

102. Hoorfar, J., K. Buschard & F. Dagnaes-Hansen. 1993. Prophylactic nutritional modification of the incidence of diabetes in autoimmune non-obese diabetic (NOD) mice. *Br. J. Nutr.* **69:** 597–607.

103. Funda, D.P., A. Kaas, H. Tlaskalova-Hogenova & K. Buschard. 2008. Gluten-free but also gluten-enriched (gluten+) diet prevent diabetes in NOD mice; the gluten enigma in type 1 diabetes. *Diabetes Metab. Res. Rev.* **24:** 59–63.

104. Schmid, S., K. Koczwara, S. Schwinghammer, *et al.* 2004. Delayed exposure to wheat and barley proteins reduces diabetes incidence in non-obese diabetic mice. *Clin. Immunol.* **111:** 108–118.

105. Locke, N.R., S. Stankovic, D.P. Funda & L.C. Harrison. 2006. TCR gamma delta intraepithelial lymphocytes are required for self-tolerance. *J. Immunol.* **176:** 6553–6559.

106. Scott, F.W., H.E. Cloutier, R. Kleemann, *et al.* 1997. Potential mechanisms by which certain foods promote or inhibit the development of spontaneous diabetes in BB rats: dose, timing, early effect on islet area, and switch in infiltrate from Th1 to Th2 cells. *Diabetes* **46:** 589–598.

107. Maurano, F., G. Mazzarella, D. Luongo, *et al.* 2005. Small intestinal enteropathy in non-obese diabetic mice fed a diet containing wheat. *Diabetologia* **48:** 931–937.

108. Chakir, H., D.E. Lefebvre, H. Wang, *et al.* 2005. Wheat protein-induced proinflammatory T helper 1 bias in mesenteric lymph nodes of young diabetes-prone rats. *Diabetologia* **48:** 1576–1584.

109. Turley, S.J., J.W. Lee, N. Dutton-Swain, *et al.* 2005. Endocrine self and gut non-self intersect in the pancreatic lymph nodes. *Proc. Natl. Acad. Sci. USA* **102:** 17729–17733.

110. Ejsing-Duun, M., J. Josephsen, B. Aasted, *et al.* 2008. Dietary gluten reduces the number of intestinal regulatory T cells in mice. *Scandinavian J. Immunol.* **67:** 553–559.

111. Hansen, A.K., F. Ling, A. Kaas, *et al.* 2006. Diabetes preventive gluten-free diet decreases the number of caecal bacteria in non-obese diabetic mice. *Diabetes Metab. Res. Rev.* **22:** 220–225.

112. Laparra, J.M. & Y. Sanz. 2010. Bifidobacteria inhibit the inflammatory response induced by gliadins in intestinal epithelial cells via modifications of toxic peptide generation during digestion. *J. Cell Biochem.* **109:** 801–807.

113. Oliares, M., M. Laparra & Y. Sanz. 2011. Influence of Bifidobacterium longum CECT 7347 and gliadin peptides on intestinal epithelial cell proteome. *J. Agric. Food Chem.* **59:** 7666–7671.

114. Cinova, J., G. De Palma, R. Stepankova, *et al.* 2011. Role of intestinal bacteria in gliadin-induced changes in intestinal mucosa: study in germ-free rats. *PLoS One* **6:** e16169–e16179.

115. Matsuzaki, T., Y. Nagata, S. Kado, *et al.* 1997. Prevention of onset in an insulin-dependent diabetes mellitus model, NOD mice, by oral feeding of Lactobacillus casei. *APMIS* **105:** 643–649.

116. Chen, Q., Y.C. Kim, A. Laurence, *et al.* 2011. IL-2 controls the stability of Foxp3 expression in TGF-{beta}-induced Foxp3+ T cells in vivo. *J. Immunol.* **186:** 6329–6337.

117. Calcinaro, F., S. Dionisi, M. Marinaro, *et al.* 2005. Oral probiotic administration induces interleukin-10 production and prevents spontaneous autoimmune diabetes in the non-obese diabetic mouse. *Diabetologia* **48:** 1565–1575.

118. Johansson, M.L., G. Molin, B. Jeppsson, *et al.* 1993. Administration of different Lactobacillus strains in fermented oatmeal soup: in vivo colonization of human intestinal mucosa and effect on the indigenous flora. *Appl. Environ. Microbiol.* **59:** 15–20.

119. Mack, D.R., S. Michail, S. Wei, *et al.* 1999. Probiotics inhibit enteropathogenic *E. coli* adherence in vitro by inducing intestinal mucin gene expression. *Am. J. Physiol.* **276:** G941–G950.

120. Giongo, A., K.A. Gano, D.B. Crabb, *et al.* 2010. Toward defining the autoimmune microbiome for type 1 diabetes. *ISME J.* **5:** 82–91.

121. TEDDY Study Group. 2008. The Environmental Determinants of Diabetes in the Young (TEDDY) Study. *Ann. N.Y. Acad. Sci.* **1150:** 1–13.

122. Carratu, R., M. Secondulfo, L. de Magistris, *et al.* 1999. Altered intestinal permeability to mannitol in diabetes mellitus type I. *J. Pediatr. Gastroenterol. Nutr.* **28:** 264–269.

123. Kuitunen, M., T. Saukkonen, J. Ilonen, *et al.* 2002. Intestinal permeability to mannitol and lactulose in children with type 1 diabetes with the HLA-DQB1∗02 allele. *Autoimmunity* **35:** 365–368.

124. Sapone, A., L. de Magistris, M. Pietzak, *et al.* 2006. Zonulin upregulation is associated with increased gut permeability in subjects with type 1 diabetes and their relatives. *Diabetes* **55:** 1443–1449.

125. Bosi, E., L. Molteni, M.G. Radaelli, *et al.* 2006. Increased intestinal permeability precedes clinical onset of type 1 diabetes. *Diabetologia* **49:** 2824–2827.

126. Brown, C.T., A.G. Davis-Richardson, A. Giongo, *et al.* 2011. Gut microbiome metagenomics analysis suggests a functional model for the development of autoimmunity for type 1 diabetes. *PLoS One* **6:** e25792–e25801.

127. Westerholm-Ormio, M., O. Vaarala, P. Pihkala, *et al.* 2003. Immunologic activity in the small intestinal mucosa of pediatric patients with type 1 diabetes. *Diabetes* **52:** 2287–2295.

128. Secondulfo, M., D. Iafusco, R. Carratu, *et al.* 2004. Ultrastructural mucosal alterations and increased intestinal

permeability in non-celiac, type I diabetic patients. *Digest. Liver Dis.* **36:** 35–45.

129. Auricchio, R., F. Paparo, M. Maglio, *et al.* 2004. In vitro-deranged intestinal immune response to gliadin in type 1 diabetes. *Diabetes* **53:** 1680–1683.

130. Tiittanen, M., M. Westerholm-Ormio, M. Verkasalo, *et al.* 2008. Infiltration of forkhead box P3-expressing cells in small intestinal mucosa in coeliac disease but not in type 1 diabetes. *Clin. Exp. Immunol.* **152:** 498–507.

131. Cinova, J., L. Palova-Jelinkova, L.E. Smythies, *et al.* 2007. Gliadin peptides activate blood monocytes from patients with celiac disease. *J. Clin. Immunol.* **27:** 201–209.

132. Ziegler, A.G., S. Schmid, D. Huber, *et al.* 2003. Early infant feeding and risk of developing type 1 diabetes-associated autoantibodies. *JAMA* **290:** 1721–1728.

133. Smyth, D.J., V. Plagnol, N.M. Walker, *et al.* 2008. Shared and distinct genetic variants in type 1 diabetes and celiac disease. *N. Engl. J. Med.* **359:** 2767–2777.

134. Karczewski, J., F.J. Troost, I. Konings, *et al.* 2010. Regulation of human epithelial tight junction proteins by Lactobacillus plantarum in vivo and protective effects on the epithelial barrier. *Am. J. Physiol. Gastrointest. Liver Physiol.* **298:** G851–G859.

135. Ljungberg, M., R. Korpela, J. Ilonen, *et al.* 2006. Probiotics for the prevention of beta cell autoimmunity in children at genetic risk of type 1 diabetes—the PRODIA study. *Ann. N.Y. Acad. Sci.* **1079:** 360–364.

Ann. N.Y. Acad. Sci. ISSN 0077-8923

ANNALS OF THE NEW YORK ACADEMY OF SCIENCES

Issue: *The Year in Diabetes and Obesity*

Making progress: preserving beta cells in type 1 diabetes

Mary Pat Gallagher,[1] Robin S. Goland,[1] and Carla J. Greenbaum[2]

[1]Naomi Berrie Diabetes Center, Columbia University, College of Physicians and Surgeons, New York, New York. [2]Diabetes Program, Benaroya Research Institute, Seattle, Washington

Address for correspondence: Carla J. Greenbaum, M.D., Benaroya Research Institute, 1201 9th Ave, Seattle, WA 98101. cjgreen@benaroyaresearch.org

The clinical care of patients with type 1 diabetes (T1D) has greatly improved over the past few decades; however, it remains impossible to completely normalize blood sugar utilizing currently available tools. Research is underway with a goal to improve the care and, ultimately, to cure T1D by preserving beta cells. This review will outline the progress that has been made in trials aimed at preserving insulin secretion in T1D by modifying the immune assault on the pancreatic beta cell. Although not yet ready for clinical use, successful trials have been conducted in new-onset T1D that demonstrated utility of three experimental agents with disparate modes of action (anti-T cell, anti-B cell, and costimulation blockade) to preserve insulin secretion. In contrast, prevention studies have so far failed to produce positive results but have shown that such studies are feasible and have identified new promising agents for study.

Keywords: type 1 diabetes; prevention; autoimmune; beta cell

Introduction

Immune-mediated type 1 diabetes (T1D) affects an estimated 900,000 people worldwide, and its frequency is increasing throughout the developed world.[1] Several studies point to a particular increase in children under the age of five years, and others demonstrate an increase among those without "high-risk" human leukocyte antigen (HLA) genotypes, suggesting a changing phenotype of disease.[2] Despite significant advances in diabetes management over the past two decades, it is not yet possible to completely normalize glucose levels, and episodes of hypoglycemia and hyperglycemia are essentially unavoidable. Although decreasing in frequency with recent improvements in clinical care, the risks for severe hypoglycemia and microvascular and macrovascular complications of diabetes have not been abolished. The successful clinical management of T1D requires daily uncomfortable, time-consuming, expensive, and often frustrating self-monitoring and self-management skills. Management is burdensome at best and often impossible to accomplish for patients and families, particularly those with psychosocial or financial barriers to care. Clearly, new approaches are needed.

The description of islet cell autoantibodies and the presence of insulitis in pancreata from people with T1D led to the consensus that T1D was caused by an immune-mediated assault on the pancreatic beta cells, thus paving the way for clinical trials to determine if the disease course could be altered by modulation of the immune system, preserving beta cell function before or after clinical disease onset. The clinical course of T1D, from genetic risk and development of autoantibodies through years after diagnosis, as illustrated in Figure 1, was conceptualized in print as early as 1984. The initial marker of immune system activation against the islet is the presence of autoantibodies. Subsequently, impaired beta cell function can be identified in the earliest stages via intravenous glucose tolerance tests that demonstrate diminishing insulin responses. More significant impairment can later be identified via an oral glucose tolerance test and subsequently to an oral "mixed meal" stimulus (e.g., "mixed meal" of fat, carbohydrate, and protein). Although earlier models of the natural history of T1D depicted complete absence of C-peptide soon after diagnosis and recent data suggest that detectable C-peptide may be present for many years, there is not yet a full understanding of the clinical relevance of these

doi: 10.1111/j.1749-6632.2011.06321.x

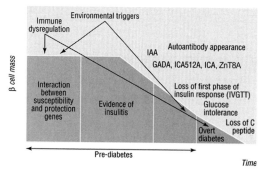

Figure 1. Models of pathogenesis and natural history of type 1 diabetes. Schematic representation of gradual decline in beta cell function over time in T1D. Printed with permission from Ref. 88.

observations.[3] In individuals progressing to T1D, abnormal postprandial glucose values are the first glycemic abnormality detected, and essentially all such individuals eventually cross the threshold to the diagnosis of clinical disease. In the early stages of evolving T1D, postprandial glucose values >200 mg/dL are often present at a time when fasting glucose and HbA1c values are normal. Symptoms of hyperglycemia are usually absent until fasting hyperglycemia occurs. Thus, one could consider that T1D is present in antibody-positive individuals with abnormal glucose tolerance, in essence shifting the line for "diagnosis" earlier in the disease course. Although not illustrated in Figure 1, it is of interest that the underlying cause of the honeymoon period, characterized by a transient diminished requirement for exogenous insulin postdiagnosis, is not known. It may be the result of exogenous insulin relieving the effect of "glucose toxicity" on beta cell function and/or insulin action. Whatever the mechanism, this is a transient event in the course of the disease but does support the concept that beta cell dysfunction rather than death is a component of the early disease process.

Preserving beta cell mass and/or function before diagnosis would provide a clear clinical benefit in preventing hyperglycemia and clinical disease. Less well known, but important to understand, is the clinical benefit of preserving beta cells after diagnosis. As shown in the Diabetes Control and Complications Trial (DCCT), subjects in the intensively treated group who had endogenous insulin secretion, characterized by stimulated C-peptide values ≥0.2 pmol/mL, had a 50% reduction in retinopathy progression and 62% less severe hypoglycemia

than intensively treated subjects without residual insulin secretion (Fig. 2).[4] These data echo results from studies in islet cells transplantation in which even a limited amount of endogenous secretion from transplanted cells results in a significant reduction in hypoglycemia even if insulin independence is not achieved.[5] Because hypoglycemia is the limiting problem in achieving strict glucose control and reduction in vascular complications, preservation of beta cells is clinically important to those with diabetes as well as to those at risk for disease.

The first generation of T1D studies, those performed before the year 2001, demonstrated that intervention may alter the disease course, highlighted the potential risks involved, and fostered new considerations in study design. The next generation of studies, largely conducted since 2001, built upon this framework and was also able to use increasingly sophisticated information about the immune system to test new therapies.

In this review, we will highlight the new information gained from clinical trials in T1D performed in the past decade. We will critically examine these results in both a scientific and clinical context, focusing on questions to address for the next generation of studies aimed at prevention or reversal of T1D.

First-generation T1D studies

More than 30 studies testing the concepts of immunosuppression, immunostimulation, beta cell rest, and antigen therapy, as well as other mechanisms on preservation of insulin production in T1D, were conducted and reported from the 1980s to 2001 (reviewed in 2002).[6] Most were pilot studies using varying outcome measures, making interpretation somewhat difficult. Nonetheless, lessons from these studies inform the current generation of trials. For example, cyclosporine was the immunosuppressive agent most extensively studied in the 1980s and 1990s. Several trials, which included a total of approximately 500 patients, demonstrated an increase in "clinical remissions" (most often defined as fasting glucose <140 mg/dL, postprandial glucose <200 mg/dL, and HbA1c <7.5% without exogenous insulin) but also an unacceptable incidence of drug-induced nephrotoxicity.[7–16] Although not formally tested in these studies, there were no apparent long-lasting effects of therapy after treatment was discontinued. Several other non-specific immunosuppressant drugs, such as anti-thymocyte

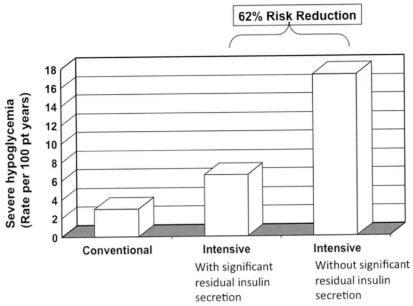

Figure 2. Subjects receiving intensive insulin therapy in the DCCT had fewer micro- and macrovascular complications compared to those receiving conventional therapy. Within the intensively treated group, subjects with residual insulin secretion (C-peptide > 0.2 pmol/mL) had a marked reduction in severe hypoglycemia. Adapted with permission from Ref. 4.

globulin, prednisone, and azathioprine, were also evaluated with mixed results.[17–19] In adequately powered, randomized trials, no effect was seen of immunostimulation (BCG),[20] antigen therapy,[21,22] or nicotinamide[23] in subjects with recently diagnosed T1D. In contrast, aggressive glucose control at the time of diagnosis did seem to preserve beta cell function one year after of diagnosis. Shah *et al.* randomized subjects immediately after T1D diagnosis to usual care or a bedside closed-loop glucose-controlled insulin infusion system. After one year, stimulated C-peptide was significantly higher in the treatment group.[24] The results of this trial were consistent with the observations made in the DCCT. In the DCCT, the group of T1D subjects who received more intensive insulin therapy early in the course of the disease had higher stimulated C-peptide levels than subjects who received less intense metabolic control.[4] A trial to further assess whether intensive diabetes control in the immediate post-diagnosis period can preserve beta cell function is currently recruiting patients through the NIH Type 1 Diabetes TrialNet (TrialNet; an NIH-sponsored clinical trial network).[25] Although many improvements have been made since 1998 with respect to intensive metabolic control of T1D, the mechanisms by

which controlling hyperglycemia leads to better beta cell function are not well understood.

Great strides have been made over the last few decades in identifying individuals at risk for T1D, thus enabling trials to prevent autoimmunity (primary prevention) or to prevent hyperglycemia in subjects in whom beta cell destruction is already underway (secondary prevention). Moreover, although fully powered prevention studies require large screening efforts and a long period of follow-up, the accuracy of prediction estimates and the ability to conduct such studies has been clearly demonstrated in multiple settings (Table 1). Three such fully powered trials were completed by 2001. The European Nicotinamide Diabetes Intervention Trial (ENDIT) tested whether oral nicotinamide would prevent or delay disease onset in antibody-positive individuals. Although the treatment was found to be safe, no effect on disease onset was found (approximately 30% after five years in both groups).[26] The North American Diabetes Prevention Trial-Type 1 (DPT-1) evaluated the effect of both parenteral and oral insulin administration in relatives of T1D patients who were at risk for T1D. Parenteral insulin (IV insulin for four continuous days annually and ultralente insulin 0.25 u/kg administered BID) was

Table 1. Summary of fully powered T1D prevention trials to date

Study	European Nicotinamide Diabetes Intervention Trial (ENDIT)	Diabetes Prevention Trial-1 (DPT-1)	Diabetes Prevention Trial-1 (DPT-1)	T1D Prediction and Prevention Study (DIPP)
Study centers	Europe, N. America	North America	North America	Finland
Primary or secondary	Secondary; antibody-positive relatives	Secondary; antibody-positive relatives with low insulin secretion or abnormal glucose tolerance	Secondary; antibody-positive relatives	Secondary; antibody-positive children
Experimental therapy	Nicotinamide	Parenteral insulin	Oral insulin	Nasal insulin
Dates	1990–1998	1994–2000	1994–2002	1994–2008
Number screened	30,000	84,228	103,391	116,720
Number eligible	1,004	372	388	328
Number enrolled	552	339	372	224
Primary endpoint	Diagnosis of diabetes	Diagnosis of diabetes	Diagnosis of diabetes	Diagnosis of diabetes
Outcome	~30% developed T1D; no effect of therapy	~65% developed T1D; no effect of therapy	~35% developed T1D; overall no effect of therapy. *Post hoc* analysis suggests effect in subgroup with high IAA	~60% developed T1D; no effect of therapy

ineffective in delaying or preventing disease in high-risk subjects; 15% of subjects in both the experimental and control groups developed T1D annually.[27] In a separate arm of the DPT-1 study, oral insulin was administered (7.5 mg/day) daily in relatives at intermediate risk for diabetes development. Although the overall results of the oral insulin intervention study were negative (~7% progressed to diabetes annually in both groups), a post-hoc analysis revealed that subjects with very high titers of antibody to insulin demonstrated up to a four-year delay in diabetes onset in those given oral insulin as compared to placebo (Fig. 3).[28] The hypothesis that oral insulin could delay or prevent the onset of disease in individuals with high levels of insulin autoantibodies and moderate risk of T1D is currently being evaluated in a randomized, placebo-controlled trial

through TrialNet.[29] Lessons learned from the first generation of trials include the following:

1. Adverse effects of immunosuppressant therapies may limit their chronic use in T1D (e.g., nephrotoxicity for cyclosporine).
2. Immunosuppressant therapies do not seem to have lasting effects on insulin secretion in T1D after treatment is discontinued.
3. To effectively study and compare the effects of experimental agents on preservation of insulin secretion in new-onset T1D, standardized study design and outcome measures are important.
4. Large numbers of subjects must be screened to identify those at increased T1D risk for potential participation in T1D prevention studies. Although feasible and critically important,

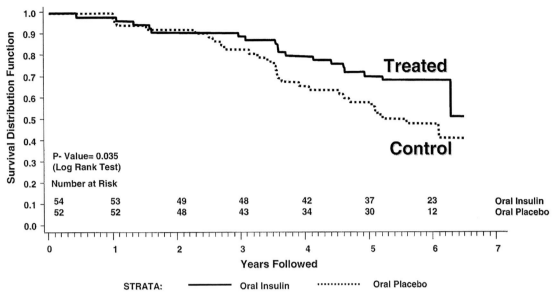

Figure 3. Data from *post hoc* analysis of the DPT-1 Oral Insulin Trial demonstrating the delay in diabetes among those treated with oral insulin who had high levels of insulin autoantibodies. The number of subjects at risk in each group at each year of follow-up is enumerated at the bottom of the figure. The log-rank test was used for comparison between the groups, with the P-values as indicated. Printed with permission from Ref. 28.

these prevention studies are logistically difficult, labor-intensive, and long in duration. Because of these limitations, only very few studies can be conducted at any one time and it is perhaps not surprising that the first efforts were not successful.

Recent trials

Building on previous work, the next generation of trials aimed to exploit new information about the immune response and in most cases, to standardize key aspects of study design. Standardized variables now shared by many new-onset T1D trials include the primary outcome measure of C-peptide after mixed meal stimulation test as the marker for beta cell function; and common subject characteristics (time after diagnosis, subject age, and level of glucose control). Adequately powered, randomized trials have demonstrated three therapies with distinct mechanisms of action (anti-T cell, anti-B cell, and costimulation blockade) that can preserve beta cell function in recently diagnosed subjects for a period of months. Other well-designed studies using other agents have shown no effect on the T1D disease process. However, a key point is that negative trials are nonetheless successful trials when they enable us

to answer the question posed. This past decade has seen results from multiple successful trials teaching us about the pathophysiology of T1D and suggesting new avenues to pursue. To that end, selected trials that illustrate important points have been chosen for discussion below.

Anti-CD3

CD3 is a protein complex located on the surface of T cells and is integral to the initiation of T cell activation. The toxicity of the first anti-human CD3 monoclonal antibody, OKT3, used for the treatment of organ transplant rejection, was reduced by elimination of FcR-binding portion of the molecule in the development of two different humanized antibodies, teplizumab (hOKT31(Ala-Ala)) and otelixizumab (ChAglyCD3). Elegant preclinical studies suggested several mechanisms by which FcR-nonbinding CD3-specific antibodies may produce a state of "tolerance" to self. These include "antigenic modulation," partial phosphorylation of the T cell receptor complex resulting in decreased production of IL-2 and inactivation of T helper 1 (Th1) cells, and promotion of T regulatory cells.[30–32]

In the first trial with hOKT3(Ala-Ala), 24 subjects with new-onset T1D were randomized to receive 14 days of drug or were assigned to a control group.[33] In this open-label study, 9 of the 12 subjects in the treatment group had stable insulin secretion at one year as compared to 2 of 12 controls. Subsequently, additional data from this open-label study including a total of 42 subjects (21 drug-treated) were reported.[34] Stimulated C-peptide response (compared to baseline) was greater one year after diagnosis in subjects treated with drug compared to control subjects (97 ± 9.6% vs. 53 ± 7.6% of response at study entry, $P < 0.01$; Fig. 4A). HbA1c and insulin requirements were both lower in the treatment group as well. During the second year, C-peptide levels declined at a similar rate in treatment and observation groups. Nonetheless, the marked effect in the first year resulted in a significantly greater percentage of drug-treated individuals with stimulated C-peptide of 0.2 pmol/mL at 24 months compared to controls (67% vs. 26%; $P = 0.01$); recall that C-peptide of 0.2 pmol/mL was identified as a clinically important cutoff in the DCCT study (Fig. 2).[4]

Side effects of drug treatment included transient lymphopenia that occurred initially in all subjects. In most subjects, lymphocyte counts returned to >80% of baseline levels within several weeks. In rare cases, more prolonged lymphopenia has been observed.[35] Despite these transient laboratory abnormalities, no serious infections were reported, making the clinical importance of these changes uncertain. Additional adverse events included symptoms associated with cytokine release such as fever, headache, and arthralgias. Rash was present in almost all subjects and a transient grade 3 cytopenia resulted in one subject stopping therapy.

The marked effect of anti-CD3 treatment on beta cell function was also seen in a placebo-controlled trial with the other therapeutic, otelixizumab. In this study, 80 subjects with new-onset T1D, ages 12–39, received six days of active drug or placebo.[36] Insulin secretion (assessed by C-peptide release during a glucose clamp and after glucagon stimulation) was significantly improved in the drug-treated group at 6, 12, and 18 months as measured by change in C-peptide from baseline and an equivalent HbA1c was observed in the context of less insulin dosing. Side effects of drug treatment included transient reactivation of Epstein Barr virus associated with a "mono-like" illness as well as transient infusion reactions, rash, and lymphopenia. *Post hoc* analysis suggested that there was a more pronounced effect in subjects with higher C-peptide levels at study en-

try. Long-term follow-up demonstrated continued effects on insulin dose up to four years after treatment with no long-term adverse effects reported.[37]

These positive findings in the context of manageable adverse events led to several subsequent studies of anti-CD3 drugs aimed to move toward clinical use. Two Phase 3 trials were initiated in new-onset T1D: the Protégé Study of teplizumab (Macrogenics, Inc.) and the DEFEND Study of otelixizumab (ToleRx, Inc). In addition, the AbATE study, sponsored by the NIH Immune Tolerance Network (ITN; an NIH sponsored clinical trial group), was launched to test whether repeat dosing of teplizumab would prolong its effect on insulin secretion, and the Delay study tested whether treating subjects with teplizumab further out from diagnosis would be effective. Finally, the Anti-CD3 Prevention Study was initiated by TrialNet to study whether teplizumab could delay onset of T1D in high-risk individuals with dysglycemia.

The Protégé Study involved more than 100 sites worldwide and reported no effect of teplizumab as measured by the study's primary endpoint of a HbA1c level of <6.5% with an insulin dose of <0.5 units/kg/day.[38] This result was perhaps not surprising considering the diversity of subjects, health care systems, and clinicians encompassed in the study. In addition, C-peptide was not different between treatment and placebo groups overall. Post-hoc analysis suggested an effect of C-peptide secretion in selected subgroups of subjects (younger children and those treated in the United States), but these observations can only be considered as hypothesis generating, not as true evidence of efficacy in these subgroups. The DEFEND-1 study results revealed that there was no difference in C-peptide between subjects treated with otelixizumab or placebo at one year.[39] It is likely that this lack of effect was related to the fact that the dose of otelixizumab used in this trial was markedly lower than in the original study. The investigators chose the lower dose with the aim of reducing short-term side effects.

The AbATE study was an open label trial of 83 subjects randomized within three months of diagnosis to 14 days of IV drug administration or observation. As in previous studies, the drug-treated subjects had significantly greater C-peptide production in response to a mixed meal at one and two years compared to those in the observation group. However, it is unclear whether the second dose of drug

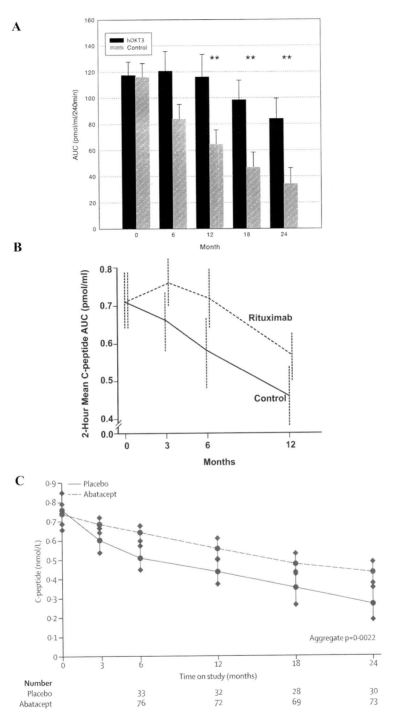

Figure 4. (A) C-peptide responses to a MMTT in control and h-OKT3–treated subjects. Total C-peptide during a 4 h MMTT over 24 months is shown. Black, h-OKT3–treated; gray, control. $**P < 0.02$. Printed with permission from Ref. 34. (B) C-peptide responses to a MMTT in control and anti-CD20–treated subjects. Mean C-peptide AUC during first 2 h of 4 h MMTT over 12 months are shown. Printed with permission from Ref. 32. (C) C-peptide responses to a MMTT in control and abatacept-treated subjects. Mean stimulated C-peptide 2 h AUC during first 2 h of 4 h MMTT over 24 months are shown. Printed with permission from Ref. 44.

contributed to the preservation of C-peptide seen at two years. It is worthwhile to note that approximately one-third of subjects were unable to complete their full dose due to pre-specified stopping rules or adverse events.[40]

Together these results highlight a current conundrum in the clinical development of anti-CD3 therapies to preserve beta cells; too low a dose may be ineffective, yet a higher dose may lead to short-term safety concerns in a significant number of subjects. Carefully administered, however, a clinical role of anti-CD3 remains possible, particularly if a population of individuals with diabetes can be identified who have a prolonged clinical response or if the anti-CD3 (teplizumab) TrialNet Prevention Study is able to demonstrate a clinically significant delay in disease onset (further discussed in section on ongoing trials below).

Anti-CD20

Initially considered an unlikely candidate for immunotherapy in a T cell–mediated disease such as T1D, the B cell–depleting anti-CD20 monoclonal antibody, rituximab, was evaluated in subjects with recently diagnosed T1D largely on the basis of its effectiveness in other autoimmune disease (the FDA has approved rituximab for use in rheumatoid arthritis and it is commonly used off-label for multiple sclerosis, systemic lupus erythematosus, and autoimmune hemolytic anemia).[41] Rituximab is the second agent that has shown positive results in preserving insulin secretion in new-onset T1D.

In a randomized, double blind, Phase 2 study led by the late Mark Pescovitz, M.D., and sponsored by TrialNet, 87 patients with recently diagnosed T1D between 8 and 40 years of age were randomized to receive four weekly infusions of rituximab or placebo. At one year, the stimulated C-peptide was 20% higher in the rituximab group than in the placebo group (or 0.56 pmol/mL vs. 0.47 pmol/mL; Fig. 4B). The rituximab group also had significantly lower levels of HbA1c and required less insulin to achieve better glycemic control.[42] Infusion reactions to the first dose of rituximab were common, likely due to the omission of glucocorticoid routinely used as a pre-treatment when rituximab is given in other autoimmune diseases. Nonetheless, infusion reactions were generally mild and rarely prevented further rituximab dosing. Indeed, after the first dose, there was no difference in "reactions" between placebo-

and rituximab-treated subjects—thus highlighting the importance of placebo-controlled trials. As reported in other rituximab studies, B cells reached a nadir at about six months after therapy, IgG levels were unaffected, and IgM levels remained lower in treated subjects at one year. No increase in infection or neutropenia was noted in the rituximab treatment group. As with anti-CD3 therapy, however, the drug effect was most apparent early, with the slope of C-peptide declining in parallel with the placebo-treated patients after six months. Importantly, rituximab is in widespread clinical use for other indications; therefore, much is known about adverse effects. Thus it is reasonable to test whether repeated rituximab dosing, as is used in other autoimmune disease, would prolong C-peptide preservation in those with disease, or whether this therapy would delay disease onset in at-risk subjects.

CTLA-4

Cytotoxic T lymphocyte antigen 4 (CTLA-4) is a homologue of CD28, a high-affinity receptor that down-regulates T cells. Abatacept, a CTLA-4-immunoglobulin fusion protein that modulates the costimulation of immature T cells and prevents full T lymphocyte activation,[43] was also recently found to be effective in preserving insulin secretion in new-onset T1D.

The effect of abatacept in recent-onset T1D was evaluated in a multicenter, double-blinded, randomized controlled trial sponsored by TrialNet.[44] The placebo-controlled study recruited 112 subjects with recently diagnosed T1D, ages 6 to 36. The stimulated C-peptide was 59% higher at two years in the abatacept treatment group compared to placebo (Fig. 4C). Hemoglobin A1c was lower in the treatment group but insulin use was not different. Adverse events were minimal and there was no increase in infections or neutropenia. Strikingly, however, as in the anti-CD3 and anti-CD20 studies, the major drug effect was seen early despite continued administration of drug. After six to nine months, the rate of C-peptide fall in the treatment group was parallel to the decline in the placebo group. As in the AbATE trial, this result was unexpected because there was continued infusion of abatacept throughout the two-year study period. This result hints that perhaps a shorter course of drug would have similar benefits. Testing abatacept in T1D prevention is being considered to determine whether treatment during an earlier stage of the disease process can change the duration of therapeutic effect.

Other studies

The DIPP study aimed at secondary prevention, delaying or preventing antibody-positive children from developing clinical diabetes. After screening more than 100,000 infants and children for high-risk HLA types in Finland, 264 individuals with two or more autoantibodies were randomly assigned to 1 u/kg of nasal insulin per day. Presentation of antigen (insulin) to the nasal mucosa was thought to have potential to induce a toleragenic response.[45] No safety concerns were identified and compliance was high; however, there was no effect of this therapy on development of clinical disease, which occurred at a rate of about 15% per year in both groups.[46] In contrast to testing the immune effect of insulin as an antigen, another group evaluated the effect of twice daily subcutaneous regular insulin titrated to avoid postprandial hyperglycemia in a small study of ICA-positive high-risk relatives of T1D patients and also found no effect.[47] Following up epidemiologic data suggesting an impact of gluten-containing foods on the development of diabetes,[48] 150 infants who had first-degree relatives with T1D and who also had high-risk HLA genes were randomized to initial gluten exposure at 6 months or 12 months in the BABYDIET study, conducted in Germany. This primary dietary prevention trial had no effect on appearance of islet antibodies, with about 12% of children in both groups developing antibodies over three years.[49]

Two other primary prevention studies also involved nutritional interventions but were designed as pilot studies. The Finnish Trial to Reduce Diabetes in the Genetically at Risk (Finnish TRIGR Trial) was undertaken to test the hypothesis that protein in cow's milk contributes to the development of islet autoimmunity and T1D. A total of 230 infants with high-risk HLA genes were randomly assigned to standard baby formula (with cow's milk proteins) or hydrolyzed protein formula as a supplement to breast feeding and followed for the development of islet antibodies and T1D. The pilot study results suggested that there may be an effect, but the small numbers involved and imbalance in follow-up lessen the strength of the observations reported.[50] Importantly, however, the fully powered TRIGR Study, testing this hypothesis, has completed

recruitment and results should be available to answer this question more definitively in a few years.[51] In the Nutritional Intervention to Prevent (NIP) Diabetes Trial, sponsored by TrialNet, infants with a high genetic risk for T1D and pregnant women carrying a fetus with high genetic risk for T1D were randomized to receive docosahexaenoic acid (DHA) or placebo to see if supplementation in infancy or prenatally might prevent or delay the autoimmunity leading to T1D. As a pilot trial, this study was not powered to determine whether the therapy had an effect on autoimmunity; however, preliminary reports from this study suggest a reduction in inflammatory cytokine levels in infants receiving the DHA, providing a rationale for this approach in future large-scale primary prevention trials.[52]

Additional studies have yielded negative results in new-onset T1D. The 65-kD isoform of glutamic acid decarboxylase (GAD) is a major autoantigen in T1D. Initial human studies suggested that treatment with GAD might provide a very low-risk approach to help preserve beta cell function.[53,54] However, the TrialNet GAD study found no significant differences in stimulated C-peptide levels, HbA1c, or insulin use at one year in GAD or placebo-treated subjects with new-onset T1D.[55] Similarly, a Phase 3 study of GAD in Europe failed to meet its primary endpoint of preserving insulin secretion.[56] Although disappointing, it is premature to abandon antigen therapy as an approach to alter beta cell destruction. It is possible that using different doses of antigen, different adjuvants, different routes of administration, using peptide fragments instead of whole protein, or using antigens other than GAD would be more effective. The additional data from studies examining the effects of GAD administration on immune markers and other biomarkers may provide some answers. Such data may also support testing GAD in conjunction with other therapies or earlier in the disease process (before clinical onset), particularly because of the good safety record to date even in subjects as young as age three years.

In addition to anti-T cell or anti-B cell therapy, anticytokine therapy is another approach to altering the immune response. Widely used in rheumatoid arthritis, etanercept is a tumor necrosis factor-alpha (TNF-α) antagonist tested in a pilot study of 18 subjects with T1D (ages 7–18 years) in a placebo-controlled study. At week 24, C-peptide had increased by 39% in the etanercept group and had decreased by 20% in the placebo group. HbA1c and insulin dose were also both lower in the etanercept group compared with the placebo group.[57] Although the treatment was well tolerated in this study, the FDA recently issued a warning regarding the use of this drug due to risk of tuberculosis and other infections, thus any potential future trials of etanercept in T1D will need careful patient selection and monitoring.

Interleukin 2 (IL-2; proleukin) is a proinflammatory cytokine used to stimulate the immune response in HIV and cancer. By combining this drug, which augments both T effector and T regulatory cells, with rapamycin (sirolimus) to block the proliferation and survival of T effector cells, beta cell destruction might be halted by shifting the balance to T regulatory cells.[58] Although effective in mouse models, results recently presented from a Phase 1 trial of IL2 and rapamycin in T1D, sponsored by the NIH Immune Tolerance Network, were perplexing.[59] Combining one month of therapy with IL-2 and sirolimus resulted in a marked increase in T regulatory cells. Further, defects in T cell signaling previously described in individuals with T1D were improved. However, there was an unexpected drop in C-peptide at three months. This was transient, as C-peptide subsequently increased in almost all subjects. Although the mechanism of the untoward transient effect on beta cell function is not clear, preliminary data show that both an increase in eosinophils and NK cells occurred.[60,61] These data highlight the difficulties in extrapolating from mouse to human and emphasizes the caution needed in evaluation of novel approaches.

The use of a bone marrow reconstitution as a "reset" for the immune system has been considered for autoimmune diseases. However, the risk of morbidity (secondary malignancy, opportunistic infection, and metabolic syndrome) and potential for mortality with even the safest conditioning regimens for autologous hematopoietic stem cell transplant (AHSCT) have limited the use of this therapy. As discussed in a thoughtful review article, expert clinicians and investigators generally agree that at this time, the study of AHSCT in autoimmune disease should be reserved for patients with severe, debilitating disease that is refractory to standard therapies and for whom there is a poor prognosis.[62] It is therefore surprising that a group of investigators nevertheless tested this approach in subjects with

T1D and reported that 20/23 patients became insulin free for variable periods of time.[63,64] This was a small uncontrolled study and the results reported excluded data from some patients. The investigators reported an overall positive effect on C-peptide response at 36 months. Though there were no deaths in this small series, significant toxicities were seen, including severe respiratory disease, hypogonadism, and oligospermia. Although not minimizing the difficulties of living with T1D, given the significant morbidity reported and the fact there is no evidence that AHSCT therapy consistently results in a permanent cure of any autoimmune disease, it is our opinion that such high-risk therapy should not be pursued in the new-onset T1D population at this time.

Ongoing T1D trials: prevention

Individuals at risk for diabetes can now be clearly identified and enrolled in studies according to their degree of risk.

New information gathered from analysis of the DPT-1 has now identified a group of individuals at extremely high risk of T1D. As illustrated in Figure 5, autoantibody-positive relatives of patients with T1D, who have abnormal glucose tolerance, have a greater than 75% risk of diabetes.[65] The identification of this subgroup is extremely important. First, because the rate of progression in this group is so high, a trial to delay or prevent the onset of disease can be carried out with smaller numbers of subjects

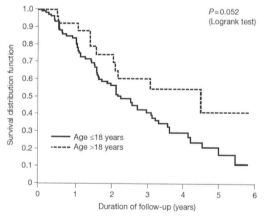

Figure 5. Marked risk of progression to diabetes in antibody-positive relatives of T1D patients with indeterminate or impaired glucose tolerance whether above or below age 18. Printed with permission from Ref. 65.

and over a shorter period of time. Second, a therapy that would delay the onset of clinical disease by even a few years would be clinically important. This group is now being enrolled in a TrialNet study using teplizumab in a single 14-day course of drug with the aim of delaying or preventing diabetes onset.[66]

First-degree relatives with two antibodies and normal glucose tolerance have a five-year risk of developing T1D of 30–50%. Two prevention studies in this population are ongoing. The first is the INIT II study in Australia, in which intranasal insulin is delivered in an attempt to induce immune tolerance, as discussed above. Although the Finnish DIPP trial failed to demonstrate a benefit of intranasal insulin in young antibody-positive children, the INIT II study is evaluating different dosing regimens (40 IU and 440 IU IN daily for seven days then weekly for 12 months) and includes older subjects (ages 4–30 years). In subjects with latent autoimmune diabetes in adults (LADA), nasal insulin was associated with a decreased T cell response to insulin, supporting that there may be some immunologic effect of intranasal insulin that warrants further investigation.[67]

The second ongoing trial for T1D relatives with normal glucose tolerance and positive antibodies is the TrialNet study to determine if insulin delivered orally will delay or prevent the onset of T1D. As discussed above, this is the trial to address the *post hoc* observation seen in the original oral insulin trial conducted by the Diabetes Prevention Trial (DPT-1). This study population's five-year estimated risk of diabetes is approximately 35% at the time of study entry. Recruitment is ongoing for this study.

Newborn infants with a first-degree relative with T1D and an at-risk HLA type are estimated to have a 10-year risk of developing T1D of $\geq 7.6\%$.[50] As discussed above, the fully powered TRIGR study, testing whether casein hydrolysate formula, rather than cow's milk–based formula, can prevent autoantibodies and diabetes in this group of children with high genetic risk has completed recruitment and results are anticipated within the next several years.[51]

Ongoing T1D trials: intervention

Several studies are underway that focus on the concept that "inflammation" plays a large role in beta cell dysfunction (Table 2). The IL-1 pathway is known to play a key role in the inflammatory response. Two therapies designed to block this pathway are under investigation. The Anti-Interleukin-1 in Diabetes Action (AIDA) Study (sponsored by the JDRF) is testing Anakinra, a selective antagonist of the IL-1 receptor in 18–35-year-old subjects within 12 weeks of T1D diagnosis.[68] A trial of Canakinumab, a human anti-interleukin-1-beta (anti-IL-1β) monoclonal antibody, sponsored by TrialNet, has fully enrolled the planned 66 subjects (ages 6–45) with new-onset T1D within 100 days of diagnosis.[69] Canakinumab has been evaluated and shown benefit in patients with Rheumatoid Arthritis and Systemic Juvenile Idiopathic Arthritis (SJIA).[70] Results of these trials should be available within a year and will lay important groundwork for consideration of combination therapies.

Another anti-inflammatory approach is the use of Alpha-1 antitrypsin (AAT; Aralast). AAT is a serine proteinase inhibitor found in high concentrations in the serum that decreases cytokine production, complement activation, and immune cell infiltration. The ITN is currently evaluating the safety and efficacy of AAT in patients (ages 8–45) with recently diagnosed T1D.[71]

A randomized, placebo-controlled trial of thymoglobulin soon after diagnosis sponsored by the ITN is currently underway.[72] This study of about 55 subjects has completed enrollment with results expected in the next year. Another phase I/II pilot trial is investigating the safety and efficacy of combination therapy with Thymoglobulin® (ATG) and Neulasta® (GCSF) in a randomized, placebo-controlled trial in subjects with T1D.[73] This combination of agents has shown some effect in the NOD mouse model. The effect of ATG may be partially from its ability to deplete T cells but ATG may also induce an immunoregulatory shift from a Th1 to a Th2 cytokine phenotype. Previous small studies using ATG were stopped due to toxicities;[17,74] differences in drug, dose, and the use of steroids are hoped to ameliorate most of these concerns.

The REPAIR-T1D (Restore Pancreatic Insulin Response in type 1 diabetes) trial is a randomized, controlled, trial evaluating the effect of combination therapy with sitagliptin (a dipeptidyl peptidase-4 inhibitor [DPP-4]) and lansoprazole (a proton pump inhibitor) in subjects with recently diagnosed T1D, ages 11–45 years.[75] Though not yet convincingly demonstrated in humans, several animal studies have suggested that GLP-1 agonists

Table 2. Selected T1D beta cell preservation trials open for recruitment at the time of publication

Experimental agent	Sponsor	Subject ages	Entry criteria	Phase of trial	Website
Intervention trials					
Alefacept (T1DAL Study)	NIH/Immune Tolerance Network	12–35	Within 100 days of diagnosis	II	http://clinicaltrials.gov/ ct2/show/NCT00965458
Aralast (RETAIN Study)	NIH/Immune Tolerance Network	8–35	Within 100 days of diagnosis	II	http://clinicaltrials.gov/ ct2/show/NCT01183468
Neulasta	JDRF/NIH	12–46	Within six months of diagnosis	I–II	http://clinicaltrials.gov/ ct2/show/NCT00662519
Sitagliptin and lanso-prazole (REPAIR Study)	Sanford Health and JDRF	11–45	Within six months of diagnosis	II	http://www.clinicaltrials.gov/ ct2/show/NCT01155284? term=NCT01155284&rank =1
T regulatory cells	JDRF	18–35	Between three and 24 months of diagnosis	I	http://www.clinicaltrials.gov/ ct2/show/NCT01210664? term=Tregs&cond=Diabe- tes&rank=1
Thymoglobu-lin and Neulasta	Helmsley Trust	16–64	Between four months and two years of diagnosis	I–II	http://www.clinicaltrials.gov/ ct2/show/NCT01106157? term=thymoglobulin+and+ neulasta&rank=1
Prevention trials					
Anti-CD3	NIH/Type 1 Diabetes TrialNet	16–45	Antibody positive; dysglycemia	II	http://www.diabetestrialnet. org/studies/ACD3.htm
Oral insulin	NIH/Type 1 Diabetes TrialNet	3–45	Antibody positive	III	http://www.diabetestrialnet. org/studies/oral-insulin.htm
INIT II	Diabetes Research Centre	4–30	Antibody positive	III	http://www.diabetestrials.org/ initii.html

such as sitagliptin or exenatide enhance beta cell growth.[76–78] Two studies in the NOD mouse model demonstrated restoration of euglycemia when used in combination with gastrin or proton pump inhibitor therapy, agents that are also purported to support beta cells.[79,80]

Given that T regulatory lymphocytes (T_{reg} cells) are thought to have a role in shaping the body's immune reactions, the ability to modify T_{reg} cell

behavior has been identified as a potential therapy. A phase I trial is currently ongoing to evaluate the safety and potential efficacy of the administration of an expanded pool of T_{reg} cells that have been harvested from the subjects (ages 18–35 years) and then expanded before being re-infused.[81]

Umbilical cord blood (UCB) is also a potential source of regulatory T lymphocytes, and infusion of autologous-banked UCB in subjects with T1D has

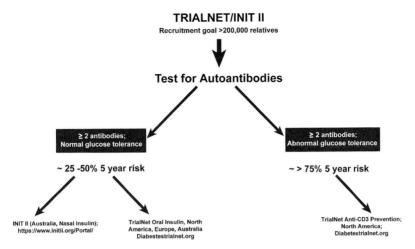

Figure 6. Prevention trials available for relatives of patients with T1D.

been evaluated in a small pilot study demonstrating the feasibility and safety of this approach.[82] These investigators are now evaluating the effect of UCB infusion coupled with administration of vitamin D and omega 3 fatty acid supplementation in a randomized, controlled pilot trial.[83]

Looking toward the future

Although a new therapy has not yet been identified that is ready for clinical use in T1D patients or those at risk for disease, much progress has been made toward the important goal of beta cell preservation. In prevention, stratification of risk groups continues to allow for testing of multiple agents (Fig. 6). As the newer sciences of genomics, proteomics, and metabolomics are applied, we anticipate the development of better tools to help dissect the heterogeneity of the disease and target therapies more selectively in at-risk individuals. Several immunomodulatory agents have been found to slow the rate of beta cell deterioration during the early stages of T1D when compared to placebo. These studies were well designed, well powered, and because similar outcome measures were studied, easily compared. It is not clear why experimental drugs with different mechanisms, including targeting T cells, B cells, and costimulation, all had their major effect on insulin secretion soon after treatment. It is also not clear why the salutary drug effect waned with time so that, with time, the fall in insulin secretion in both drug- and placebo-treated subjects became parallel.

In other autoimmune diseases, such as rheumatoid arthritis or systemic lupus erythematosus, immunomodulatory drugs are often given in repeated doses to control clinical "flares" of the disease. However, as demonstrated in the abatacept trial, despite continued drug dosing for 24 months, the rate of fall in C-peptide in the drug-treated group eventually paralleled the decline seen in the placebo group. It is possible that the immune and inflammatory mechanisms underlying beta cell loss are distinct early in the course of T1D from those that occur later. Studies targeting inflammation as well as immune modulation may address this possibility.

Antigen-based therapy, such as GAD, did not have a significant effect on beta cell function when administered to subjects within three months of diagnosis. It is possible that antigen-based therapy would be more successful earlier in the course of the disease and should be evaluated in the prevention of T1D. Similarly, rituximab and abatacept could be considered in prevention trials, for use at a time when beta cell mass is more substantial than at clinical diagnosis of new-onset T1D. More novel approaches to antigen delivery, including administration via a plasmid, have undergone early trials and await publication.[84]

The engagement and collaboration of patients, families, funding and regulatory agencies, and industry along with a large number of clinicians and clinical investigators has resulted in marked successes this past decade in that T1D trials have provided clear answers. It takes 10 to 15 years for a typical drug to be developed successfully from dis-covery to registration with the FDA,[85] and in early phases of research, the chance of a drug reaching patients is small—approximately 1 in 10.[86] More-over, at least 45% of all pivotal trials have a negative outcome.[87] The stakeholders must not lose sight of the significant progress made. The message to pa-tients and families living with T1D, as well as to the clinicians providing their care, is that carefully conducted and rigorous clinical trials are being per-formed and are providing critical information that will provide the path forward to new treatments (Table 2). Through their awareness of active clini-cal trials and their willingness to encourage patients to participate, clinicians play a critical role in the success of moving this field forward.

The autoimmune response will continue to present a threat to the patient's own islets or any new beta cells transplanted into a patient with a history of beta cell autoimmunity. Thus, therapies to stop beta cell destruction will continue to be necessary even when beta cell replacement is a viable clinical option made possible through stem cell research or other advances in transplantation.

Clinical trials testing experimental treatments singly and in combination in T1D are feasible and can be done relatively expeditiously and across sites. In particular, planning and recruitment for such studies can be done rapidly and with careful monitoring in clinical trial networks with experi-enced research teams. The goal continues to be to identify therapies with clinical benefit to patients with T1D, and building upon the very important data obtained in earlier studies; the next generation of clinical studies will bring us closer to this goal.

Acknowledgments

We gratefully acknowledge Ellen Greenberg, M.S., for her invaluable assistance with manuscript prepa-ration and review; Daniel Casper, M.D., Ph.D., for his creation of graphics and illustrations; and Kelly Smith for her editorial assistance.

Conflicts of interest

The authors declare no conflicts of interest.

References

1. Unwin, N., D. Gan & D. Whiting. 2010. The IDF Diabetes Atlas: providing evidence, raising awareness and promoting action. *Diabetes Res. Clin. Pract.* **87:** 2–3.

2. Fourlanos, S., M.D. Varney, B.D. Tait, *et al.* 2008. The ris-ing incidence of type 1 diabetes is accounted for by cases with lower-risk human leukocyte antigen genotypes. *Dia-betes Care* **31:** 1546–1549.

3. Garcia-Webb, P., P. Zimmet, A. Bonser, *et al.* 1984. Factors affecting fasting serum C-peptide levels in Micronesians: comparison with a Caucasoid population. *Diabetologia* **27:** 23–26.

4. The Diabetes Control and Complications Trial Study Group. 1998. Effect of intensive therapy on residual beta-cell func-tion in patients with type 1 diabetes in the diabetes control and complications trial. A randomized, controlled trial. *Ann. Intern. Med.* **128:** 517–523.

5. Takita, M., S. Matsumoto, H. Qin, *et al.* 2011. Secretory Unit of Islet Transplant Objects (SUITO) Index can pre-dict severity of hypoglycemic episodes in clinical islet cell transplantation. *Cell Transplant.* In press.

6. Greenbaum, C.J. 2002. Type 1 diabetes intervention trials: what have we learned? A critical review of selected interven-tion trials. *Clin. Immunol.* **104:** 97–104.

7. Feutren, G., L. Papoz, R. Assan, *et al.* 1986. Cyclosporin increases the rate and length of remissions in insulin-dependent diabetes of recent onset. Results of a multicentre double-blind trial. *Lancet* **2:** 119–124.

8. The Canadian European Randomized Control Trial Group. 1988. Cyclosporin-induced remission of IDDM after early intervention. Association of 1 yr of cyclosporin treatment with enhanced insulin secretion. *Diabetes* **37:** 1574–1582.

9. Skyler, J.S. & A. Rabinovitch. 1992. Cyclosporine in recent onset type I diabetes mellitus. Effects on islet beta cell func-tion. Miami Cyclosporine Diabetes Study Group. *J. Diabetes Complicat.* **6:** 77–88.

10. Jenner, M., G. Bradish, C. Stiller & P. Atkison. 1992. Cyclosporin A treatment of young children with newly-diagnosed type 1 (insulin-dependent) diabetes mellitus. London Diabetes Study Group. *Diabetologia* **35:** 884–888.

11. Pozzilli, P., N. Visalli, M.L. Boccuni, *et al.* 1994. Random-ized trial comparing nicotinamide and nicotinamide plus cyclosporin in recent onset insulin-dependent diabetes (IM-DIAB 1). The IMDIAB Study Group. *Diabet. Med.* **11:** 98–104.

12. Pozzilli, P., N. Visalli, R. Buzzetti, *et al.* 1995. Adjuvant ther-apy in recent onset type 1 diabetes at diagnosis and insulin requirement after 2 years. *Diabete. Metab.* **21:** 47–49.

13. Rakotoambinina, B., J. Timsit, I. Deschamps, *et al.* 1995. Cyclosporin A does not delay insulin dependency in asymp-tomatic IDDM patients. *Diabetes Care* **18:** 1487–1490.

14. De Filippo, G., J.C. Carel, C. Boitard & P.F. Bougneres. 1996. Long-term results of early cyclosporin therapy in juvenile IDDM. *Diabetes* **45:** 101–104.

15. Bougneres, P.F., J.C. Carel, L. Castano, *et al.* 1988. Factors associated with early remission of type I diabetes in children treated with cyclosporine. *N. Engl. J. Med.* **318:** 663–670.

16. Assan, R., J. Timsit, G. Feutren, *et al.* 1994. The kidney in cyclosporin A-treated diabetic patients: a long-term clinico-pathological study. *Clin. Nephrol.* **41:** 41–49.

17. Eisenbarth, G.S., S. Srikanta, R. Jackson, *et al.* 1985. Anti-thymocyte globulin and prednisone immunotherapy of re-cent onset type 1 diabetes mellitus. *Diabetes Res.* **2:** 271–276.

18. Silverstein, J., N. Maclaren, W. Riley, *et al.* 1988. Immunosuppression with azathioprine and prednisone in recent-onset insulin-dependent diabetes mellitus. *N. Engl. J. Med.* **319:** 599–604.

19. Cook, J.J., I. Hudson, L.C. Harrison, *et al.* 1989. Double-blind controlled trial of azathioprine in children with newly diagnosed type I diabetes. *Diabetes* **38:** 779–783.

20. Allen, H.F., G.J. Klingensmith, P. Jensen, *et al.* 1999. Chase. Effect of Bacillus Calmette-Guerin vaccination on new-onset type 1 diabetes. A randomized clinical study. *Diabetes Care* **22:** 1703–1707.

21. Chaillous, L., H. Lefevre, C. Thivolet, *et al.* 2000. Oral insulin administration and residual beta-cell function in recent-onset type 1 diabetes: a multicentre randomised controlled trial. Diabete Insuline Orale group. *Lancet* **356:** 545–549.

22. Pozzilli, P., D. Pitocco, N. Visalli, *et al.* 2000. No effect of oral insulin on residual beta-cell function in recent-onset type I diabetes (the IMDIAB VII). IMDIAB Group. *Diabetologia* **43:** 1000–1004.

23. Pozzilli, P., N. Visalli, A. Signore, *et al.* 1995. Double blind trial of nicotinamide in recent-onset IDDM (the IMDIAB III study). *Diabetologia* **38:** 848–852.

24. Shah, S.C., J.I. Malone & N.E. Simpson. 1989. A randomized trial of intensive insulin therapy in newly diagnosed insulin-dependent diabetes mellitus. *N. Engl. J. Med.* **320:** 550–554.

25. http://clinicaltrials.gov/ct2/show/NCT00891995?term=metabolic+control+in+new+onset+diabetes&rank15.

26. Gale, E.A., P.J. Bingley, C.L. Emmett & T. Collier. 2004. European Nicotinamide Diabetes Intervention Trial (ENDIT): a randomised controlled trial of intervention before the onset of type 1 diabetes. *Lancet* **363:** 925–931.

27. Diabetes Prevention Trial—Type 1 Diabetes Study Group. 2002. Effects of insulin in relatives of patients with type 1 diabetes mellitus. *N. Engl. J. Med.* **346:** 1685–1691.

28. Skyler, J.S., J.P. Krischer, J. Wolfsdorf, *et al.* 2005. Effects of oral insulin in relatives of patients with type 1 diabetes: the Diabetes Prevention Trial–Type 1. *Diabetes Care* **28:** 1068–1076.

29. http://www.diabetestrialnet.org/studies/oral-insulin.htm.

30. Chatenoud, L., M.F. Baudrihaye, H. Kreis, *et al.* 1982. Human in vivo antigenic modulation induced by the anti-T cell OKT3 monoclonal antibody. *Eur. J. Immunol.* **12:** 979–982.

31. Chatenoud, L., E. Thervet, J. Primo & J.F. Bach. 1994. Anti-CD3 antibody induces long-term remission of overt autoimmunity in nonobese diabetic mice. *Proc. Natl. Acad. Sci. U.S.A.* **91:** 123–127.

32. You, S., B. Leforban, C. Garcia, *et al.* 2007. Adaptive TGF-beta-dependent regulatory T cells control autoimmune diabetes and are a privileged target of anti-CD3 antibody treatment. *Proc. Natl. Acad. Sci. U.S.A.* **104:** 6335–6340.

33. Herold, K.C., W. Hagopian, J.A. Auger, *et al.* 2002. Anti-CD3 monoclonal antibody in new-onset type 1 diabetes mellitus. *N. Engl. J. Med.* **346:** 1692–1698.

34. Herold, K.C., S.E. Gitelman, U. Masharani, *et al.* 2005. A single course of anti-CD3 monoclonal antibody hOKT3gamma1(Ala-Ala) results in improvement in C-peptide responses and clinical parameters for at least 2 years after onset of type 1 diabetes. *Diabetes* **54:** 1763–1769.

35. Herold, K.C., S. Gitelman, C. Greenbaum, *et al.* 2009. Treatment of patients with new onset Type 1 diabetes with a single course of anti-CD3 mAb Teplizumab preserves insulin production for up to 5 years. *Clin. Immunol.* **132:** 166–173.

36. Keymeulen, B., E. Vandemeulebroucke, A.G. Ziegler, *et al.* 2005. Insulin needs after CD3-antibody therapy in new-onset type 1 diabetes. *N. Engl. J. Med.* **352:** 2598–2608.

37. Keymeulen, B., M. Walter, C. Mathieu, *et al.* 2010. Four-year metabolic outcome of a randomised controlled CD3-antibody trial in recent-onset type 1 diabetic patients depends on their age and baseline residual beta cell mass. *Diabetologia* **53:** 614–623.

38. Sherry, N., W. Hagopian, J. Ludvigsson, *et al.* 2011. Teplizumab for treatment of type 1 diabetes (Protege study): 1-year results from a randomised, placebo-controlled trial. *Lancet* **378:** 487–497.

39. http://www.diabetesincontrol.com/articles/diabetes-news/10641-otelixizumab-developed-by-gsk-and-tolerx-fails-in-type-1-diabetes-study.

40. AbATE Study (hOKT3γ1(Ala-Ala); teplizumab; Treatment of Type 1 Diabetes-Update on Clinical Trials [Symposia]. 2011. In *Proceedings of the 71st Scientific Sessions American Diabetes Association*. San Diego, CA.

41. Manno, R. & F. Boin. 2010. Immunotherapy of systemic sclerosis. *Immunotherapy* **2:** 863–878.

42. Pescovitz, M.D., C.J. Greenbaum, H. Krause-Steinrauf, *et al.* 2009. Rituximab, B-lymphocyte depletion, and preservation of beta-cell function. *N. Engl. J. Med.* **361:** 2143–2152.

43. Marelli-Berg, F.M., K. Okkenhaug & V. Mirenda. 2007. A two-signal model for T cell trafficking. *Trends. Immunol.* **28:** 267–273.

44. Orban, T., B. Bundy, D.J. Becker, *et al.* 2011. Co-stimulation modulation with abatacept in patients with recent-onset type 1 diabetes: a randomised, double-blind, placebo-controlled trial. *Lancet* **378:** 412–419.

45. Harrison, L.C. 2008. Vaccination against self to prevent autoimmune disease: the type 1 diabetes model. *Immunol. Cell. Biol.* **86:** 139–145.

46. Nanto-Salonen, K., A. Kupila, S. Simell, *et al.* 2008. Nasal insulin to prevent type 1 diabetes in children with HLA genotypes and autoantibodies conferring increased risk of disease: a double-blind, randomised controlled trial. *Lancet* **372:** 1746–1755.

47. Vandemeulebroucke, E., F.K. Gorus, K. Decochez, *et al.* 2009. Insulin treatment in IA-2A-positive relatives of type 1 diabetic patients. *Diabetes Metab.* **35:** 319–327.

48. Knip, M. 2009. Diet, gut, and type 1 diabetes: role of wheat-derived peptides? *Diabetes* **58:** 1723–1724.

49. Hummel, S., M. Pfluger, M. Hummel, *et al.* 2011. Primary dietary intervention study to reduce the risk of islet autoimmunity in children at increased risk for type 1 diabetes: the BABYDIET study. *Diabetes Care* **34:** 1301–1305.

50. Knip, M., S.M. Virtanen, D. Becker, *et al.* 2011. Early feeding and risk of type 1 diabetes: experiences from the Trial to Reduce Insulin-dependent diabetes mellitus in the Genetically at Risk (TRIGR). *Am. J. Clin. Nutr.* **94:** 1814S–1820S.

51. Akerblom, H.K., J. Krischer, S.M. Virtanen, *et al.* 2011. The Trial to Reduce IDDM in the Genetically at Risk (TRIGR) study: recruitment, intervention and follow-up. *Diabetologia* **54:** 627–633.

52. http://www.diabetestrialnet.org/studies/nutritional.htm.

53. Ludvigsson, J., M. Hjorth, M. Cheramy, *et al.* 2011. Extended evaluation of the safety and efficacy of GAD treatment of children and adolescents with recent-onset type 1 diabetes: a randomised controlled trial. *Diabetologia* **54:** 634–640.

54. Agardh, C.D., C.M. Cilio, A. Lethagen, *et al.* 2005. Clinical evidence for the safety of GAD65 immunomodulation in adult-onset autoimmune diabetes. *J. Diabetes Complicat.* **19:** 238–246.

55. Wherrett, D.K., B. Bundy, D.J. Becker, *et al.* 2011. Antigen-based therapy with glutamic acid decarboxylase (GAD) vaccine in patients with recent-onset type 1 diabetes: a randomised double-blind trial. *Lancet* **378:** 319–327.

56. GAD65; Treatment of Type 1 Diabetes-Update on Clinical Trials [Symposia]. 2011. In *Proceedings of the 71st Scientific Sessions American Diabetes Association.* San Diego, CA.

57. Mastrandrea, L., J. Yu, T. Behrens, *et al.* 2009. Etanercept treatment in children with new-onset type 1 diabetes: pilot randomized, placebo-controlled, double-blind study. *Diabetes Care* **32:** 1244–1249.

58. Rabinovitch, A. & J.S. Skyler. 1998. Prevention of type 1 diabetes. *Med. Clin. North Am.* **82:** 739–755.

59. http://clinicaltrials.gov/ct2/show/NCT00525889?term=il +2+rapa&rank2.

60. FOCIS. 2011. Rapamycin plus IL-2 combination therapy in T1D subjects enhances IL-1 responsiveness in CD25+ Treg, but also NK and effector T cells [Abstract]. Federation of Clinical Immunology Societies. Washington, DC.

61. American Diabetes Association. 2011. Rapamycin plus IL-2 combination therapy in subjects with T1D results in a sustained increase in IL-2 responsiveness and a transient decrease in C-peptide levels [Abstract]. *American Diabetes Association 71st Scientific Sessions.* San Diego, CA.

62. Annaloro, C., F. Onida & G. Lambertenghi Deliliers. 2009. Autologous hematopoietic stem cell transplantation in autoimmune diseases. *Expert. Rev. Hematol.* **2:** 699–715.

63. Voltarelli, J.C., C.E. Couri, A.B. Stracieri, *et al.* 2007. Autologous nonmyeloablative hematopoietic stem cell transplantation in newly diagnosed type 1 diabetes mellitus. *JAMA* **297:** 1568–1576.

64. Couri, C.E., M.C. Oliveira, A.B. Stracieri, *et al.* 2009. C-peptide levels and insulin independence following autologous nonmyeloablative hematopoietic stem cell transplantation in newly diagnosed type 1 diabetes mellitus. *JAMA* **301:** 1573–1579.

65. Sherr, J., J. Sosenko, J.S. Skyler & K.C. Herold. 2008. Prevention of type 1 diabetes: the time has come. *Nat. Clin. Pract. Endocrinol. Metab.* **4:** 334–343.

66. http://clinicaltrials.gov/ct2/show/NCT01030861?term= teplizumab&rank = 1.

67. Fourlanos, S., C. Perry, S.A. Gellert, *et al.* 2011. Evidence that nasal insulin induces immune tolerance to insulin in adults with autoimmune diabetes. *Diabetes* **60:** 1237–1245.

68. http://clinicaltrials.gov/ct2/show/NCT00711503?term=aida +diabetes&rank1.

69. http://clinicaltrials.gov/ct2/show/NCT00947427?term= canakinumab+diabetes&rank1.

70. Breda, L., M. Del Torto, S. De Sanctis & F. Chiarelli. 2011. Biologics in children's autoimmune disorders: efficacy and safety. *Eur. J. Pediatr.* **170:** 157–167.

71. http://clinicaltrials.gov/ct2/show/NCT01183468?term=aat +diabetes&rank1.

72. http://www.clinicaltrials.gov/ct2/show/NCT00515099?term =atg+diabetes &rank2.

73. http://www.clinicaltrials.gov/ct2/show/NCT01106157?term =thymoglobulin+and+neulasta&rank1.

74. Saudek, F., T. Havrdova, P. Boucek, *et al.* 2004. Polyclonal anti-T-cell therapy for type 1 diabetes mellitus of recent onset. *Rev. Diabet. Stud.* **1:** 80–88.

75. http://www.clinicaltrials.gov/ct2/show/NCT01155284?term =NCT01155284&rank1.

76. Xu, G., D.A. Stoffers, J.F. Habener & S. Bonner-Weir. 1999. Exendin-4 stimulates both beta-cell replication and neogenesis, resulting in increased beta-cell mass and improved glucose tolerance in diabetic rats. *Diabetes* **48:** 2270–2276.

77. Li, Y., T. Hansotia, B. Yusta, *et al.* 2003. Glucagon-like peptide-1 receptor signaling modulates beta cell apoptosis. *J. Biol. Chem.* **278:** 471–478.

78. Drucker, D.J. 2003. Glucagon-like peptides: regulators of cell proliferation, differentiation, and apoptosis. *Mol. Endocrinol.* **17:** 161–171.

79. Suarez-Pinzon, W.L., R.F. Power, Y. Yan, *et al.* 2008. Combination therapy with glucagon-like peptide-1 and gastrin restores normoglycemia in diabetic NOD mice. *Diabetes* **57:** 3281–3288.

80. Suarez-Pinzon, W.L., G.S. Cembrowski & A. Rabinovitch. 2009. Combination therapy with a dipeptidyl peptidase-4 inhibitor and a proton pump inhibitor restores normoglycaemia in non-obese diabetic mice. *Diabetologia* **52:** 1680–1682.

81. http://clinicaltrials.gov/ct2/show/NCT01210664?term=t+ reg+diabetes& rank1.

82. Haller, M.J., H.L. Viener & C. Wasserfall. 2008. Autologous umbilical cord blood infusion for type 1 diabetes. *Exp. Hematol.* **36:** 710–715.

83. http://www.clinicaltrials.gov/ct2/show/NCT00873925?term =diabetes+umbilical+cord&rank7.

84. Solvason, N., Y.P. Lou, W. Peters, *et al.* 2008. Improved efficacy of a tolerizing DNA vaccine for reversal of hyperglycemia through enhancement of gene expression and localization to intracellular sites. *J. Immunol.* **181:** 8298–8307.

85. DiMasi, J.A., R.W. Hansen & H.G. Grabowski. 2003. The price of innovation: new estimates of drug development costs. *J. Health Econ.* **22:** 151–185.

86. Institute of Medicine (US) Forum on Drug Discovery, Development, and Translation. 2011/01/07 ed. Washington, DC, 2010:85.

87. Kola, I. & J. Landis. 2004. Can the pharmaceutical industry reduce attrition rates? *Nat. Rev. Drug. Discov.* **3:** 711–715.

88. Devendra, D., Liu, E. & Eisenbarth, G.S. 2004. Type 1 diabetes: recent developments. *BMJ.* **328:** 750–754.